EMS

IN THE UNITED STATES

Fragmented Past, Future of Opportunity

A DESK REFERENCE FOR EMS LEADERS & STATE OFFICIALS

DONNIE WOODYARD, JR

FOREWORD BY DOUGLAS M. WOLFBERG

EMS in the United States: Fragmented Past, Future of Opportunity
by Donnie Woodyard, Jr

The views expressed in this book are solely those of the author and do not necessarily reflect the views of any employer or organization that the author is affiliated with or may have previously been affiliated with. This book represents the author's personal opinions and should not be construed as official statements or positions of any employer or organization.

Additionally, any discussion of law in this book is for informational purposes only and should not be considered legal advice or an interpretation of the law. Every attempt has been made to verify and present factually accurate information, and complete citations to prior works have been provided. However, the author and publisher assume no responsibility for errors or omissions in the citations or the content of the book. Please consult appropriate legal professionals or experts for specific advice related to your situation.

For more information and to view many of the historic records referenced in this book, visit www.EMS-History.com

Library of Congress Control Number: 2023911112

Woodyard Jr, Donnie R.
EMS In the United States:
Fragmented Past, Future of Opportunity
Includes indexes.
LCCN: 2023911112
ISBN 979-8-9885254-0-0 (pbk. book)
ISBN 979-8-9885254-2-4 (hardback)
ISBN 979-8-9885254-1-7 (digital)
1. Ambulances - History 2. Ambulance service - History. 3. Emergency Medical Technicians – History. 4. Paramedics – History. 5. EMS Regulation. 6. EMS Management & Leadership.

Cover Graphic Design By: J. A. B. Warna Perera
Foreword By: Douglas M. Wolfberg, JD

Med1 Technology LLC
1942 Broadway St. STE 314C
Boulder CO 80302

For all the EMS leaders and today's visionaries working together to advance our profession.

#WeAreEMS

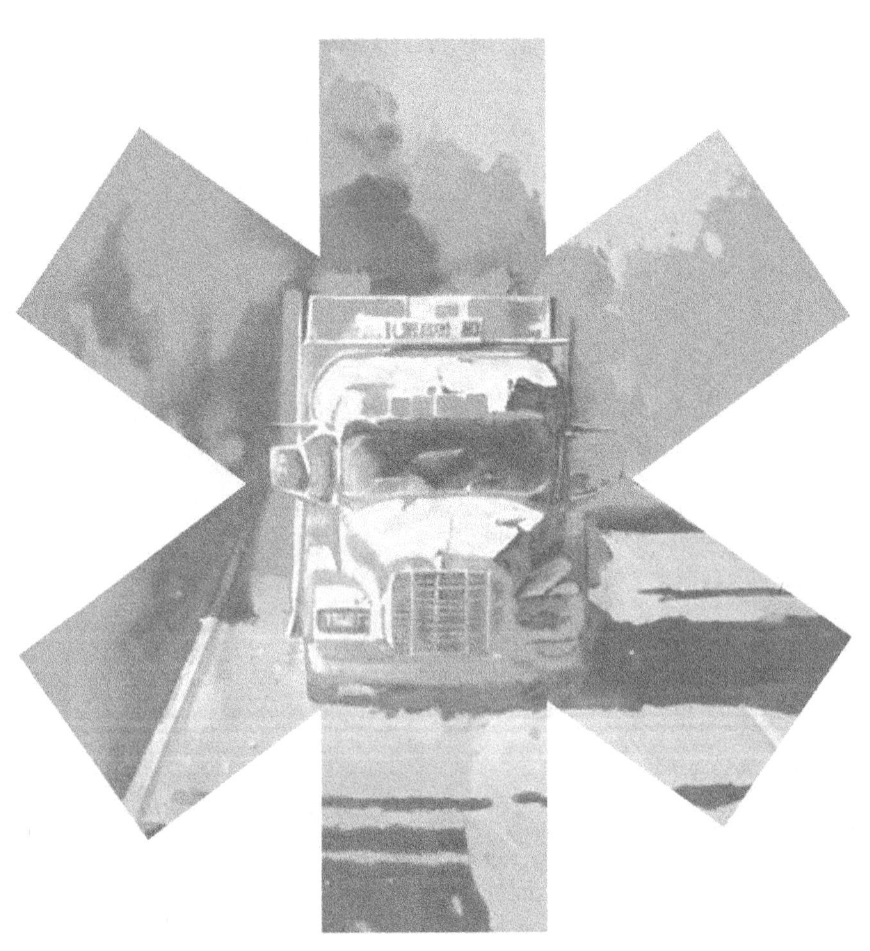

CONTENTS

Please note that each chapter of this book is designed to serve as an independent reference and resource. As a result of this intentional design, you may observe some topics being revisited across multiple chapters, though the depth of detail may vary. This recurrent mention is designed to enrich your understanding and provide comprehensive perspectives on critical subjects.

FOREWORD

By Douglas M. Wolfberg

President John Quincy Adams said that a leader is anyone who inspires others to do more, dream more and become more. EMS is highly regimented and often focused on levels of licensure, supervisory vs. field provider status and other indicia of rank and title. But leadership need not be constrained by such classifications. Any EMS professional can be an EMS leader under the formula handed down to us by President Adams.

Anyone who is a leader or aspires to leadership in this profession must read this important work. EMS owes Donnie Woodyard a debt of gratitude for documenting our history and illuminating the future course for the profession. *EMS in the United States: Fragmented Past, Future of Opportunity* is a magnificent and monumental work.

Those who have been involved in EMS for a long time often refer to themselves (and are often referred to by others) as "EMS dinosaurs." Though EMS dinosaur status does not have a precise unit of measurement, as someone who has been involved in EMS for 45 years as of this writing, I suppose I qualify. I've also had the privilege of close associations with the generation of EMS dinosaurs that came before me, some of whom were acknowledged "founding fathers" of the EMS profession. So, I have had a front row seat, either as a direct participant, or as a recipient of firsthand accounts, of EMS throughout almost its entire modern history. I've come to terms with my EMS dinosaur status, largely because it allows for an unparalleled vantage point from which to assess the state of affairs of a profession to which I have dedicated my entire working life.

I answered my first ambulance call in 1978. For the first 30 years, I can say with the benefit of hindsight that the pace of progress in EMS was glacial at best. Nothing, it seemed, was *revolutionary* – it was barely *evolutionary* – and painfully so. Many practices – both operationally and clinically – were done simply because "we've always done it this way" (which Admiral Grace Hopper correctly said was "the most dangerous phrase in the language"). While EMS still clings to some of these anachronisms (red lights and sirens, anyone?), we've entered, and are firmly entrenched in, the era of evidence-based practices. The implications have been profound.

In comparison to the snail's pace of progress in EMS I witnessed in my first 30 years, I believe that the past 15 years have been a time of breathless and exciting change. How energizing it has been to see the unflinching gaze of data and evidence topple so many sacred cows. Everything we do deserves fresh scrutiny. Why does everyone who calls 911 require a full EMS response? Why do we run "hot"? Why does every response require transport to an acute care hospital? Can some conditions be effectively managed outside the hospital? Can some patients be transported to destinations other than acute care hospitals to effectively manage their conditions? Can telehealth play a role in more appropriately providing out of hospital care?

EMS outwardly looks like public safety. Our vehicles have markings, lights and sirens – and our people wear uniforms - that connect us by appearance to our fire and police counterparts. But make no mistake: EMS is healthcare. Some EMS systems over the past 15 years have reengineered themselves as participants in the broader community healthcare system. And herein is the exciting future that lies ahead. For a profession that started modestly as a "ride to the hospital" with minimally trained first-aid attendants, EMS is becoming community-based healthcare. "EMS providers" are becoming *practitioners*. "Crew members" are becoming *clinicians.*

These are truly momentous times in EMS. To use a golf metaphor (strange, since I'm not a golfer), I often wish I wasn't already on the "back nine" of my career. I'd like to help shape the next 45 years of our profession. I've always thrived on change, and what's in store for EMS is exciting. Being an EMS leader in such times of change can be enthralling and satisfying.

Though I hope I have a bit more to contribute, the future belongs to the next generation of EMS leaders, and the ones after that. But past is prologue. To build a future we must understand the past. We must learn from our failures as well as from our successes. The future of EMS will be what you – our future leaders - make it. This book is your roadmap. Study our history and then go out and make EMS history anew.

Mechanicsburg, Pennsylvania
July 2023

ACKNOWLEDGEMENTS

I would like to convey my deepest gratitude for the steadfast support and invaluable guidance I have received from countless mentors, friends, supervisors, and EMS leaders throughout my life. The myriad opportunities for learning and leadership, generously provided by various managers, have played a pivotal role in my development. For this, I remain profoundly thankful.

Looking back, I recognize that I often didn't fully appreciate the significance of the opportunities given to me. The privilege of engaging in meaningful dialogues, receiving mentorship, attending conference sessions, or simply sharing a cup of coffee with many visionaries who were instrumental in shaping my career and the modern EMS system, has been an inspiring journey. These luminaries, mentors, friends, and guides include numerous individuals, but I want to specifically acknowledge and appreciate Jeanne-Marie Bakehouse, Jeff Beckman, Gary Brown, Drew Dawson, Wayne Denny, Tim Dienst, Dia Gainor, Jon Krohmer, Debra McDonald, Scott Hayes, Susan McHenry, Norman McSwain, Rocco Morando, Jim Page, Rick Patrick, Peter Safar, Joe Schmider, Keith Wages, and Gam Wijetunge. I will forever be thankful for their willingness to generously share their time, historical insights, advice, and profound wisdom.

I am particularly grateful to the volunteers at Giles Rescue Squad who devoted their time to teach my first EMT class and initiate my journey into EMS. I'm also thankful to Cedarville University for entrusting me as the EMS Chief, which marked my first EMS leadership position. I extend my gratitude to numerous additional EMS agencies that provided me experience, opportunities, and guidance along the way: Cedarville University EMS, Cedarville Township Fire Department, Hamilton County EMS System, Riverview Hospital, Ivy Tech Community College, Westfield Fire Department, Med1, Falck, and the statewide system stakeholders in Louisiana and Colorado for their ongoing support and collaboration.

My appreciation also extends to the National Registry of EMTs for the opportunity to serve as the Chief Operating Officer and gain insights into national EMS leadership, the nuances of examinations and certification, and the chance to develop a national perspective on EMS. To the EMS Compact Commissioners, I extend my respect and gratitude for their pioneering efforts in setting a modern example of unity, professionalism, and standards in our field and the opportunity to learn and collaborate to make a difference.

I also wish to convey my heartfelt thanks to stakeholders and colleagues who have demonstrated remarkable understanding and grace during my moments of error. Your steadfast support and the learning opportunities offered have played a vital role in both my personal and professional development. I am extremely thankful to the many leaders who placed their trust in me, offering a novice like me an opportunity to contribute.

This book would not have been possible without the relentless efforts of those working tirelessly behind the scenes, providing invaluable fact-checking, guidance, and unwavering encouragement. To everyone who played a key role in this transformative journey, I extend my deepest gratitude. Your steadfast support has fostered my evolution in unimaginable ways.

While recognizing everyone's contribution is an impossible task, I want to express my heartfelt thanks to the following individuals who shared their invaluable feedback on this manuscript: Shawn Baird, Jeff Beckman, MD, David Bump, Sean Caffrey, Dia Gainor, John Moon, and Don Stanton. I would like to express special appreciation to Marc Pagan, Bill Seifarth, Joseph Schmider, and Douglas Wolfberg for their significant time devoted to feedback, edits, and critiques on the full manuscript.

I owe a profound debt of gratitude to my family as well. The sacrifices my parents made to ensure my access to education and the opportunity to chase my dreams have been nothing short of monumental.

Lastly, I must acknowledge my first employer, Burgess. His decision to hire a teenager evolved into an invaluable life lesson on problem-solving and overcoming preconceived limitations. His investment in me helped me understand the critical importance of investing in others. He taught me that by creating an environment conducive to success, minimizing the repercussions from failures, and prioritizing learning, one can indeed turn the impossible into the possible. This empowering approach enables individuals to reach previously unattainable heights. I am forever grateful for these lessons, which have profoundly influenced my outlook and actions.

Thank you, everyone, for being an integral part of this extraordinary journey and for contributing to my personal and professional growth.

PREFACE

Today's Emergency Medical Services system operates as a critical cornerstone of the United States' healthcare infrastructure. It serves communities around the clock, demonstrating extraordinary dedication, resilience, and adaptability, particularly during the recent COVID-19 pandemic. Each day, the EMS system proves instrumental in saving countless lives and providing a healthcare safety net for millions of Americans, notably those without consistent access to primary care.

However, the current EMS system is traversing challenging terrain. Many see the system teetering on the brink of crisis, with states nationwide rigorously questioning its sustainability and seeking for new solutions to ensure its long-term viability. These challenges are not sudden anomalies but are rather the repercussions of a series of decisions and events deeply rooted in its multifaceted history.

This history includes significant contributions from visionaries like Dr. J.D. 'Deke' Farrington, a leading orthopedic surgeon, and Dr. Pete Safar, the father of critical care medicine and modern resuscitation science. It also highlights the ironic circumstance where ambulance services, once predominantly provided by funeral homes, underwent a significant transition. In the 1960s and 1970s, many funeral homes ceased these services, not predominately due to regulatory changes, but due to a failing financial model.

Pivotal moments included the attempts by the federal government to establish two parallel, yet unfortunately uncoordinated, nationalized EMS systems in the 1970s. These initiatives, backed by over $2 Billion (valued in 2023 dollars), led to federal agencies providing conflicting requirements to state officials. This lack of coordination, along with the military's considerable influence on EMS design and progression, has left enduring impressions on today's EMS landscape.

EMS pioneers strove to align the system's development with the conventional growth paths of other allied health professions. Yet, this aspiration was not consistently achieved nationwide. National standard curriculums and certification bodies established as early as the 1970s often found their influence overshadowed by local champions, who developed EMS agencies at the community level, fostering an aversion to national standards.

The abrupt changes and significant reduction in federal funding in 1981 forced communities to pursue alternative resources for their local ambulance services. This transition heightened skepticism towards any federal or national program. In "EMS in the United States: Fragmented Past, Future of Opportunity," these historical trends and their implications on the current state of EMS are thoroughly examined.

Despite these challenges, EMS remains a critical element of the healthcare system today. The future holds opportunities to further unify the profession, leveraging tools such as the EMS Compact. With new technological advancements and the emergence of telehealth, there exists a new frontier for EMS to enhance health provision and perhaps create a sustainable financial model.

This book aims to serve as a comprehensive resource for aspiring EMS leaders and managers. It offers a detailed understanding of EMS's roots, the challenges it has faced, and the opportunities that lie ahead. The book explores historical developments, the roles of visionaries, the influence of Hollywood, and the significance of the emblematic Star of Life. It also scrutinizes systemic issues such as financial structures and disparities in access that underscore EMS operations.

Moreover, the book elucidates the certification, licensure, and credentialing processes, state sovereignty implications, and the promising prospects of telehealth and health equity in EMS. By tracing EMS's complex trajectory from its fragmented past to its opportunity-rich future, it invites readers to participate in informed discussions about the future of EMS.

"EMS in the United States: Fragmented Past, Future of Opportunity" provides an essential roadmap for aspiring EMS leaders and managers. It fosters a comprehension of the past to better manage the present and envision the future. This historical overview serves as a blueprint for understanding the present challenges and shaping the future of EMS. It advocates for a system that is efficient, equitable, and sustainable, thereby continuing its vital service to the American people.

Through this exploration, readers will gain insight into how the EMS system has evolved in the face of adversity and change. This knowledge equips future EMS leaders and managers with a historical perspective, vital for making informed decisions as they navigate the challenges and opportunities ahead.

In the age of technology and telehealth, EMS stands on the cusp of a new era. With the opportunity to further unify the profession through mechanisms such as the EMS Compact, there is potential for substantial growth and improvement. This book aims to highlight these opportunities and stimulate meaningful conversations about how to seize them effectively.

As we venture forward, it is important to remember that the history of our EMS holds the blueprint for its revival. Its future lies in the lessons learned from its past, the ingenuity of its present leaders, and the promise held by innovations yet to come. The EMS system's ongoing commitment to the well-being of the American people is a testament to its resilience and importance.

In the face of current challenges, we should be emboldened by the fact that the EMS system has always risen to meet every trial it has faced. Its fragmented past, marked by struggle and triumph, has forged a resilient system that continues to serve as a bedrock of our healthcare infrastructure.

The opportunity-rich future of EMS beckons, and this book invites all aspiring EMS leaders and managers to play a part in shaping it. It is a call to understand the past, manage the present, and envision a future where the EMS system continues to serve everyone with increased efficiency, equity, and sustainability.

A Letter to Today's EMS Visionaries and Leaders,

Throughout my more than thirty-year EMS career, I have come to appreciate the significance of having experienced mentors and dependable resources to navigate the intricacies of our complex EMS system. When I initially assumed leadership roles at both the state and national levels, I was struck by the scarcity of resources that could bridge the knowledge gap between local EMS leadership and the broader state or national leadership--understanding the history, grasping an overview of the organization, and possessing a guide to traverse the layers of influence. I was fortunate enough to have exceptional mentors, yet I witnessed many ambitious emerging leaders falter, in part, due to gaps in their knowledge and resources.

To help address this gap, I authored this book as a resource to provide a historical context for pivotal decisions that have shaped contemporary EMS systems. It is conceived as a desk reference, with each chapter functioning independently. You may notice some repeated information across different chapters, but this is intentional, serving to provide additional context in relation to the specific issue or historical event being discussed. Furthermore, I impart some insights drawn from my personal experience in leadership and management.

From the birth of EMS in the United States to current challenges such as health equity and COVID-19, my objective is to offer you an overview of key historical decisions and demonstrate how they persistently influence the design and operations of EMS in our country.

It is my hope that this book will not only act as a resource for budding EMS leaders, but also enable you to comprehend the historical underpinnings as the EMS system continues to modernize and evolve. By illuminating key facets of our history that are often neglected, we can delve deeper into understanding how EMS has developed, recognizing that our current state is inherently linked to past decisions. Each historical decision was made with purpose, and understanding this context will help guide us in shaping the future.

I am eager for you to embark on this journey with me, exploring the rich history, complex present, and opportunity-laden future of EMS in the United States. The work you undertake is critical for the health and safety of our communities. I am optimistic that this guide will prove to be an asset to you as you work tirelessly to enhance emergency medical care in the United States.

Sincerely,

Donnie W. Woodyard, Jr.

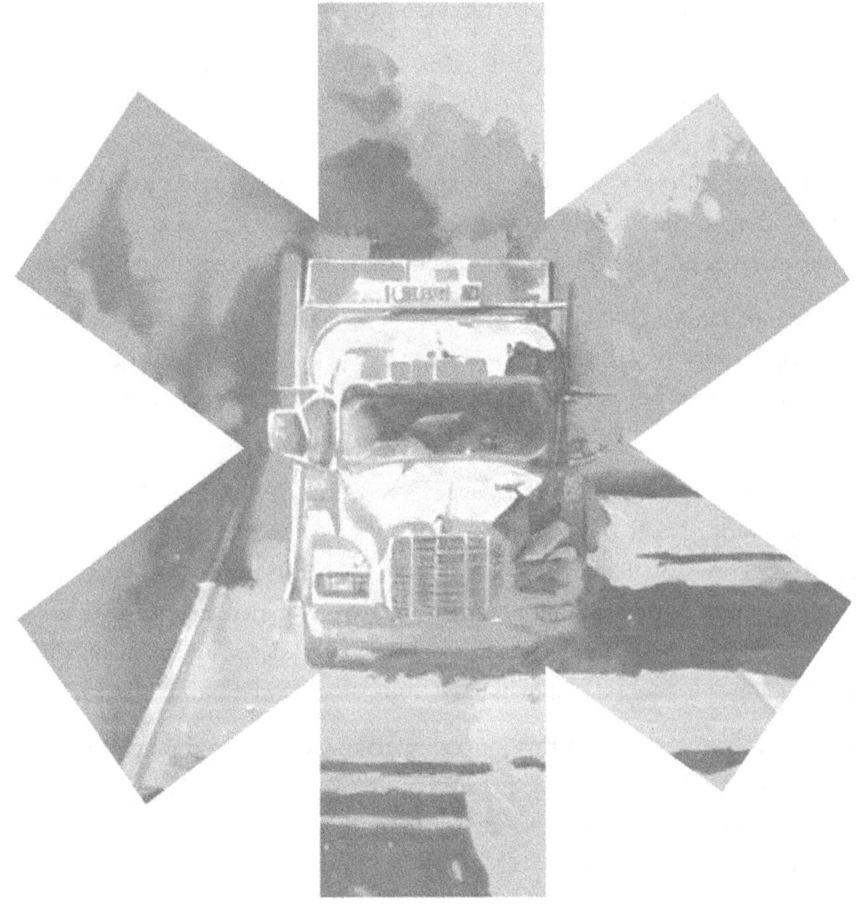

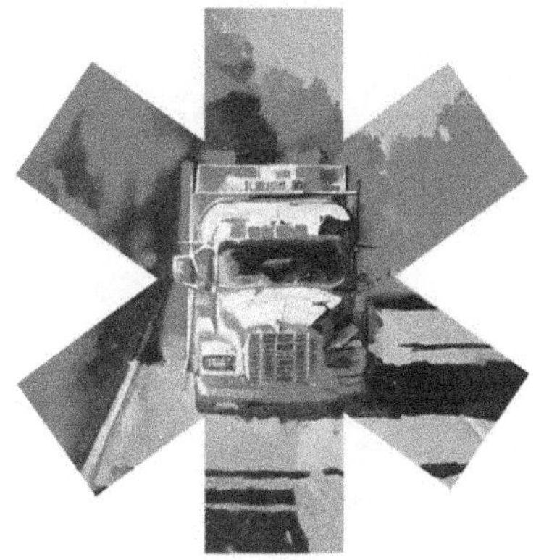

Section 1

FOUNDATIONS

"History is the witness that testifies to the passing of time;
it illumines reality, vitalizes memory, provides guidance in daily life
and brings us tidings of antiquity."
-Marcus Tullius Cicero

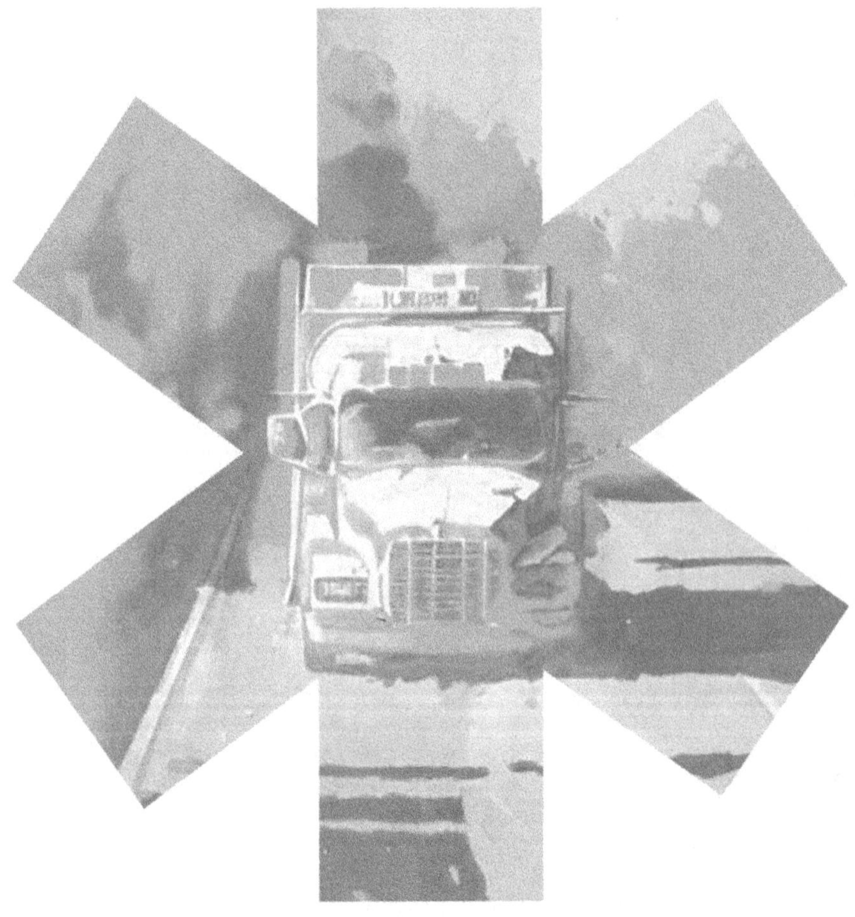

1

The Origins of EMS In The United States

"The army which goes forth to battle, equipped with ambulance wagons, will have its material strength increased by one-third. "

THE IDEA OF TRANSPORTING THE SICK AND INJURED TO PLACES OF healing has been a part of human society since its inception. The Biblical parable of the Good Samaritan (Luke 10:25-37), in which care and transportation are provided for an injured individual, is the inspiration and foundation for modern "Good Samaritan" laws nationwide. It was during the Napoleonic wars when a French Surgeon, Baron Dominique-Jean Larrey, established a formalized system complete with specialized equipment to aid the sick and injured.[1] Often credited with the creation of the first ambulances, Larrey's horse-drawn "Flying Ambulances" included bandages to treat wounds and transport wounded soldiers to field hospitals. Following stabilization, patients would then be moved to convents or monasteries for further care.

This system was later adopted in the United States during the American Civil War. In 1865, the first hospital-based ambulance service was introduced at the Commercial Hospital in Cincinnati, Ohio, which is presently known as the University of Cincinnati Medical Center.[2] Substantial enhancements in ambulance-related transportation technology were observed from the initial part of the 20th century to the mid-century. The horse-drawn ambulances were superseded by motorized vehicles, aircraft were used for patient transport during the two World Wars, and the Dodge Ambulance was established as the standard for the U.S. military.

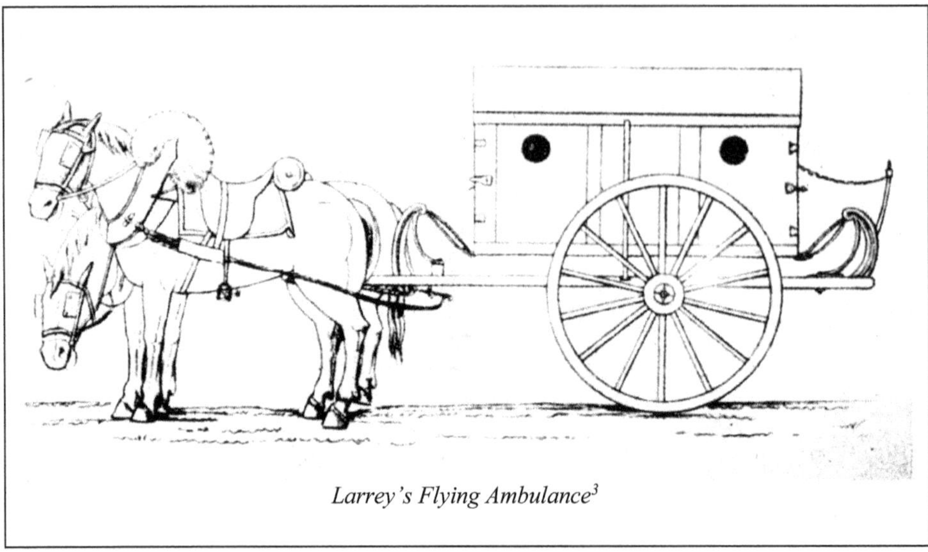

Larrey's Flying Ambulance[3]

Nevertheless, up until the 1960s, transportation of the sick and injured was the primary purpose of ambulance services. As a transportation service, ambulances had minimal regulation, and this resulted in significant disparities in their availability and quality. Ambulances, mainly owned and managed by local hospitals and funeral homes, were equipped with a stretcher, basic first aid supplies, and a driver who typically lacked medical training. Hearses, despite being ill-equipped for patient comfort, safety, or in-transit medical care, were often used as ambulances. As a result, patients frequently did not receive necessary medical attention during transport, leading to considerable variations in the quality of care provided.

The early 20th century brought about significant advancements in transportation technology, including the use of motor vehicles and airplanes for patient conveyance. These developments substantially contributed to the modernization of EMS systems. Motor vehicles offered quicker and more efficient transportation, while airplanes facilitated speedy transport of patients across vast distances, especially during wartime.

However, despite these advances in transportation, there was minimal progression concerning the quality of out-of-hospital medical care. Consequently, patients often did not receive any medical attention during their transit to the hospital. The public's demand for improved emergency medical services began to rise significantly during the 1950s, spurred by military advancements in emergency medical care and the development of the U.S. interstate highway system.

MILITARY INNOVATIONS THAT SHAPED CIVILIAN EMS

Historically, military conflicts have served as crucibles for medical innovation, propelling advancements in Emergency Medical Services through necessity and urgency. The U.S. military's role in these advancements began with World War I's trench warfare, where nonphysicians were deployed to treat casualties at the front lines. This early application of first aid by nonphysicians became the bedrock upon which the roles of the modern corpsmen and combat medics were built. It was also during World War I that airplanes were specifically designed for the evacuation of the wounded. French medical officer Eugene Chassaing pioneered this concept by transforming military airplanes into air ambulances. In April 1918 at Flanders, Belgium, a modified Dorand II was flown, carrying two patients in the fuselage. Similarly, U.S. Army Major Nelson Driver and Captain William Ocker converted a Curtiss JN-4 Jenny into a flying ambulance by the war's end.

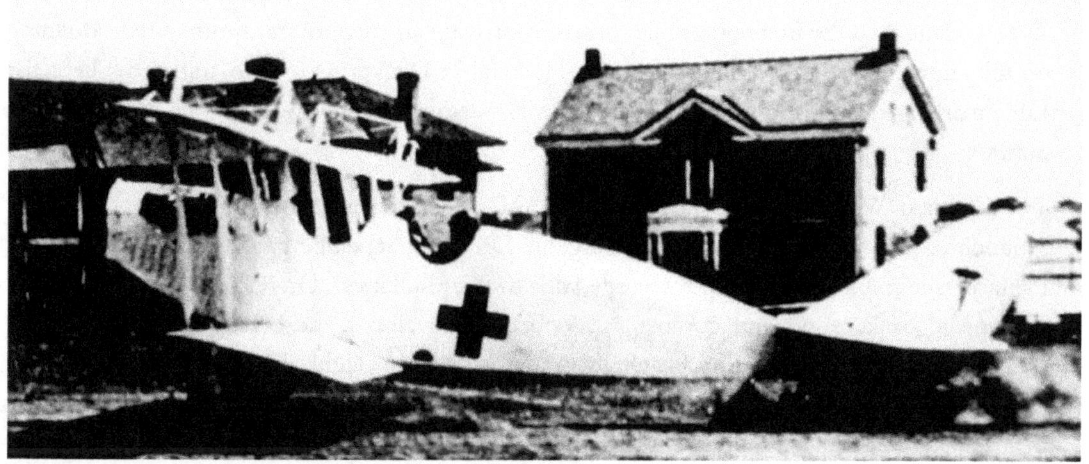

Curtiss JN-4D Jenny aircraft configured as an air ambulance.[4]

The practice of air evacuation was further enhanced during World War II, thanks to advancements in aircraft size, range, and reliability. U.S. Army Air Forces C-47s evacuated large numbers of casualties from combat theaters, including the Mediterranean campaigns in Sicily and at Anzio. In a landmark moment in 1943, Lieutenant Elsie Ott, an Army Air Forces nurse, oversaw the first intercontinental evacuation flight, transporting five critically ill patients from India to Washington, D.C. This milestone prompted the creation of a flight nurses training program at Bowman Field in Kentucky, graduating its first class the same year.

In the post-war period, Schaefer Air Service emerged in 1947 as the first FAA-certified air ambulance service in the U.S., founded by J. Walter Schaefer in Los Angeles, California. Another significant milestone was achieved in 1960, when Lincoln Ragsdale and his wife, who were African-American business owners, expanded their funeral-ambulance service in Phoenix, Arizona, to include an airplane ambulance. Notably, Lincoln Ragsdale was a commercial pilot and a veteran of World War II, where he had served with distinction in the 99th Pursuit Squadron.[5] This marked what was likely the inception of the first African American owned aeromedical service in the United States.

These advancements continued into the Korean War and the Vietnam War, where helicopter evacuation directly from the scene of injury to the hospital became standardized practice. These 'DUSTOFF' operations, as initiated by the U.S. Army in 1962, dramatically cut the time to treatment, reinforcing the critical concept of the 'Golden Hour'.

In the mid-1950s, physicians began advocating for the application of combat-derived emergency strategies in the civilian realm. Influenced by these lessons, physicians such as J.D. "Deke" Farrington and Sam Banks developed a trauma training program for the Chicago Fire Department. This program eventually evolved into the EMT-Ambulance course, bringing military-inspired emergency response strategies into civilian use.

By 1969, military helicopter evacuation principles were also being translated into civilian practice. The Department of Transportation funded a pilot project operating three civilian helicopter ambulances in Mississippi. One of these services, known as 'Rescue 7', continues to operate in Hattiesburg, MS, even today. The following year, the Maryland Police Aviation Division launched the first community-based rotor-wing air-medical transport system. Building on this momentum, in 1972, St. Anthony's Hospital in Denver, Colorado, initiated 'Flight for Life', marking the first hospital-based rotor-wing air-medical transport service in the United States. [6]

The Vietnam War also gave birth to the SAM (structural aluminum malleable) splints, a groundbreaking invention by trauma surgeon Dr. Sam Scheinberg. Having observed that military issue splints were often disregarded due to their bulkiness, Dr. Scheinberg leveraged his orthopedic background and combat experience to develop a more practical solution. His creation, inspired by a foil bubblegum wrapper, was lightweight, malleable, and adaptable, capable of immobilizing a wide range of bone and soft tissue injuries. The SAM splint is now a mainstay in first aid kits, trauma kits, and ambulances worldwide.

The Global War on Terror in Iraq and Afghanistan further streamlined the integration of military and civilian EMS. Tactical Combat Casualty Care (TCCC) was developed and validated, offering comprehensive guidelines for controlling hemorrhage, managing respiratory distress, and hypotensive resuscitation. Tourniquets, hemostatic agents, and needle chest decompression techniques emerged as significant life-saving tools from these conflicts, and their successful application on the battlefield led to their incorporation into civilian EMS protocols.

The symbiotic relationship between military conflicts and EMS has consistently driven medical innovation. Each war has spurred a wave of change, from the advent of the combat medic to the implementation of air evacuation, the creation of the practical SAM splints, and the adoption of life-saving techniques. This cross-pollination of ideas has profoundly shaped civilian EMS, ensuring that those in critical need receive the highest standard of emergency medical care.

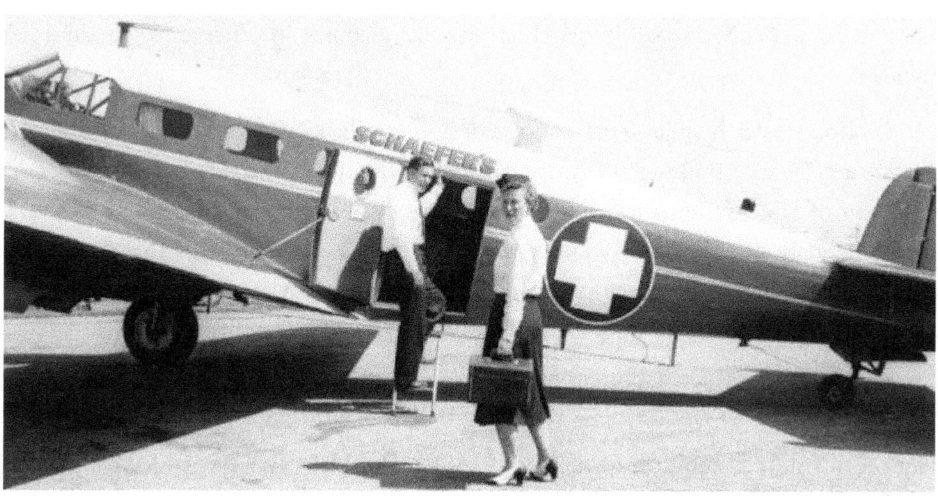

The Schaefer Air Service was the first FAA-certified air ambulance service in the United States.

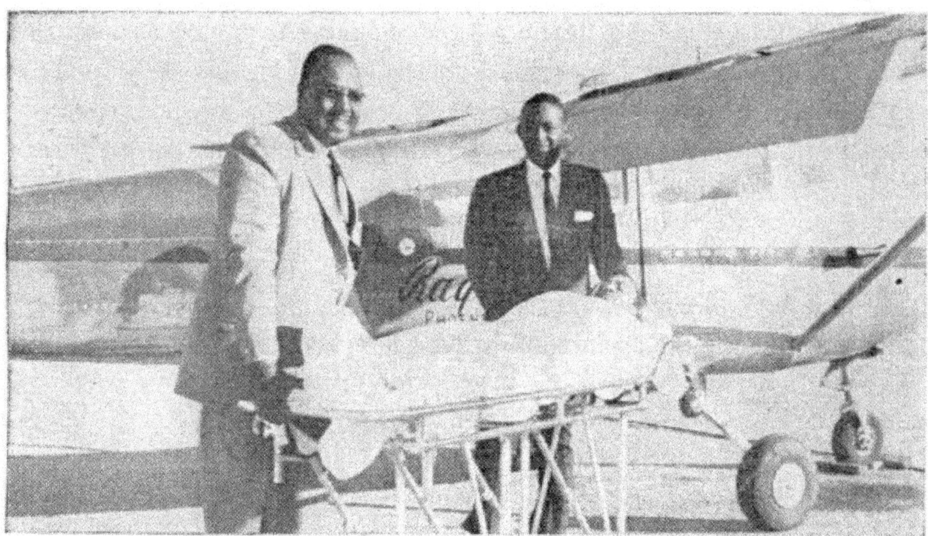

In 1960, Mr. and Mrs. Lincoln J Ragsdale added an airplane ambulance to their funeral home-based ambulance service.

Injuries, Interstate Highways & Motor Vehicle Deaths

The construction of the Interstate Highway System in the United States, which began in the 1950s, was intended to improve transportation and commerce across the country. However, one unintended consequence was a dramatic increase in road deaths. The highways encouraged people to drive more frequently and for longer distances, and the lack of safety features in vehicles, such as seat belts and airbags, contributed to a rise in traffic fatalities.

In response to the increase in road deaths, the President's Committee for Traffic Safety[7] released a report in 1966, recommending the establishment of a national program aimed at reducing highway fatalities and injuries. The following year, the National Academy of Sciences (NAS) and National Research Council (NRC) published a report titled "*Accidental Death and Disability: The*

Neglected Disease of Modern Society,'[8] which prompted changes in emergency medical services nationwide.

The NAS/NRC report highlighted the poor design and lack of equipment in ambulances, as well as the insufficient training for ambulance drivers and attendants. It recommended the establishment of EMS systems to provide pre-hospital care for the injured, with eleven of the 29 recommendations directly related to creating a national EMS system. These recommendations included developing federal standards for ambulances, adopting state ambulance regulations, and initiating pilot programs to evaluate automotive and helicopter ambulance services in sparsely populated areas. The report additionally presented a vision for the creation of trauma systems as they exist in their current form.

Building on this momentum, on September 9, 1966, President Lyndon B. Johnson signed the National Traffic and Motor Vehicle Safety Act[9] and the Highway Safety Act[10]. These acts created the Department of Transportation (DOT) and required this new government agency to establish guidelines and standards for EMS systems. The *Highway Safety Act* required states to develop EMS plans while the DOT was responsible for developing ambulance specifications, equipment standards, communications, educational requirements, and staffing. The decision of Congress to assign the development of EMS to the Department of Transportation, rather than the Department of Health, Education, and Welfare (DHEW), reinforced the perspective that EMS was primarily a transportation service and not a medical service.

"In this century, more than 1,500,000 of our fellow citizens have died on our streets and highways: nearly three times as many Americans as we have lost in all our wars."
– President Johnson

Nevertheless, the national highways were becoming more and more dangerous, and the administration had to address the public's concern. As President Johnson signed the *Highway Safety Act,* he reminded the nation that nearly three times as many Americans had died in traffic accidents in the 20th century as had died "in all our wars" and this Act was a step in addressing the issue.[11]

Although Congress clearly viewed ambulances as a transportation service that provided first aid, physicians had a different vision for the emerging EMS system. In 1967, Dr. J.D. "Deke" Farrington, a leading trauma surgeon, published an article titled "*Death in a Ditch*".[12] Dr. Farrington, in detail, again highlighted the dangers of automobile crashes on America's highways and outlined his vision for preventing the growing epidemic of fatalities. He called for a new approach to providing emergency medical care at the scene of emergencies and during transport, introduced the concept of vehicle extrication to manage spinal injuries and emphasized the importance of emergency medical care and bleeding control. He also noted the need for specialized training and education, that went far beyond the Red Cross's first aid course and recognized the need for the "certification of ambulance attendants."

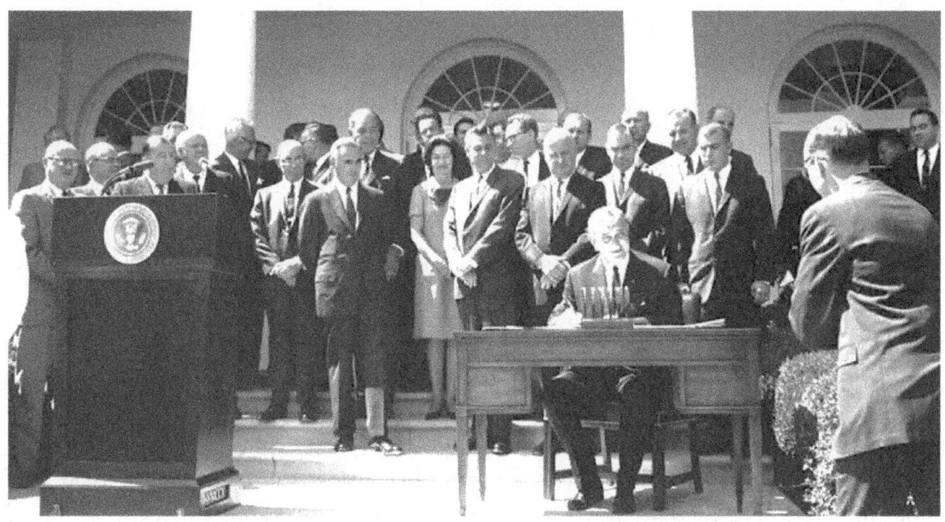

President Johnson signing the Highway Safety Act of 1966.

By the time Dr. Farrington wrote "*Death in a Ditch*", he already had nearly a decade of experience in training Chicago fire fighters in a prototype medical care course. That course would later evolve into the first nationally recognized EMT-Ambulance course. Concurrently, as Dr. Farrington was training and advancing an early form of modern EMS in the Midwest, Peter Safar, MD, (the founder of critical care medicine) was working with colleagues to establish the Freedom House Ambulance Service in Pennsylvania, Dr. Norman McSwain was developing an EMS system in Kansas, and Dr. Eugene Nagel was working with the Miami-Dade Fire Department to develop an advanced life support ambulance.

As these visionary physicians were pioneering innovative strategies in emergency medical care—strategies that greatly surpassed basic first aid and transportation—the ambulance service sector faced numerous considerable challenges. In the debates centered on the *Highway Safety Act*, the federal government was focused on addressing traumatic injuries related to motor vehicle crashes in predominately rural America. Consequently, the EMS-specific components of the Highway Safety Act were centered around enhancing "communication and transportation" for victims of traffic crashes. [13] However, influential physicians were already striving to establish a new category of medical professional—one that extended the care provided by emergency departments into ambulances for both medical and trauma patients. These visionaries capitalized on the funding, awareness, and opportunities provided by the *Highway Safety Act*.

A notable shortfall of the *Highway Safety Act* was that the Department of Transportation, and not the Department of Health, Education and Welfare (later known as the Department of Health and Human Services) emerged as the de facto lead entity for Emergency Medical Services in the United States. Although treatment for motor vehicle crash victims is crucial, the medical emphasis of EMS has not historically been a core focus of the Department of Transportation. (In 2020, motor vehicle crashes accounted for ~3.5% of EMS activations nationally.)[14] Some believe this has hampered the development of EMS as a healthcare service. As such, a tension began to emerge between EMS being categorized as a transportation service versus its fundamental role within the healthcare system.

The journey towards a comprehensive national EMS system took time to fully unfold. A significant milestone in this journey was the publication of the 1972 NAS-NRC "Roles and Resources" report.[15] This report, co-authored by Dr. J.D. Farrington and Dr. Peter Safar, played a pivotal role in shaping the future of EMS by emphasizing the need for a more integrated and proactive approach to emergency care. It underlined the importance of federal government involvement, which had previously fallen behind the efforts of professional and lay health organizations, in improving and providing EMS agencies. The report called for legislative and executive actions to ensure universal access to high-quality emergency care. It recommended the integration of federal resources, the establishment of a dedicated division within the Department of Health, Education, and Welfare (DHEW) to oversee the EMS program, and the coordination of efforts through regional EMS programs.

These recommendations paved the way for significant developments in the field of EMS, including the enactment of the *EMS Systems Act* and a surge of federal investment during the 1970s. These initiatives aimed to foster the development of robust EMS systems throughout the United States, bringing the comprehensive vision of universal access to emergency medical services closer to reality.

CASE STUDY: FREEDOM HOUSE AMBULANCE[a]

Established in Pittsburgh, Pennsylvania, in 1967, the Freedom House Ambulance Service not only dismantled racial, ethnic, nationality, and gender barriers but also served as an official incubator for testing innovative ideas related to ambulance services before they were formally proposed to President Johnson's Committee on Emergency Medical Services[16] and later was the model Paramedic service used when the Department of Transportation created the first national standard curriculum for EMT-Paramedic. This transformative initiative, largely overlooked in history until recently, not only formed the groundwork for the "systems approach" to Emergency Medical Services but also the foundations of modern paramedic practice.

This project resulted from a shared vision of numerous individuals from Freedom House Enterprises combined with EMS system visionaries including Jerry Esposito,[b] Dr. Donald Benson, Dr. Peter Safar, and Dr. Nancy Caroline. Although its primary objective was to deliver professional prehospital care to underprivileged African American communities, it also served as the conceptual foundation for a new medical profession.

The influence of the Freedom House Ambulance Service is still difficult to comprehend. For example, in a 1971 letter to F. J. Lewis, the Acting Chief of the Emergency Medical Programs Division at the National Highway Traffic Safety Administration (NHTSA), the chair of the National Academy of Sciences' Committee on EMS highlighted the necessity for the DOT to develop a more comprehensive EMT curriculum. This new national curriculum would *mimic* the

---

[a] A special appreciation to Mr. John Moon, one of the Freedom House Ambulance Service members and one of America's first paramedics for reviewing this section. Also, readers are strongly encouraged to read the full history of Freedom House Ambulance as captured in a book by Kevin Hazzard: "American Sirens: The Incredible Story of the Black Men Who Became America's First Paramedics"

[b] Jerry (Gerald) Esposito later co-authored with Dr. Peter Safar the first outline describing the purpose, structure, and organization of the National Registry of EMTs.

Freedom House's education model, demanding a minimum of 480 hours, encompassing clinical rotations, the utilization of mannequins and live animals, and a designated period for field exercises.

Then in 1973, Dr. Benson, a ranking member of President Johnson's Committee on EMS, and one of the physician medical directors for the Freedom House Ambulance Service, published a seminal paper elucidating the need for a "Systems Approach" to implementing Emergency Medical Services (While this is likely the first publication to use a Systems Approach to describe EMS, the phrase would be rediscovered nearly three decades later when the *EMS Agenda for the Future* was written). He emphasized that EMS extended beyond mere ambulance services. Building on Dr. Safar's prior work and his own experience with the Freedom House Ambulance Service, Dr. Benson articulated,

> "Necessary components include recognizing an emergency, providing first aid, communicating with emergency treatment facilities, transporting patients in appropriate vehicles, availing well-trained emergency care personnel, categorizing emergency care facilities, and collecting data and auditing. It is vital that dynamic, informed civic and professional leaders undertake the responsibility to transform comprehensive emergency medical services from an often discussed but unfulfilled 'plan' into a tangible reality."

A few years into its operation, when the service had demonstrated the ability of non-physicians to provide innovative medical care, Dr. Safar recognized the service required more dedicated time and attention from a physician medical director. He appointed Dr. Nancy Caroline, a resident studying under his tutelage, as the new medical director of the service. This appointment marked her as one of the inaugural Paramedic medical directors in the United States, and the first female physician EMS Medical Director.

Nancy Caroline, MD, under Safar's mentorship, further refined the intensive training program for the Freedom House Ambulance paramedics, amalgamating classroom instruction, hospital-based learning, and field training. Immediately following her experience with Freedom House Ambulance Service, she authored “Emergency Care in the Streets.” This was the first-ever paramedic textbook, which stood as the sole comprehensive educational resource for paramedics for many years.

Staffed almost exclusively by African American paramedics, the Freedom House Ambulance Service offered rapid, superior advanced life support care for all types of emergencies, including medical, trauma, obstetric, and cardiac events. Dr. Caroline, a Jewish female physician, also recognized the importance of this initiative in breaking down social, religious, racial, and economic barriers.

Despite being recognized as the model EMS service in the nation, and confronting racial discrimination, limited resources and minimal backing from mainstream medical institutions, the paramedics of the Freedom House Ambulance Service provided compassionate, high-quality care to their communities for nearly a decade. However, due to political opposition and fiscal challenges, Freedom House was eventually closed. The mayor of Pittsburgh proposed cutting social welfare programs, citing the expenses of Freedom House as justification, but paradoxically replaced it with a more expensive ambulance service. Freedom House Ambulance officially ceased operations on September 22, 1975.

Nonetheless, the impactful legacy of the Freedom House Ambulance Service continues to radiate, leaving a national and international imprint on Emergency Medical Services. Dr. Safar, a distinguished anesthesiologist, placed paramount importance on efficient airway management, resulting in the development of the pioneering rear-facing airway seat and wall-mounted suction unit in ambulances. Moreover, it was a Freedom House paramedic – John Moon – who achieved the milestone of the first recorded non-physician field intubation. Through the collective endeavors of Drs. Safar and Caroline, alongside the dedicated paramedics, community-oriented EMS models were forged, influencing the ongoing evolution of modern EMS systems. An essential lesson gleaned early on was that Dr. Safar effectively demonstrated that non-physicians, with appropriate training, could proficiently administer advanced life support measures such as medication, airway management, and cardiac defibrillation.

Significantly, in 1975 the Department of Transportation designated the Freedom House Ambulance Service as the national model for EMT-Paramedic education and system design. During this period, other paramedic pilot projects were also in development. However, it was the Freedom House Ambulance Service that distinguished itself by not only providing comprehensive Advanced Life Support for all types of emergencies with highly skilled specialized allied health professionals but also implementing a "systems approach" to EMS.

In 1977, when the U.S. Department of Transportation published the first National Standard Curriculum for EMT-Paramedic, Dr. Caroline aptly encapsulates the spirit of the Freedom House Ambulance Service project: "A special debt is owed to the trainees from the Freedom House Ambulance Service... who participated in a pilot program and were not hesitant to offer advice and criticism during the development of the modular curriculum and text. These skilled and dedicated personnel effectively unveiled and demonstrated the challenging world of emergency care outside the hospital and taught enormous respect for the skills and compassion of emergency medical technicians."

Today, the Freedom House Ambulance Service stands as a notable landmark in the field of EMS. It underscores the crucial role of education, training, and community involvement in shaping prehospital care. Even in its absence, it serves as a powerful testament to what can be achieved in the face of adversity, illuminating the path forward for future initiatives in emergency medical services. The Freedom House Ambulance Service remains a testament to the power of inclusivity, perseverance, and innovative thinking in healthcare.

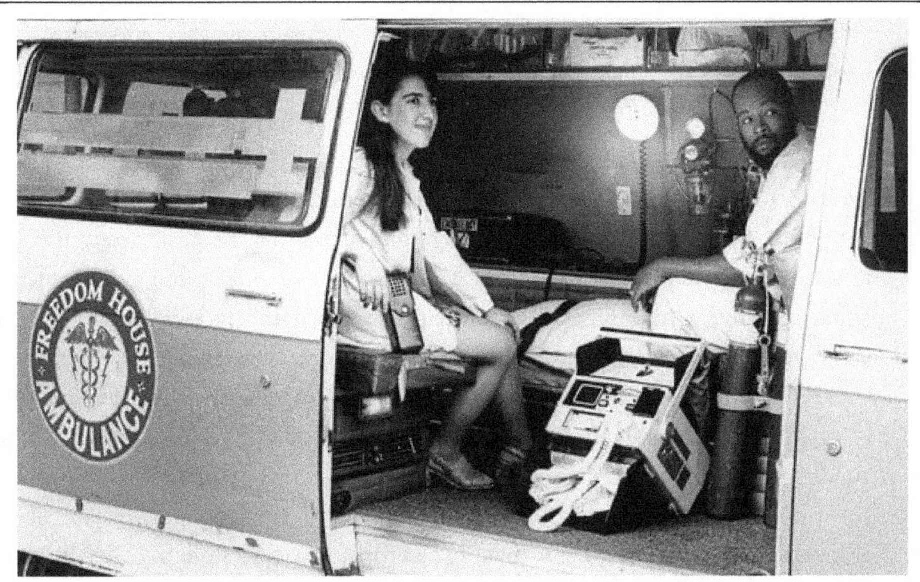

Dr. Caroline in the Freedom House Ambulance[17].

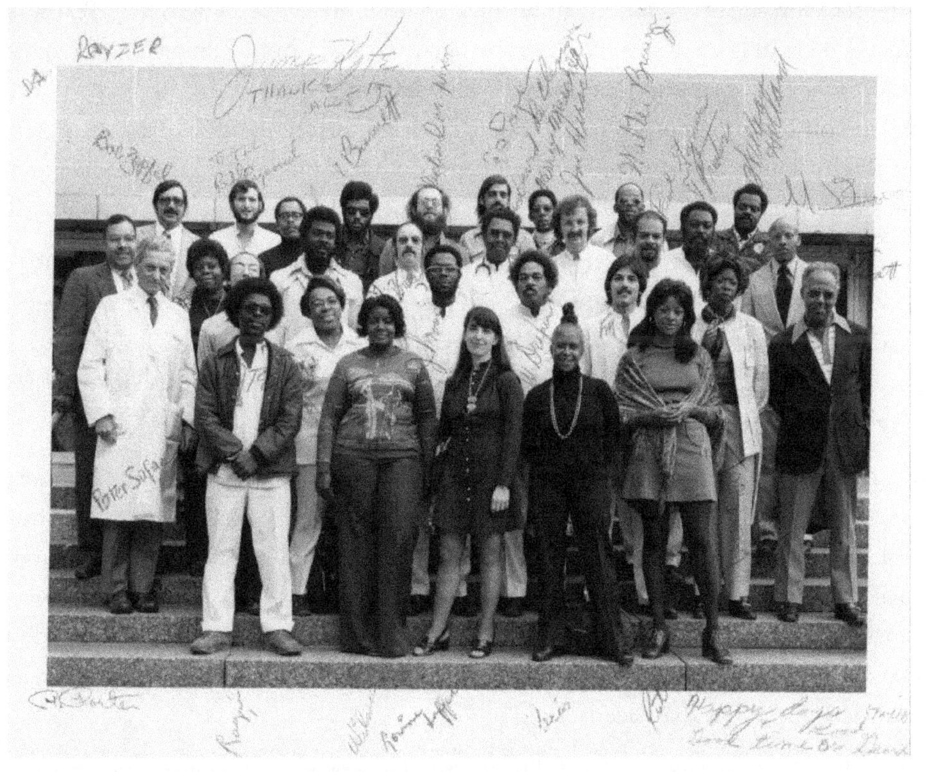

Members of the Freedom House Ambulance Service:
The pioneers of the modern EMS system in the United States.[18]

EMS: TRANSPORTATION OR HEALTH?

"The present predominating view of ambulances is that they are transportation services… existing standards for ambulance personnel are outdated in terms of present and emerging concepts of medical science."
-1975 NHTSA Report[19]

As physician-led EMS pilot programs were successfully operating around the nation, the vision was becoming clear: lives could be saved by bringing professional medical care to the sick and injured, and this would require a new type of medical professional. Providing medicine outside of the hospital required a new type of medical professional that could incorporate vehicle extrication and rescue services with advanced training in trauma, medicine, anesthesiology, cardiology, and obstetrics. On December 8, 1969, the Los Angeles Fire Department launched "Squad 51" at Harbor General Hospital with two paramedics. However, this pilot project outpaced medical regulation and legislation. At that time, only physicians or nurses were authorized to provide medical care. On July 14, 1970, Governor Ronald Reagan signed the *Wedworth-Townsend Paramedic Act* into law, making California the first state to officially recognize paramedics.[20]

Concurrently, President Lyndon Johnson's Committee on Highway Traffic Safety recommended creating a national certification agency for uniform training and examination of emergency ambulance service personnel. This led the American Medical Association's Commission on EMS to appoint a Task Force studying the feasibility of such an organization. In 1970, this Task Force established a new independent national organization to meet President Johnson's requirement. In June 1970, the Registry of EMTs was formed.

Meanwhile, the U.S. Department of Health, Education, and Welfare (DHEW) began researching existing state legislation related to emergency care. In June, 1969, the Department published a "*Compendium of State Statutes on the Regulation of Ambulance Services, Operation of Emergency Vehicles and Good Samaritan Laws.*"[21] Then in 1972, they published a summary of "*State Statutes on Emergency Medical Services.*"[22]

As federal agencies were striving to establish a national system, the TV show "Emergency!" debuted showcasing the cutting-edge paramedic program in Los Angeles, California. This portrayal sparked nationwide demands for improved EMS agencies. As demand grew, policymakers and regulators grappled with escalating needs. To address this, grassroots ambulance services formed nationwide, and state health departments began tracking individuals with first aid certifications working on ambulances, which started the tradition of states issuing EMS certifications rather than licenses.

While the 1966 *Highway Safety Act* had directed the Department of Transportation to improve EMS systems by administering grants for ambulance purchases, communications systems, and training programs, tensions grew between local governments, states, and federal agencies. Visionary physicians were transforming EMS into a medical service and shows like Emergency! were portraying the potential of EMS to communities across the nation. Meanwhile, despite federal mandates, funding, and DOT's enforcement powers granted by the *Highway Safety Act*, states were not developing consistent EMS systems. These frustrations catalyzed demands for additional Congressional action. In 1973, Congress passed the *Emergency Medical Services Systems Act (EMS Act)*.[23]

The *EMS Act* identified and defined fifteen components of an EMS system and established a federal lead agency for EMS in the Division of EMS of the Department of Health, Education and Welfare (DHEW, later reorganized as the Department of Health and Human Services). This office was directed to establish coordinated local, regional, and state EMS systems. DHEW planned a network of 303 regional EMS systems to ensure equitable access to EMS nationwide.[24]

DHEW region and State	Regional EMS system		Number of systems [1]
	HSA	Other	
Region I:			
Connecticut		X	5
Maine		(2)	5
Massachusetts		X	8
New Hampshire		(2)	3
Rhode Island	•	--------	1
Vermont	•	--------	5
Region II:			
New Jersey	X	--------	5
New York	X	--------	8-1
Puerto Rico		(3)	1
Virgin Islands			
Region III:			
Delaware	•	--------	1
District of Columbia	•	(4)	1-1
Maryland		(4)	4-1
Pennsylvania	†	†	
Virginia		(4)	6-2
West Virginia	†	†	
Region IV:			
Alabama		(3)	6
Florida	X	--------	9
Georgia		(6)	11-1
Kentucky		X	9
Mississippi		(2)	4
North Carolina	X	--------	6
South Carolina		(1)	4
Tennessee		(8)	5-2
Region V:			
Illinois		(9)	8
Indiana	X	--------	3
Michigan	X	--------	8
Minnesota		(10)	7-3
Ohio		(11)	10
Wisconsin	X	--------	7-1
Region VI: [13]			
Arkansas		X	8
Louisiana		X	8
New Mexico		X	7
Oklahoma		X	11
Texas		X	25
Region VII:			
Iowa		X	5-2
Kansas		X	7-3
Missouri		X	8-3
Nebraska		(13)	7-2
Region VIII:			
Colorado		X	4
Montana		(2)	3
North Dakota		(14)	4-2
South Dakota		(2)	2
Utah		(15)	1
Wyoming	X	--------	1
Region IX:			
American Samoa			
Arizona		X	4
California		(5)	12
Guam			
Hawaii	•	--------	1
Nevada		X	3
Trust Territory			
Region X:			
Alaska		(17)	3
Idaho		(2)	2
Oregon	X	--------	3
Washington		X	8

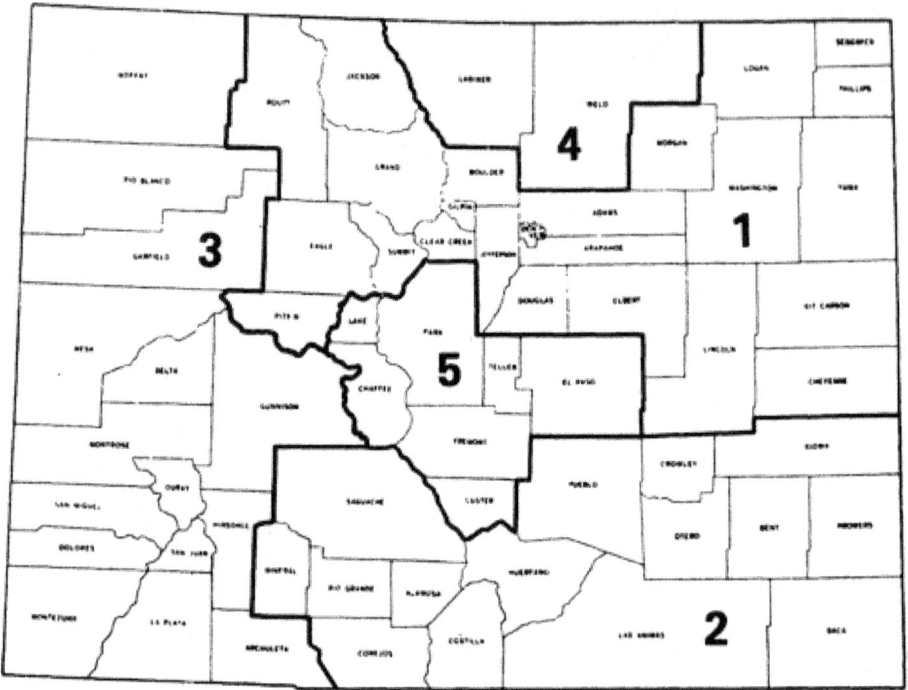

COLORADO

6/30/76

Figure 5. Project regions within the state of Colorado.

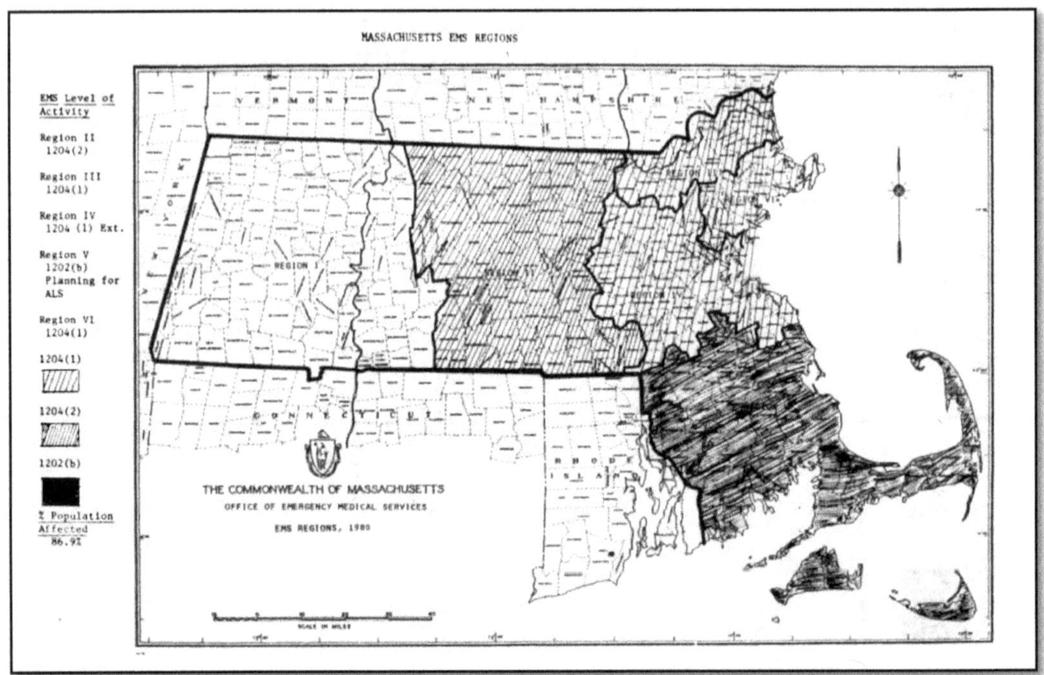

The Department of Health, Education and Welfare identified over 300 Regional EMS Systems, identified in the table above.[25] Maps above demonstrate Colorado's proposed regions (1976)[26] and Massachusetts regions(1980).

Although the *EMS Act* defined a lead federal agency for EMS and provided over $300 million in federal support ($2.1 billion in 2023 dollars), Congress failed to clarify the relationship between the Department of Transportation's ongoing EMS system development work (under the 1966 *Highway Safety Act*) and the new mandates for the DHEW. The new Act also failed to provide adequate staffing within the DHEW to implement the legislative requirements, nor did the Act address sustainable funding for EMS systems. While the *EMS Act* intended to implement a nationwide "*Systems*" approach to Emergency Medical Services, it inadvertently hastened conflicting and uncoordinated development of isolated local initiatives without sustainable funding mechanisms.

While the *EMS Act* was being implemented, state governors now had two competing mandates to establish EMS: one directive from the DOT (tied to highway safety funding) and a separate directive from the DHEW. A 1977 congressional investigation report bluntly described the dysfunction:

> "The DOT required each state to submit for approval a comprehensive emergency medical services plan…that imposed a different planning requirement on State Health Departments in conflict and inconsistent with the plans required by the U.S. DOT"[27]

Despite the coordination challenges, the major shortfall of the *EMS System Act* was the lack of long-term sustainable financing for EMS. The federal government, in collaboration with organizations like the Robert Wood Johnson Foundation[28], established grants to aid states and local governments in enhancing their EMS systems. While these grants initiated regional EMS systems, the fatal assumption was that once established, local governments would maintain them. This oversight left EMS systems nationwide facing substantial community expectations and unsustainable financial burdens. The lack of a clear funding strategy hindered EMS growth and progress, creating a financial burden that continues to impact many systems today – fifty years later.

The scarcity of long-term, sustainable funding persisted despite considerable contributions from grants. These grants made crucial advancements possible, including training EMS personnel, procuring state-of-the-art ambulance equipment and vehicles, and constructing robust EMS communication networks. However, the absence of a comprehensive funding strategy remained a significant barrier.

Moreover, these federal EMS programs helped establish the first national standards for EMS education and training. This standardization was part of the vision to ensure communities had access to ambulances and that EMS practitioners nationwide received the same high-quality training.

The federal EMS programs and grants also significantly boosted public awareness of EMS and the importance of emergency medical care. This increased awareness resulted in greater demand for EMS agencies and helped solidify EMS as a vital component of the healthcare system. However, the persistent issue of insufficient funding continued to hinder the full potential of

EMS development and the realization of a truly national, coordinated approach to emergency medical services.

While Congress recognized the need for the United States to have a coordinated Emergency Medical Services system, defining EMS as either a component of the Department of Transportation or the Department of Health, Education and Welfare, both had shortcomings. Ironically, the nation is still struggling with the same question fifty years later: Is EMS transportation, health, public safety, fire…?

Perhaps rather than a continuous attempt to align Emergency Medical Services into another predefined government agency or technical field, EMS is best categorized as itself: Emergency Medical Services.

15 Components of an EMS System (1973)

The *Emergency Medical Services Systems Act* of 1973 identified and defined the following 15 components of an EMS system:

1. **Regulation and policy**: The EMS system should be regulated and governed by appropriate laws, regulations, and policies.
2. **Resource management**: EMS systems should be designed to efficiently and effectively manage available resources.
3. **Human resources and training**: EMS personnel should be appropriately trained, certified, and licensed to perform their roles.
4. **Transportation**: EMS systems should have appropriate vehicles, including ambulances, helicopters, or other modes of transportation.
5. **Communications**: EMS systems should have effective communication systems to ensure rapid response and coordination between EMS personnel, hospitals, and other emergency services.
6. **Trauma systems**: EMS systems should have a trauma system in place that provides for the rapid identification, triage, and transport of patients with traumatic injuries.
7. **Public information and education**: EMS systems should provide public information and education programs to promote community awareness of emergency medical services.
8. **Medical direction**: EMS systems should be under the direction of a licensed physician who is responsible for medical oversight and quality assurance.
9. **Patient care:** EMS personnel should provide high-quality care to patients based on established medical protocols and standards.
10. **Communications with medical facilities**: EMS personnel should have the ability to communicate with medical facilities to provide patient information and receive medical advice.

11. **Information systems**: EMS systems should have appropriate information systems to collect and manage patient data, as well as to track system performance.
12. **Evaluation**: EMS systems should regularly evaluate their performance and use the results to improve the system.
13. **Public access**: EMS systems should provide a system for public access to emergency medical services, including a universal phone number (such as 911) for emergency calls.
14. **Disaster planning**: EMS systems should have a disaster plan in place to respond to large-scale emergencies.
15. **Mutual aid**: EMS systems should have the ability to provide mutual aid to neighboring EMS systems during emergencies.

While the 15 elements listed above—identified by the visionaries of EMS systems—remain relevant, Sustainable System Finance was not included. Without a robust system for financing, the efficiency, reliability, and sustainability of EMS systems are compromised. Hence, sustainable financing becomes a cornerstone to the effective operation and longevity of these services.

14 Attributes of an EMS System (1996)

The 14 attributes of an EMS system as identified in the 1996 *EMS Agenda for the Future* are as follows:

1. **Integration of Health Services**: This attribute emphasizes the coordination and integration of emergency medical services with other healthcare entities and services, such as hospitals, public health agencies, and specialty care providers.
2. **EMS Research**: It highlights the importance of conducting research in the field of EMS to improve patient outcomes, enhance system effectiveness, and develop evidence-based practices.
3. **Legislation and Regulation**: This attribute focuses on the need for appropriate laws and regulations to govern EMS systems, ensuring standards, quality control, and accountability.
4. **System Finance**: It refers to the financial aspects of an EMS system, including funding sources, reimbursement mechanisms, and cost-effective resource allocation.
5. **Human Resources**: This attribute recognizes the significance of having well-trained and qualified EMS personnel, including emergency medical technicians and paramedics, as well as addressing issues related to recruitment, retention, and career development.
6. **Medical Direction**: It emphasizes the role of medical directors in providing oversight, guidance, and medical control for EMS systems, ensuring that patient care is delivered in accordance with established protocols and standards.

7. **Education Systems**: This attribute highlights the need for comprehensive and standardized EMS education programs, including initial training, continuing education, and ongoing professional development for EMS personnel.
8. **Public Education**: It emphasizes the importance of educating the public about EMS systems, including how to access emergency care, perform basic life support techniques, and recognize the signs of emergencies.
9. **Prevention**: This attribute underscores the role of EMS in injury and illness prevention through activities such as community outreach, public health campaigns, and safety education.
10. **Public Access**: It focuses on improving public access to emergency care through initiatives such as enhanced 9-1-1 systems, community-based first response programs, and the placement of automated external defibrillators (AEDs) in public locations.
11. **Communication Systems**: This attribute highlights the need for reliable and effective communication systems to facilitate prompt and accurate information exchange among EMS practitioners, dispatch centers, hospitals, and other healthcare entities.
12. **Clinical Care**: It emphasizes the delivery of high-quality patient care in the prehospital setting, including standardized protocols, evidence-based practices, and ongoing quality improvement initiatives.
13. **Information Systems**: This attribute recognizes the importance of utilizing information technology and data systems to support EMS operations, clinical documentation, performance measurement, and system evaluation.
14. **Evaluation**: It underscores the need for ongoing evaluation and continuous quality improvement of EMS systems, including outcome measurement, benchmarking, and data-driven decision-making.

These attributes collectively provide a framework for the development and improvement of EMS systems, promoting effective and efficient emergency medical care.

DOT & EMS DEVELOPMENT (1977)

In December 1977, Robert E. Motley[c] of the Department of Transportation summarized, in the *Journal of Emergency Care & Transportation* from his perspective, the Department of Transportation's role in EMS development:

> The need for the development of Emergency Medical Technician as a professional in the field of allied health was first identified in the September 1966 report, "*Accidental Death and Disability: The Neglected Disease of Modern Society*", developed by the National Academy of Sciences. At that time, 48% of the nation's ambulance personnel had

[c] NHTSA described Robert Motley as "a noteworthy force in the development of EMT training… and adviser in the development of national EMS." He was actively involved with the NREMT and in 1977 he was presented with the Joseph D. Farrington, MD, Award of Excellence from the National Association of Emergency Medical Technicians.

standard Red Cross training or no formal training. Fifty-two percent had advanced Red Cross training. The majority of personnel were poorly paid technicians operating commercial or funeral director ambulance services or were volunteers. The turnover rate exceeded 40% annually.

The Department of Health, Education and Welfare established an emergency medical services program in the Division of Accident Prevention in early 1960. The program lacked departmental support or interest and was transferred by Congress to the U.S. Department of Transportation with the passage of the Highway Safety Act of 1966. The Act mandated the establishment of highway safety standards, one of which was Standard 11, "Emergency Medical Services." During the first two or three years, the efforts of DOT were directed to in-depth research on the recommendations of findings of the National Academy of Sciences 1960 report. The first national training course directed to ambulance personnel was published by the DOT in October 1969.

A national EMT training program cannot be put into effect without a state organizational structure and authority. In 1966, only four states had an established EMS program or personnel identified as having an EMS responsibility; three were offering a formal state training program for ambulance personnel. Over the next 11 years, highway safety funds between $9 and $15 million annually were spent on a matching grant basis and development of an effective prehospital care system. [29]

THE END OF FEDERAL GRANTS AND A STALLED SYSTEM

In 1981, the *Omnibus Budget Reconciliation Act*[30] consolidated EMS funding into state administered preventive health and health services block grants, dissolved the designated 'lead federal EMS office' in the Department of Health and Human Services (HHS, formerly DHEW), and repealed most of the Emergency Medical Services Act[31]. These changes had a devastating impact on the systemic and directed development of EMS systems. Under the new block grant funding model, states were given broad discretion to allocate funds for preventive health and health services, including EMS. Unfortunately, this change quickly resulted in a sharp decrease in total funding for state-level EMS programs, as most states chose to spend the money on other areas of need.

"With all that has been accomplished over the past five years in EMS (1975-1980), a setback of this dimension is unthinkable."
-ACEP Testimony to Congress, April 22, 1980

Despite the elimination of the designated HHS EMS program, the Department of Transportation's programs remained intact, including the Section 402 *State and Community Highway Safety Grant Program.*[d] However, the changes in federal funding left the newly formed

[d] Section 402 and 405 funding remain a significant source of federal funding for many state EMS programs.

EMS regions and state EMS offices without financial support and the associated federal system development resources.

The development of EMS systems varied greatly from state to state after these changes. Some states increased their involvement in EMS, while others delegated more authority to cities and counties. Additionally, the absence of accountability and objective scientific evidence regarding optimal models for EMS organization and delivery left many systems in a quandary about the most appropriate steps to take.

The repercussions of the changes to federal funding were especially severe in rural areas, where funding was already very scarce. Many state EMS offices struggled to maintain existing programs, let alone develop new ones. This destabilized the systematic development of EMS, leading to inconsistencies and gaps in EMS agencies across the country. Some states were simply unable to perform the core coordination and system development functions.

In the early 1990s, the Department of Health and Human Services oversaw a modest renaissance of dedicated federal EMS leadership. This renewal was largely facilitated by the enactment of the *Trauma Care Systems Planning and Development Act.*[32] The Act led to the establishment of the Division of Trauma and Emergency Medical Systems within the Health Resources and Services Administration (HRSA), an arm of the U.S. Public Health Service. Even though the division had limited funding and a brief existence, it signified a crucial revival of EMS under the authority of HHS.

However, by the mid-1980s, numerous regional EMS systems that had federal designation were deteriorating and not economically viable. In the face of sporadic leadership at the federal, state, or regional levels, local systems showcasing resilience initiated their solutions, thereby preserving the continuity of EMS agencies. Determined efforts at the individual level helped many community EMS agencies to endure, amplifying the sentiment of community-centric pride that pervades EMS today. Yet, the process of establishing alternate funding sources and rebuilding state EMS offices in the aftermath of federal support withdrawal spanned several decades.

Moreover, even now—many decades later—several EMS offices across the nation are grappling with substantial challenges. They are bereft of dedicated funding, consistently plagued by understaffing, and inadequately positioned within the state government to exercise necessary influence or access resources aligned with public expectations and responsibilities. The challenges at hand are firmly rooted in the historical fragmentation and fractures within the EMS system. This stark reality underscores the dire need for an exhaustive evaluation and reform to rectify these enduring systemic inadequacies.

PERSISTENCE AND GROWTH

Despite challenges faced by EMS systems due to the loss of federal funding, the national movement of EMS system development had begun, marked by remarkably rapid growth and development. Local ambulance services and rescue squads continued to emerge in urban, rural, and frontier communities across the nation, fostering a strong sense of local community and identity. Yet, for some, these challenges also seeded distrust and resentment towards national EMS programs, sentiments that have been passed down from generation to generation.

During this transformative period, multiple professional organizations, such as the National Registry of EMTs, the National Association of Emergency Medical Technicians and the National Association of State EMS Directors (later reorganized as the National Association of State EMS Officials – NASEMSO), continued to play crucial roles in shaping the EMS landscape. These organizations coordinated efforts across state boundaries and provided support, resources, and advocacy for EMS professionals and state EMS offices. They contributed significantly to the development and promotion of national standards and best practices for EMS.

In tandem with organizational efforts, EMS education and training evolved, introducing new technologies and techniques, and gaining an enhanced understanding of the unique challenges faced by EMS professionals in the field. This evolution led to the creation of advanced and specialized EMS training programs, such as critical care paramedic programs, community paramedic programs, flight paramedicine, and tactical EMS programs.

The modern EMS system in the United States evolved quickly, driven by visionaries, innovators, and implementers. Sentinel events in this timeline showcase the pace of innovation and the swift implementation of this new medical specialty. Milestones, significant events, and the impact of influential publications were critical to shaping the EMS landscape. Moreover, the establishment of the 911 emergency system and the formation of various EMS organizations and associations further highlighted the evolution of EMS from primarily a transportation service to an essential component of the broader healthcare system.

The EMS system in the United States progressed from conceptual pilot projects to a public expectation in just over a generation, focusing on the delivery of emergency medical care, medical oversight, and the recognition of specialized roles within the profession. Through the unwavering dedication and determination of numerous key stakeholders, the EMS system has grown, evolved, and continues to innovate, adapt, and work towards providing high-quality emergency medical care to communities across the country. This remarkable journey sets the stage for continued progress and innovation in the field of emergency medical services.

EMS Development Timeline[e]

Year	Milestone Event
1928	Julian Stanley Wise forms the Roanoke (VA) Life Saving and First Aid Crew. The first independent, all-**volunteer rescue squad** in the United States.
1958	Drs. J.D. Farrington and Sam W. Banks started training Chicago fire fighters in a prototype emergency medical care course, the precursor of the **EMT-Ambulance** course.[33] Dr. Peter Safar, who had just introduced the concept of **CPR**, established the first intensive care unit (ICU).
1959	At the request of the White House, Office of Civil Defense Mobilization, the American Medical Association publishes a "Summary Report on National Emergency Medical Care".[34] This changes the approach to emergency medicine and established the AMA's **Taskforce on Emergency Medical Care**.
1960	The Department of Health, Education and Welfare (DHEW) established an **Emergency Medical Services Program** in the Division of Accident Prevention.
1963	The American Medical Association (AMA) designed and publicized the **Universal Medical Identification Symbol**[35], which later became known as the Star of Life.
1965	On July 30, 1965, **President Lyndon B. Johnson** signed the *Medicare and Medicaid Act*, which includes a benefit for ambulance transportation and gives rise to a reimbursement structure that funds much of modern EMS.
1966	Release of the **white paper**, "*Accidental Death and Disability: The Neglected Disease of Modern Society*", raising awareness about the importance of emergency medical care. September 9, 1966 — President Lyndon B. Johnson signed the National Traffic and Motor Vehicle Safety Act[36] and the Highway Safety Act[37] creating the Department of Transportation and the initial requirements for national guidelines and standards for EMS systems.
1967	The American Medical Association hosts the **National Conference on Emergency Medical Services**, which produces recommendations for training ambulance personnel. Dr. Peter Safar and colleagues establish the **Freedom House Ambulance Service** in Pittsburgh, PA. J.D. Farrington, MD, FACS, writes "***Death in a Ditch***", the article published by American College of Surgeons presents Dr. Farrington's vision related to the safe

[e] The development of EMS included many pilot projects and seminal events. This is not an exhaustive list.

	extrication, on scene care, and the need to maintain care during the transportation of injured patients. The National Academy of Sciences and National Research Council (NAS/NRC) attempt to **standardize training** by publishing the *Training of Ambulance Personnel and Others Responsible for Emergency Care of the Sick and Injured at the Scene and During Transport*
1968	February 16, 1968 — The nation's **first call to 911** is received at a police station in Haleyville, Alabama, marking the beginning of the 911 emergency system in the United States. May 22, 1968 — The Committee on Acute Medicine of the American Society of Anesthesiologists recommends creating a "**Registry of EMTs**". St. Vincent's Hospital in New York City launches America's first **mobile coronary care** unit using physicians. David Boyd, MD, developed the "**Trauma Unit**" concept at Cook County Hospital in Chicago, Illinois. The Cedarville College Emergency Fire and Rescue Service (OH) morphed into Cedarville College Rescue Squad, the first all-student operated rescue squad in the United States.
1969	April 1969 — The Ohio State University Hospital and the Columbus Division of Fire launch the **'Heart Mobile'** with three firefighters and a cardiac physician. May 5-6, 1969 — The **Airlie House Conference** on emergency medical services takes place in Warrenton, Virginia. Dr. Peter Safar introduces the concepts of a standardized **national EMS Patient Care Report**, highlights the future need for computer analysis of EMS data, and calls for a single organization to certify EMS personnel. The Miami (FL) Fire Department starts a **paramedic program** under Dr. Eugene Nagel. Seattle, WA, quickly follows with Medic 1. New York City (NY) uses computers to assist with optimizing the positioning of 109 ambulances across the city.[38] AAOS publishes the first national standard **EMT-Ambulance curriculum**, based on the Chicago (IL) prototype course by Dr. J.D. Farrington and Dr. Sam Banks.
1970	January 21, 1970 — President Lyndon Johnson's Committee on Highway Traffic Safety established a Task Force[39] to create a **national EMS certification** agency. California's ***Wedworth Townsend Act*** is the first legislation to define paramedics under state law.

	The first **hospital-based civilian air ambulance** service, Flight for Life, is launched in Denver (CO) providing faster access to emergency medical care for patients in remote areas. March 19, 1970 "Helicopter 108," a Bell 206 JetRanger operated by the Maryland State Police completed its first **civilian medevac mission.** On June 4, 1970 — Fulfilling the requirement of President Johnson's committee, The **Registry of EMTs is created** (later renamed the National Registry of EMTs).
1971	The *Highway Safety Act* mandates that all states develop EMS programs and establishes the **National Standard Curriculum** for training Emergency Medical Technician-Ambulances (EMT-A). Rocco V. Morando is selected as National Registry's founding Executive Director and the first national EMS certification exam (EMT-Ambulance) is administered.
1972	NAS-NRC Publishes *Roles and Resources of Federal Agencies in Support of Comprehensive Emergency Medical Services* The Department of Health, Education and Welfare allocates **$16 million to EMS** demonstration programs in five states. The TV show ***Emergency!*** premieres. Due to rising concerns over the unauthorized use of the Red Cross emblem on ambulances, NHTSA requests use of the National Registry's symbol (the Universal Medical Identification Symbol, a.k.a. the **Star of Life**) as the national symbol for EMS. First **Emergency Medicine residency program** established at the University of Cincinnati. Dr. Donald Benson, medical director for the Freedom House Ambulance Service, calls for a "**systems approach**" to EMS in his publication *Elements of a comprehensive Emergency Medical Services System.*
1973	Congress passes the ***EMS Systems Act***, funding 303 regional EMS systems. The Department of Health, Education, and Welfare designated as the **lead federal agency for EMS.** The Robert Wood Johnson Foundation appropriates $15 million to fund 44 EMS pilot projects in 32 states and Puerto Rico. First Nationally Certified EMTs complete **recertification.**
1974	The federal Star of Life **ambulance purchasing specification** (KKK-A-1822) takes effect. President Ford signs the first **EMS Week** proclamation, acknowledging the importance of emergency medical services in the United States.

	The NREMT calls a meeting to develop a national standard curriculum for **EMT-Paramedic.** Dr. Norman McSwain developed **Advanced Life Support** programs in Kansas.
1975	January 8, 1975 — Rocco Morando and the NREMT calls a meeting of EMS stakeholders in Chicago to discuss creating a new **association of EMTs** (NAEMT) that could unify and advocate for the profession. The NREMT requests the American Medical Association to recognize EMT-Paramedic as an **allied health profession** and establishes national standards for continuing education for the EMS profession. The University of Pittsburgh and Nancy Caroline, MD, begin work on the first National Standard Curriculum for paramedic training. The AHA creates the **Advanced Cardiac Life Support** course. The AMA officially recognizes paramedic as an allied health occupation and establishes the "**Joint Review Committee** on Education Programs for the EMT-Paramedic". Freedom House Ambulance Service ceases operations but creates a foundation for the future development of EMS nationwide. November 15, 1975 — The **National Association of EMTs** (NAEMT) is formed and the first meeting is held at the O'Hare Hilton Hotel in Chicago.
1976	The Department of Health, Education and Welfare publishes a report to Congress titled, "***Progress, But Problems** in Developing Emergency Medical Services Systems*". Congress allocates additional funding for the development of Regional EMS systems.
1977	NHTSA publishes the first **EMT-Paramedic National Standard Curriculum**. July 11, 1977, Congress calls for an investigation and study of the Emergency Medical Services Systems and programs of the Department of Transportation (DOT) and the Department of Health, Education, and Welfare (DHEW).
1978	Dr. Jeff Clawson's initial system for triaging emergency calls and prioritizing responses is implemented in Salt Lake City. The first NREMT-Paramedic exam is administered in Minneapolis, MN. The NREMT becomes a member of the National Commission for Health Certifying Agencies. The "***Essentials for EMT-Paramedic Program Accreditation***" are approved by the AMA. March - USDOT Publishes ***Model Legislation** for Emergency Medical Services* for states.

	October - An inter-agency federal memorandum of understanding is signed between the Department of Health, Education and Welfare (the designated federal lead agency for EMS) and the Department of Transportation.
1979	**Emergency Medicine** became the 23rd recognized medical specialty for physicians. NHTSA's Crash Injury Management for the Law Enforcement Officer program is refashioned into a National Standard Curriculum for first responders. The Department of Health, Education, and Welfare was reorganized as the Department of Health and Human Services (DHHS) on October 17, 1979.
1980	The **National Association of State EMS Directors** (later NASEMSO) is created. The NREMT publishes its first national standard exam for **EMT-Intermediates**.
1981	The *Omnibus Budget Reconciliation Act* eliminated the designated lead federal agency for EMS – the Department of Health and Human Services Division of EMS – and consolidates EMS funding into state preventive health and health services **block grants**; much of the federal funding for EMS is lost.
1983	Recognizing the need for advanced level trauma training, Dr. Norman McSwain led the development of the **Prehospital Trauma Life Support** (PHTLS) curriculum. NHTSA launches a "reciprocity guidelines" project with the National Association of State EMS Directors "as a means of encouraging States to adopted uniform training".
1984	*Public Health Act* creates the federal **Emergency Medical Services for Children** (EMSC) program to add emphasis on pediatric patients.
1985	NRC publishes *Injury in America: A Continuing Public Health Problem.* This report yet again describes the gaps after 20 years of addressing **accidental death and disability**.
1988	National Registry (NREMT) Executive Director Rocco V. Morando retires. NHTSA implements a statewide EMS technical assessment program to **standardize EMS** across the nation.
1989	American College of Emergency Physicians (ACEP) launches its section membership program.
1990	Recognizing a need for standards and resources dedicated towards EMS education, NHTSA convened a Consensus Workshop on Emergency Medical Services Training Programs. Following the workshop, NHTSA awarded a contract to revise the EMT-Ambulance National Standard Curriculum.[f]

[f] Report on Activities Under the Highway Safety Act. (1990). United States: National Highway Safety Bureau.

	Trauma Care Systems Planning and Development Act of 1990 established the Division of Trauma and Emergency Medical Systems within the Health Resources and Services Administration (HRSA).
1994	The EMT-Ambulance is renamed **EMT-Basic**, and the training is shifted from a diagnosis-based approach to an assessment-based approach.
1995	**National Association of EMS Educators** (NAEMSE) is formed "to promote EMS education, develop and deliver educational resources, and advocate research and lifelong learning for the professional EMS educator."
1996	The ***EMS Agenda for the Future*** seeks to reunify the profession and connect EMS with other medical professions.
1997	NHTSA raises awareness of quality improvement and publishes *A leadership guide to quality improvement for EMS Systems.*
1999	The ***EMS Education Agenda for the Future*** is published, offering recommendations for core content and scope of practice.
2000	The **Board for Critical Care Transport Paramedic Certification** was formed.
2001	The **National EMS Information System** (NEMSIS) data standard is implemented, and the first records are created. The National Association of EMS Educators (NAEMSE) enters into a cooperative agreement with NHTSA and HRSA to revise the **EMS Instructor** Training Program.
2003	The National Registry implements the **EMS Fellowship** doctoral research program. The Indianapolis-Hamilton County, Indiana, UASI project explores linking multiple EMS agencies in a central health information exchange and the role of EMS data in homeland security.
2004	The U.S. Department of Health and Human Services, Health Resources and Services Administration Office of Rural Health Policy publishes the *Rural and Frontier EMS Agenda for the Future: A Service Chief's Guide to Creating Community Support of Excellence in EMS.*
2005	**Federal Interagency Committee on EMS** (FICEMS) is created to coordinate federal EMS efforts.
2007	Institute of Medicine published Emergency Medical Services: At the Crossroads. The **National EMS Advisory Council** (NEMSAC) is created to provide recommendations to the DOT and FICEMS. NHTSA publishes the ***National EMS Scope of Practice Model,*** a collaborative project with the National Association of State EMS Officials.

2009	NHTSA retires the National Standard Curriculum approach and replaces it with the ***EMS Education Standards.***
2010	NASEMSO passes Resolution 2010-03, titled "*National EMS Certification and Program Accreditation*" urging the National Registry of EMTs to modify their requirements and mandate graduation from a CoAEMSP accredited paramedic program as a prerequisite for National EMS Certification at the paramedic level. American Board of Medical Specialties approves **EMS as a physician** subspecialty.
2011	The National Standard Curriculum for the First Responder and EMT-Basic certification levels are retired and replaced with **Emergency Medical Responder** (EMR) and **Emergency Medical Technician** (EMT).
2013	The National Standard Curriculum for the EMT-Intermediate and EMT-Paramedic levels are retired and replaced with the **Advanced-EMT and Paramedic.** A National Advisory Panel is convened to guide the early stages of developing an interstate licensing compact for EMS.
2014	Model legislation for the **Recognition of EMS Personnel Licensure Interstate Compact (REPLICA) is released.**
2015	Colorado is the first state to pass the REPLICA compact legislation.
2016	The Board for Critical Care Transport Paramedic Certification was rebranded as the **International Board for Specialty Certifications**.
2017	The *National EMS Scope of Practice Model* is revised to enhance consistency and standardization in EMS practice across the United States. The Interstate Commission for EMS Personnel Practice, the **EMS Compact's** governing body, held its inaugural meeting on October 7-8, 2017, in Oklahoma City, OK, with 12 member states.
2020	The COVID-19 pandemic significantly impacts EMS operations, with EMS practitioners playing a crucial role in responding to the public health crisis. March 10, 2020 - The EMS Compact Commission officially activated the EMS Compact in 22 states to ensure EMS personnel could utilize the Privilege to Practice as states respond to the COVID-19 pandemic.

2

EMS VISIONARIES

"If I have seen further, it is by standing on the shoulders of Giants."
- Sir Isaac Newton, 1675

THE MODERN EMS SYSTEM IS THE RESULT OF THE TIRELESS EFFORTS of courageous and passionate visionaries who devoted their lives to improving pre-hospital care. EMS pioneers such as James O. Page, John Moon, Dr. J.D. Farrington, Dr. Peter Safar, Dr. Nancy Caroline and Rocco Morando, revolutionized emergency medical care with their contributions. Their unwavering dedication and groundbreaking work have laid the foundation for the modern EMS system, saving countless lives, and delivering critical care to those in need.

The profound impact of these visionaries is comparable to Sir Isaac Newton's quote, and it serves as a metaphor for the development of EMS. The current and future leaders in EMS bear the responsibility of building upon the knowledge and experience passed down by these trailblazers. By standing on the shoulders of these giants, they gain a broader perspective and envision an improved future for emergency medical care.

The enduring contributions of these visionaries continue to shape and influence the field of emergency medical care today. Their legacy serves as an enduring inspiration for upcoming generations of EMS leaders and visionaries. It is through their enduring contributions and visionary leadership that the EMS field can continually advance and provide optimal care to those in need.

Biographies of EMS Visionaries

David Boyd, MD (1937-)

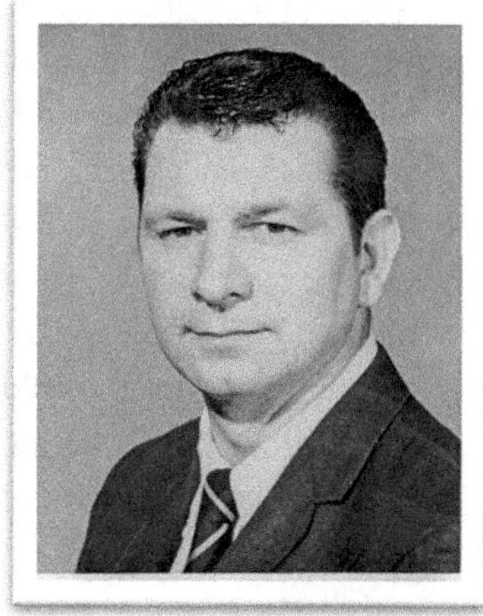

Dr. David Boyd, born and raised in Seattle, Washington, is a pioneer in emergency medicine, specifically in the realm of shock trauma and Emergency Medical Services. His groundbreaking work in these areas has shaped the national and international landscapes of trauma care and EMS.

Boyd's medical journey began at McGill University, where he pursued his medical degree. Post-graduation, he continued his education at Cook County Hospital with a rotating internship before serving as the Chief Medical Officer. He later entered the General Surgery Program at the University of Maryland, studying under the tutelage of R Adams Cowley, MD, a trailblazer in emergency medicine and shock trauma treatment. His fellowship at the R Adams Cowley Shock Trauma Center, where he was the first fellow, ignited his interest in shock trauma and paved the way for his work in EMS System design.

Inspired by his studies under Cowley, Boyd conceptualized and established a "trauma unit" at Cook County Hospital, which combined monitoring, resuscitation, and immediate surgery. This innovative approach laid the groundwork for the modern emergency medical system. Initially a local initiative under Boyd's leadership, the program developed into a statewide standard in Illinois and eventually expanded into a national program. In recognition of his transformative work, President Gerald Ford appointed Boyd as the Chief of the Department of Health, Education, and Welfare (HEW) Emergency Medical Services (EMS) Division.

Boyd is also credited with the development of specialized statewide trauma centers in Illinois for burns, spinal cord injuries, and pediatrics. Furthermore, he was instrumental in the implementation of a computerized trauma registry to streamline the trauma system by efficiently collecting and storing data.

Later in his career, he returned to clinical medicine and joined the Indian Health Service as a surgeon for the Sioux and Blackfeet Tribes. A prolific writer, Boyd authored over 150 articles and papers in his field and contributed to medical textbooks on EMS. He was instrumental in popularizing terms such as "trauma registry," "trauma center," "EMS systems," and "first responder".

In 2015, Boyd penned a professional autobiography in the Journal of Trauma and Acute Care Surgery titled "A trauma surgeon's journey,"[40] documenting his instrumental role in shaping the national and global trauma/EMS system. Dr. David Boyd's commitment and innovative approaches to emergency medical care, notably in trauma and EMS, have left a profound impact on the field. His life's work continues to resonate in the sector and inspire the generations of medical professionals that followed him.

Roddy A. Brandes (1920-2001)

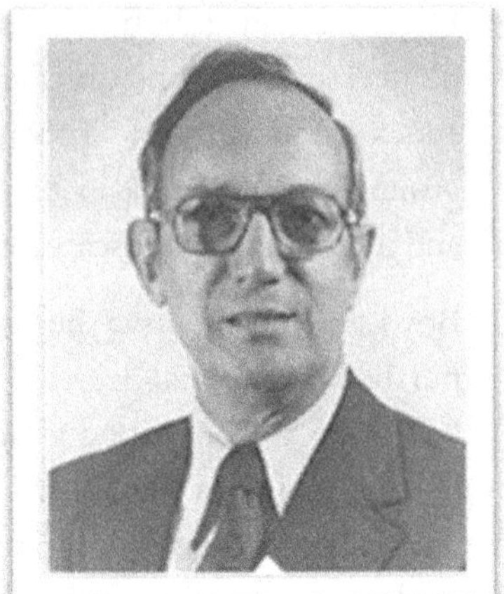

Roddy Arthur Brandes, an often under-recognized yet pivotal figure in the evolution of the modern Emergency Medical Services system, originated from Charlotte, North Carolina. Mr. Brandes rendered his services as a Captain in the United States Army Air Corps during World War II (1939-1946). After his military service, he owned and operated a truck leasing company until the City of Charlotte and Mecklenburg County sought his expertise in establishing an ambulance service for the area. In response, he instituted Mecklenburg Emergency Services in 1960.

"A major problem is that the public usually is unaware of the need for adequate ambulance services. That probably is why most local governments have failed to establish uniform standards of service…"
- Roddy A. Brandes

Considering his groundbreaking endeavors in the advancement of emergency medical services, Mr. Brandes held consultancy roles for the United States Department of Health, Education and Welfare, the National Academy of Sciences, and the American Medical Association. In 1970, while serving as President of the Ambulance Association of America,[a] he received the appointment as the first Chairman of the National Registry of Emergency Medical Technicians.

Mr. Brandes presented testimony before congressional committees on numerous occasions, advocating for the standardization and enhancement of emergency medical services throughout the United States. One particularly significant example of his contributions to modern EMS was his 1966 testimony to Congress:[41]

> "I am here as a voluntary witness respectfully asking Congress to support improvement of the quality of emergency medical services to more than 2 million victims of accidental injuries or sudden illnesses who are transported by ambulance every year to the hospital…this is one of the most sensitive public or quasi-public services in the country. Millions of Americans sooner or later will be transported in an ambulance. Their very lives sometimes will depend on the care they receive in that short period of time. Unfortunately…the chances of obtaining good care on the way to a hospital are often poor. Most of the ambulance crews in this country are untrained or ill-trained; most of the ambulances are unequipped or poorly equipped. President Johnson has called

[a] The historic records for the Ambulance Association of America end in the late 1970s. It is unclear if the Ambulance Association of America was reorganized as the American Ambulance Association.

> attention to the national disgrace of death and destruction on our highways. The question that bothers me every day is this: how many of the nearly 50,000 fatalities from automobile accidents every year - and more than 50,000 deaths from other accidents- could have been prevented by having an adequately trained ambulance crew? An injured soldier in Vietnam on the average has a better chance of surviving or having his injuries properly tended than a person hurt in an automobile accident in this country... A major problem is that the general public usually is unaware of the need for adequate ambulance services. That probably is why most local governments have failed to establish uniform standards of service...This situation is compounded by the fact that many local governmental officials accept this and are thus relieved from the responsibility of seeing that adequate service is provided... We, the concerned members of this industry, respectfully recommend that Congress support the appropriations under discussion to better enable this agency to gather information, establish guidelines, and assist local governments in setting up adequate services across this nation..."

Soon after Mr. Brandes' address to Congress, President Lyndon B. Johnson signed the National Traffic and Motor Vehicle Safety Act[42] and the Highway Safety Act.[43] These Acts culminated in the formation of the government agency later rebranded as the National Highway Traffic Safety Administration (NHTSA) and mandated the creation of guidelines and standards for a national EMS system. In 1970, as President Johnson's Committee on EMS and the American Medical Association pondered the mechanisms for standardizing EMS education and ensuring all EMS personnel met a single national standard, Roddy Brandes emerged as a central figure in these efforts.

In June 1970, Mr. Brandes was appointed as the inaugural Chairman of the board for the newly established national EMS certification body, the Registry of EMT-Ambulance. The following year, in anticipation of the rapidly expanding scope of EMS personnel beyond ambulance technicians, Mr. Brandes contributed to the rebranding of the organization as the National Registry of EMTs. The board subsequently hired its first full-time executive director, Rocco Morando, and established a permanent presence in Columbus, Ohio.

NANCY CAROLINE, MD (1944-2002)

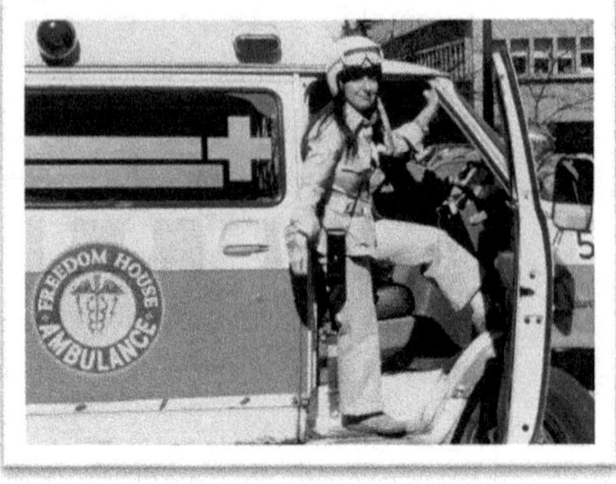

Dr. Nancy Caroline is acknowledged as a visionary and trailblazer in the advancement of the paramedic profession. Her belief in the capability of non-physicians to effectively perform emergency skills traditionally reserved for physicians was instrumental in transforming the landscape of EMS. Through her invaluable contributions, Caroline played a pivotal role in shaping the EMS field as it exists today. Her visionary mindset and dedication have not only expanded the scope of practice for paramedics but also contributed to saving numerous lives and improving patient outcomes. Dr. Nancy Caroline's impact on the development of the paramedic profession remains a testament to her innovative thinking and legacy within the EMS community.

Dr. Caroline's journey in EMS began with her mentorship under Dr. Peter Safar, a renowned figure in emergency medicine and cardiopulmonary resuscitation. While working at the University of Pittsburgh, Dr. Safar selected her as the new medical director of Freedom House Ambulance Service in Pittsburgh, making her one of the first EMS medical directors in the United States. Soon after, she and Dr. Safar collaborated on a grant-funded project by the U.S. Department of Transportation to develop a national standard curriculum for the newly emerging EMT-Paramedic.

At the time, Freedom House was on the brink of collapse; however, under Dr. Caroline's leadership, the service experienced a resurgence. Freedom House Ambulance Service became the first to train and deploy EMT-Paramedics to intubate in the field, amongst many other advanced life support skills. Despite its success, funding for the program was cut in 1975 when the city launched its own ambulance service, and Freedom House ultimately folded. Nonetheless, the program had a lasting impact on EMS in the United States, serving as a national model for city ambulances.

One of Dr. Caroline's most significant contributions to EMS was her authorship of the groundbreaking textbook, "*Emergency Care in the Streets.*" During the late 1970s, paramedics had to rely on nursing or medical textbooks that did not adequately address the unique working environments of EMS. To address this gap, Dr. Caroline wrote the first paramedic textbook tailored to their needs. For over a decade, "*Emergency Care in the Streets*" remained the only resource available for paramedic care. The textbook has since gone through multiple revisions and continues to be a vital resource for EMS educators and paramedics who began their careers with Dr. Caroline's guidance.

Dr. Caroline's impact on EMS was not limited to the United States. After her work with Freedom House, she moved to Israel and became the first medical director of Magen David Adom, the Israeli equivalent of the Red Cross. There, she developed a training program that enabled emergency workers to respond to terrorist attacks within minutes. Dr. Caroline also translated her EMS textbook into Hebrew, further broadening its impact on EMS education and practice worldwide.

Throughout her career, Dr. Caroline remained dedicated to EMS education and the advancement of the field. Her work transcended borders, as evidenced by her time spent in East Africa as the Senior Medical Officer of the African Medical and Research Foundation (AMREF) in Nairobi. In this role, she managed the Flying Doctors emergency medical service, which covered Tanzania, Uganda, Kenya, and southern Sudan. Dr. Caroline conducted medical classes for health workers in the region and wrote a weekly health column for the Kenyan newspaper, The Standard.

In addition to her work with AMREF, Dr. Caroline worked extensively with the Ethiopian Orthodox Church to improve healthcare and nutrition in over 600 orphanages. She founded a non-profit organization, Agro-Africa Limited, aimed at establishing small-scale agricultural projects to address Kenya's droughts and assist its victims. Furthermore, she served as the director of medical programs for the American Joint Distribution Committee in Addis Ababa.

Dr. Caroline continued working in EMS education until her passing in 2002. Her lifelong dedication to the field of emergency medicine, both nationally and internationally, has left an indelible mark on the EMS profession. Dr. Nancy Caroline's innovative ideas, practical approaches, and unwavering commitment to the development and delivery of high-quality emergency care have significantly impacted the EMS field in the United States and beyond. Her work has set the standard for paramedic education, training, and practice, shaping the EMS profession into what it is today.

Dr. Caroline's insistence on training non-physicians to provide emergency medical care paved the way for the modern paramedic profession. By empowering laypeople to render prehospital care, she made emergency medical care more accessible and efficient. Her hands-on approach and dedication to excellence in EMS education fostered a generation of skilled and compassionate paramedics, who have gone on to save countless lives.

Dr. Nancy Caroline's contributions to the formation of EMS in the United States cannot be overstated. She was instrumental in the development of the first paramedic training program in the country and authored the seminal EMS textbook that remains a cornerstone of paramedic education today. Through her work in the United States, Israel, and Africa, Dr. Caroline has left an indelible mark on the global EMS community. Her vision, dedication, and passion for emergency medical care have shaped the profession, improved the quality of prehospital care and in the process saved countless lives.

R. ADAMS COWLEY, MD

"The father of Trauma Medicine"

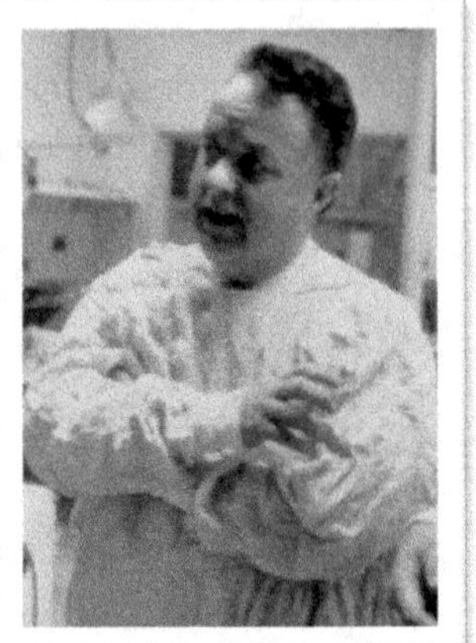

Dr. R. Adams Cowley, often hailed as the "Father of Trauma Medicine," revolutionized the realm of emergency care in the United States. Drawing from his experience with battlefield medicine during World War II, Dr. Cowley brought significant innovation to civilian trauma care. His establishment of the world's first dedicated trauma center at the University of Maryland in 1958 marked a monumental stride in the field.

A true innovator, Dr. Cowley pioneered the concept of medevac transport, introducing the use of military helicopters to expedite patients' arrival at his Shock Trauma Unit. This idea came to fruition in 1969, following the opening of his groundbreaking Center for the Study of Trauma.

Dr. Cowley had a vision beyond his Baltimore-based trauma center. He aimed to ensure no patient was denied the state-of-the-art treatment available at his institution. His aspirations were actualized in 1973, when then-Governor Marvin Mandel issued an executive order that marked the birth of the Maryland Institute for Emergency Medical Services Systems (MIEMSS) and the Division of Emergency Medical Services. Dr. Cowley was appointed as its director.

Under his leadership, Maryland's EMS and Trauma system evolved into a globally recognized model. As a strong advocate for the development of EMS systems, Dr. Cowley tirelessly testified before congress, pushing for the advancement of a systems approach to EMS. During a critical time when Congress was reallocating dedicated EMS development funds to more generalized public health block grants, Cowley implored, "In the political game of dividing the pie, you must convince the one with the knife that you deserve a fair share."[44]

Dr. Cowley's contributions have vastly expanded the skills of EMS providers, physicians, and nurses in trauma and emergency medicine. His influence helped emergency medicine to emerge as a distinct discipline. The establishment of the eight-story state-of-the-art trauma center named in his honor in 1989 is a testament to his enduring impact.

Dr. Cowley was a man of unwavering dedication, loyalty, and relentless pursuit of his vision. His tireless work ensured that the critically ill and injured were given the best chance at survival. His legacy endures in the countless lives saved and the immense strides made in trauma and emergency medicine.

J.D. 'DEKE' FARRINGTON, MD

"The father of modern EMS"

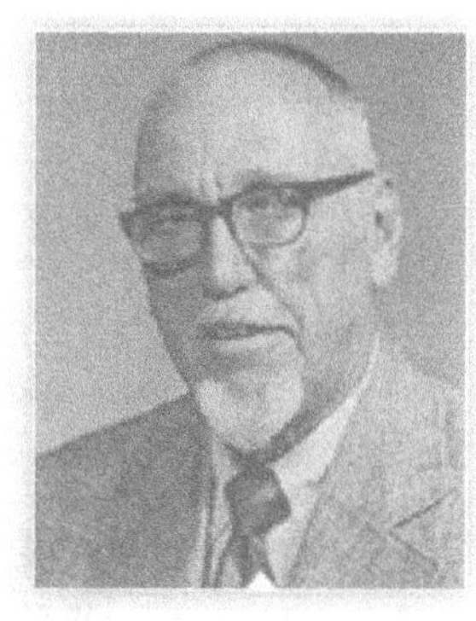

Dr. J.D. "Deke" Farrington, a respected orthopedic surgeon and an influential member of the American Academy of Orthopedic Surgeons (AAOS), is often regarded as the "father of modern EMS." Dr. Farrington significantly contributed to the design and development of emergency medical services in the United States. Starting in the 1950s, he applied lessons learned from treating combat casualties during World War II and the Korean War to civilian emergency medical care. As early as 1958, Farrington and his colleague Dr. Sam W. Banks, were training Chicago fire fighters in a prototype course that later evolved into the nationally recognized EMT-Ambulance course[45]. The training curriculum from this EMT course became known as the AAOS "Orange Book". His influence expanded over the following decades as he pursued improvements in EMS systems, training, and professionalism.

In 1966, Farrington's groundbreaking publication, *Death in a Ditch*, emphasized the dangers of car crashes on American highways and proposed a comprehensive vision for reducing fatalities through on-scene and transport emergency medical care. This work led to the establishment of the Registry of Emergency Medical Technicians (later renamed the National Registry of EMTs) in 1970, with Farrington serving on the board. Under his guidance, the NREMT conducted the first national EMT-Ambulance exam in 1971.

In his 1973 Scudder Oration speech, despite his numerous accomplishments, he famously stated:

> "We have been at war with sudden death and disability for seven years now, and must decide if we have lost, or are still in the fight. If we are still in the fight, what must we do to ensure victory?"
> - Dr. J.D. 'Deke' Farrington[46]

As the Chair of the National Registry of EMTs in 1975, Dr. Farrington sent a memo to the American Medical Association (AMA) urging them to officially recognize EMT-Paramedic as a distinct profession. His advocacy played a crucial role in gaining recognition for EMT-Paramedics, further legitimizing the EMS field. His leadership and guidance were instrumental in shaping the organization and the future of emergency medical services. His dedication to improving EMS systems, education, and professional standards has had a lasting impact on the field and has contributed to better patient care and outcomes across the United States.

Under Dr. Farrington's leadership and in collaboration with his colleagues at the American Medical Association, the Universal Medical Information Symbol (later known as the Star of Life) was chosen to represent Emergency Medical Services. As the Chair of the NREMT, Dr. Farrington also authored the letter transferring the Star of Life to NHTSA as the national symbol for EMS.

Farrington also played a key role in developing Wisconsin's state EMS system, coordinating the first recognized EMT training course in Wausau in 1969 and later serving as the medical director of the State of Wisconsin EMS program in 1971. Dr. Farrington was instrumental in establishing protocols for EMS practitioners, including standardized training and certification requirements, medical oversight, and quality assurance measures. He also worked to establish regional EMS systems to ensure that all areas of the state had access to high-quality emergency medical care.

Throughout his career, Dr. Farrington promoted the professionalization of EMS practitioners, advocating for standardized training, education, and national certification standards. He emphasized the importance of ongoing education and professional development for EMS personnel to ensure high-quality patient care in the field.

Dr. Farrington made significant contributions to EMS education, helping develop curricula and training programs. He also advocated for the inclusion of EMS education in academic settings such as medical schools and nursing programs to raise awareness and understanding of EMS among healthcare providers.

In addition to his work in EMS systems and education, Dr. Farrington was a strong proponent of research in EMS. He championed evidence-based practice and contributed to research efforts in the field, serving on committees and boards for numerous professional EMS organizations to advance the field and improve patient care.

His unwavering commitment to advancing EMS systems, promoting professionalism among providers, and advocating for evidence-based practice has played a vital role in shaping the modern EMS landscape, ultimately leading to improved patient care and outcomes.

FYI: Scudder Oration

The Scudder Oration is an annual lecture given at the American College of Surgeons (ACS) Clinical Congress in honor of Charles Locke Scudder, MD, a founding member of the American College of Surgeons and a major contributor to the surgery of trauma. The lecture is delivered by a distinguished surgeon who has made significant contributions to the field of trauma care. The Scudder Oration provides a forum for the discussion of important issues in trauma care and for the identification of new directions for research and education.

The oration series traces its origins to 1929, when Dr. Scudder himself delivered the inaugural lecture. In 1963, the series was formally renamed the "Scudder Oration on Trauma," and it remains dedicated to advancing the care of the injured patient.

Over the years, the Scudder Oration has been delivered by some of the most distinguished surgeons in the world, including Dr. J.D. Farrington (1973) and Dr. Norman McSwain (2003). These lectures have covered a wide range of topics in trauma care, including the epidemiology of trauma, the management of specific injuries, and the development of new technologies for trauma care.

The Scudder Oration is an important part of the ACS Clinical Congress and provides a valuable forum for the discussion of important issues in trauma care. The lectures delivered at the Scudder Oration have helped to shape the field of trauma care and have made a significant contribution to the improvement of patient care.

Norman McSwain, MD (1937-2015)

"What have you done for the good of mankind today?"- Dr. Norman McSwain

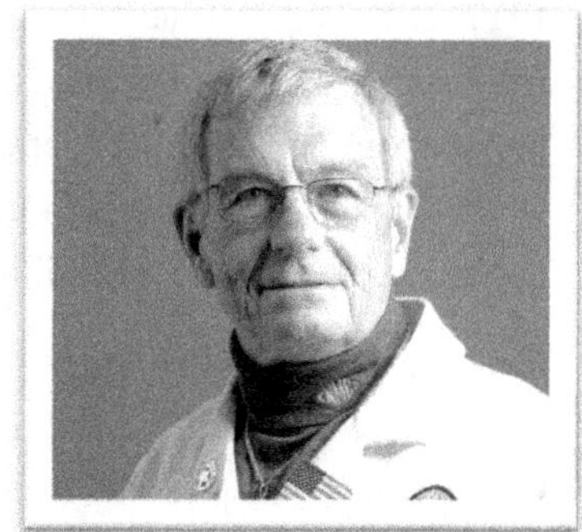

Dr. Norman McSwain made significant contributions to the Emergency Medical Services system in the United States throughout his career. As a trauma surgeon, educator, and advocate, Dr. McSwain played a pivotal role in advancing prehospital trauma care, establishing standardized training programs, and shaping the EMS landscape in the country.

Dr. McSwain's journey of contributions to EMS began in the 1960s when he recognized the critical need for timely and effective care for critically injured patients in the prehospital setting. He focused on the importance of early medical intervention and developed innovative approaches to delivering care at the scene of accidents and emergencies.

What have you done for the good of mankind today?"
- Dr. Norman McSwain

In the early 1970s, Dr. McSwain initiated the EMS expansion in Kansas, setting an ambitious goal to enable 40% of the state's population to have access to paramedics by 1976. He served as one of the nation's first Advanced Life Support (ALS) medical directors for both Johnson County Med-Act and the Kansas City Fire Department. Furthermore, in 1974, he launched an advanced life support training program, "Emergency Medical Training for the State of Kansas."

Relocating to New Orleans, Louisiana, in 1977, he joined Tulane University and played a key role in founding New Orleans EMS, the first comprehensive, integrated EMS system in the United States. Working with the city of New Orleans, he replicated and expanded the successful training programs he had initiated in Kansas. Dr. McSwain trained first responders, including paramedics and EMTs, to deliver rapid and immediate medical care to patients before they reached the hospital. Through his advocacy and training efforts, he pioneered advancements in trauma care for civilian EMS practitioners at all levels.

Dr. McSwain's dedication to improving trauma care extended beyond New Orleans. He became deeply involved in the American College of Surgeons' Committee on Trauma, both at the state and national levels. His collaboration with the National Association of Emergency Medical Technicians (NAEMT) led to the establishment of the Prehospital Trauma Life Support (PHTLS) organization. Under his leadership, a standardized curriculum was developed, training over one million providers in 64 countries to provide high-quality medical care for trauma patients before transport to medical centers.

PHTLS became a milestone for many EMS practitioners, serving as a rite of passage into the trauma care system. The program focused on essential skills such as controlling life-threatening hemorrhage, airway management, recognizing shock, and splinting fractures. Dr. McSwain's leadership ensured that PHTLS emphasized trauma patient assessment, empowering EMS practitioners to make a tangible difference in life-or-death situations.

Dr. McSwain's contributions were not limited to civilian training. His dedication to trauma care laid the groundwork for the development of Tactical Combat Casualty Care (TCCC) training. This program, inspired by his work, equipped tactical military units with the necessary skills to provide effective care in the field during combat and deployment scenarios.

Throughout his career, Dr. McSwain's impact extended beyond his direct involvement in the EMS community. He actively engaged with fellow professionals, sharing his expertise, and advocating for advancements in patient care. He mentored and welcomed newcomers, making them feel part of a larger network dedicated to improving trauma care.

Dr. McSwain's legacy goes beyond the numbers and statistics. His passion for giving back to patients and those who care for them was evident throughout his life. He consistently challenged the status quo and actively sought ways to improve the EMS system, medicine, and surgery. Dr. McSwain's unwavering dedication and love for his work kept him actively involved until his passing.

Dr. Norman McSwain's contributions to the EMS system in the United States are immeasurable. Through his work in New Orleans, he revolutionized prehospital trauma care, training EMS practitioners to deliver rapid and effective care. His involvement with the American College of Surgeons' Committee on Trauma and the establishment of PHTLS ensured standardized training and enhanced trauma care worldwide. Dr. McSwain's commitment to excellence and his legacy as a mentor, teacher, and advocate will continue to inspire generations of EMS practitioners, ultimately benefiting countless patients in critical and traumatic situations.

John Moon, Paramedic Pioneer

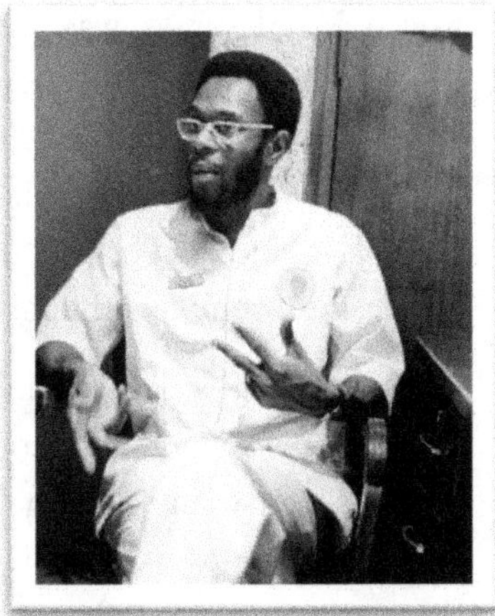

Born in Atlanta in 1949, John Moon has left an indelible mark on the history of America's paramedics. Moon faced a challenging childhood and moved to Pittsburgh's Hill District in 1963 after the tragic loss of both his parents. He completed high school and then worked as an orderly at Presbyterian Hospital in 1969.

While there, he witnessed the transformative operations of the Freedom House Ambulance Service. This pioneering organization, staffed by African Americans from Pittsburgh's urban neighborhoods, was leading the nation in training paramedics. The dedication of the Freedom House team had a profound influence on Moon and sparked his desire to join them.

It is critical to understand the history of the Freedom House. Before Seattle, Miami, and even Squad 51, the Freedom House Ambulance Service was providing cutting-edge advanced life support care to the citizens of the Hill District and greater Pittsburgh at a time when they were not considered equals in emergency services or healthcare.

Driven by determination, Moon started his Emergency Medical Services career at Freedom House Ambulance Service in 1971. He was personally mentored by pioneering physicians including Dr. Peter Safar and Dr. Nancy Caroline, who laid the foundation for modern EMS. With each patient he treated, Moon was co-developing the modern Paramedic profession. Under the tutelage of Dr. Safar, the "Father of Resuscitation," Moon made history as the first paramedic to perform an intubation on a patient, both in the operating room and in the field.

However, the innovative Freedom House Ambulance Service could not sustain its operations when the City of Pittsburgh ceased its funding and launched its own ambulance service. Although Moon and a few other paramedics were transferred to the new EMS service, their expertise and training were initially overlooked, and they were reduced to performing menial tasks. Despite these challenges, Moon proved his worth and skill, rising through the ranks to retire as the Assistant Chief of Emergency Medical Services for the City of Pittsburgh.

Moon's influence extended beyond his clinical practice in EMS. He is a strong advocate for diversity and has removed countless barriers, making the profession more accessible to minorities. Even when faced with racial prejudice, Moon's resolve remained firm, and his dedication to EMS never wavered.

After retirement, Moon has continued to serve the profession through his work with Freedom House 2.0, an organization that educates EMTs from economically disadvantaged communities.

John Moon's life and career continue to inspire. His journey from a hospital orderly to a leading figure in EMS demonstrates his exceptional dedication to public service, his community, and the EMS profession. His legacy—of dismantling racial barriers, elevating standards in emergency medical care, and mentoring numerous EMTs—still resonates in Pittsburgh and beyond. Every paramedic that has performed an intubation since Moon's initial patient intubation, and every paramedic trained on the DOT's National Standard Paramedic Curriculum (or subsequent versions), owes a debt of gratitude and honor to John Moon and his Freedom House Ambulance Service paramedic colleagues. His lifelong service to the community justifiably establishes him as one of America's first true paramedics.

Rocco Morando (1927-2023)

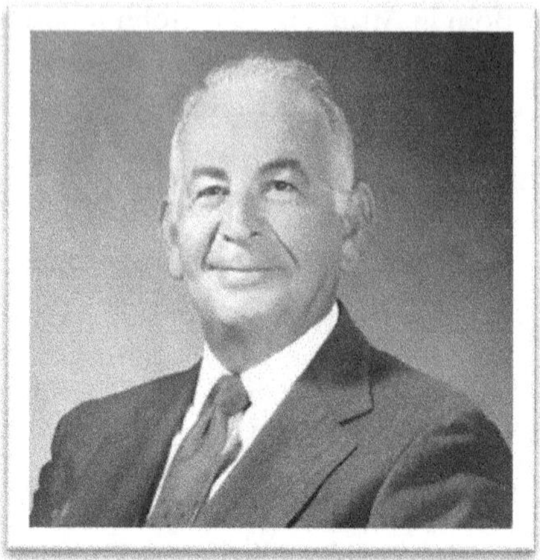

Rocco V. Morando was a pioneering figure in the development of the Emergency Medical Services system in the United States. He was born on August 19, 1927, in Martins Ferry, Ohio, and after serving in the U.S. Navy during World War II and the Korean War, he became a volunteer firefighter and first aid attendant.

In 1965, Morando joined The Ohio State University as the first consultant and coordinator for emergency rescue squad training. Five years later, following the recommendation of a task force assembled under President Lyndon B. Johnson's Committee on Highway Traffic Safety, Morando was instrumental in the founding of the National Registry of Emergency Medical Technicians and was appointed as the organization's first executive director. He served in that role for almost 20 years, during which time he oversaw many significant achievements in the field of EMS.

Under Morando's leadership, the NREMT became the standard for certification and credentialing of EMS personnel in the United States. He was a tireless advocate for improving the quality of care provided by EMS personnel and for recognizing the vital role of EMS in the healthcare system. His accomplishments started in 1971 when the NREMT administered the first EMT-Ambulance examination (administered simultaneously to 1,520 ambulance personnel at 51 test sites throughout the United States); the first recertification of Nationally Registered EMTs based on re-evaluation of skills (1973); contributions to the development of the first national paramedic curriculum in conjunction with leading EMS agencies and the University of Pittsburgh (1976-77); the first NREMT-Paramedic examination (1978); and the development of the first NREMT-Intermediate curriculum and examination (1980).

Upon his retirement in 1988, Morando was celebrated by hundreds of friends and representatives from national EMS organizations, and the NREMT headquarters in Columbus, Ohio, was renamed the Rocco V. Morando Building in his honor. Mr. Morando died February 21, 2023, at the age of 95, leaving behind a legacy that continues to improve the quality of care provided by EMS personnel and to save countless lives. The Rocco V. Morando Lifetime Achievement Award, presented by the National Association of EMTs and sponsored by the National Registry of EMTs – the two organizations he shaped - recognizes a lifetime of commitment, contributions, and leadership to Emergency Medical Services.

JAMES O. PAGE, JD (1936-2004)

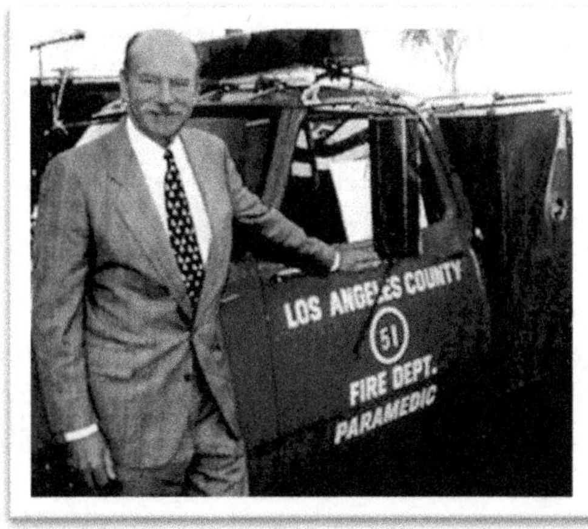

James O. Page was a visionary and influential figure in the field of emergency medical services in the United States. He played a pivotal role in shaping the modern EMS system through his leadership, innovation, and advocacy.

Born in Alhambra, CA, early in his career James Page held several jobs, including an ambulance attendant in East Los Angeles and began a career in the fire service with the Monterey Park Fire Department. He later served in the Los Angeles County Fire Department for 16 years, rising to the rank of Battalion Chief, all while studying law at Southwestern Law School.

In 1973, James Page became the first director of North Carolina's statewide EMS system, where he developed a national reputation for excellence in pre-hospital care. In 1975, he became the Executive Director of Lakes Area Emergency Medical Services in Buffalo, NY, where he spearheaded the development and implementation of the 8-county western New York EMS system.

Throughout his career, James Page made significant contributions to EMS education, practice, and policy. He championed the importance of well-trained paramedics and worked tirelessly to establish standardized paramedic education programs that met national standards. He and his colleagues Jay Fitch and Jeff Harris provided management services for the National Association of Emergency Medical Technicians (NAEMT) beginning in 1980, supporting the young organization during a formative period of its growth.

James Page was a prolific author, writing several books and magazine articles about the EMS community. He was generally recognized as the official historian of EMS, and his works were widely regarded as seminal texts in the field. Understanding the power of the written word, in 1979 he was the founding publisher of the Journal of Emergency Medical Services (JEMS), a monthly publication that became the world's most respected information source for EMS. As an attorney, prolific speaker, and innovative thinker, he realized that advocacy for emergency service organizations and their people was best carried out by communicating the facts about EMS. He championed innovations, needs, controversies, injustices, advancements, bureaucratic barricades, and groundbreaking research, essentially advocating for what was right and wrong in the profession.

In addition to his contributions to EMS education, James Page was a strong advocate for EMS policy and system development. He believed that EMS needed to be integrated into the broader healthcare system and worked towards establishing EMS as an essential component of the healthcare continuum. He was a vocal advocate for improving EMS infrastructure, including ambulance design, equipment standards, and communications systems, to enhance patient care and provider safety. In 2000, James Page co-founded the national EMS law firm Page, Wolfberg & Wirth, a firm which continues to this day as a recognized thought leader in the profession.

James Page's visionary leadership and unwavering commitment to advancing EMS education, practice, and policy have had a lasting impact on the field of EMS in the United States. His innovative ideas, advocacy efforts, and educational contributions have helped shape the modern EMS system and have influenced generations of EMS practitioners, educators, and leaders. His legacy continues to be recognized and celebrated in the EMS community, and his work continues to inspire advancements in EMS practice and policy to this day.

PETER SAFAR, MD (1924-2003)

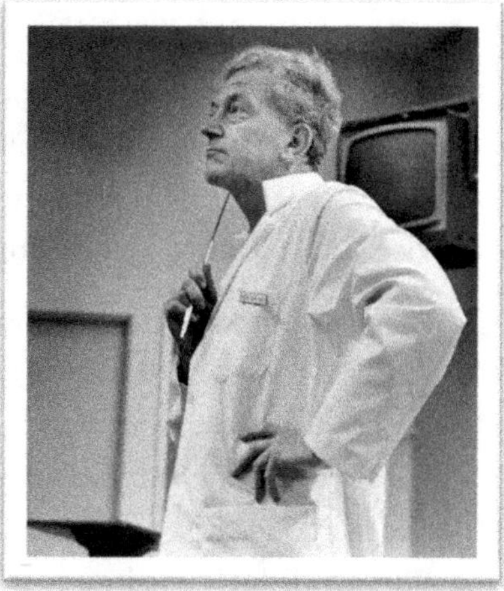

Dr. Peter Safar, an Austrian anesthesiologist, significantly advanced the fields of emergency medical services, resuscitation science, and critical care medicine, all while actively combating racial and equity disparities. Acknowledged globally as a pivotal figure in modern cardiopulmonary resuscitation (CPR), Dr. Safar conducted transformative research on mouth-to-mouth resuscitation in the 1950s during his tenure at Baltimore City Hospital. His work established this technique as a fundamental part of modern CPR. He further developed the "ABCs of CPR" (Airway, Breathing, Circulation), unifying the A (Airway) and B (Breathing) components with C (chest compressions). This methodology is now internationally recognized as the basic framework for resuscitation science. Since its inception in the 1950s, Dr. Safar's CPR methodology has preserved innumerable lives.

In 1960, Dr. Safar collaborated with Norwegian anesthesiologist Bjorn Lind and toymaker Asmund Laerdal to develop the Resusci Anne CPR mannequin. At the same time, he played a key role in establishing the first intensive care unit (ICU) in the United States in 1958 at Baltimore City Hospital, where he was the director of the department of anesthesiology. Before the ICU's establishment, medical care units specialized in treating specific ailments, but Dr. Safar envisioned a multidisciplinary unit that could provide comprehensive care for critically ill patients. This vision was grounded in his belief that coordinated and specialized care could drastically improve outcomes for patients in critical condition.

Transitioning to the University of Pittsburgh School of Medicine in 1961, Dr. Safar became the chair of the Department of Anesthesiology. Additionally, he played a significant role as a visionary, pioneer, and advocate in the development of structured EMS systems. Recognizing the crucial role of effective prehospital care in patient outcomes, his work profoundly influenced modern EMS systems. Dr. Safar was also a founding member of the National Research Council's panel on emergency medical services[47], helping to establish guidelines for ambulance design, emergency medical technician and paramedic training, and the provision of Advanced Life Support care in prehospital settings.

In 1967, Dr. Safar established the Freedom House Ambulance Service in response to significant inequities in access to emergency medical care for underserved communities, especially African Americans, in Pittsburgh, Pennsylvania. Hiring young African Americans from Pittsburgh's urban areas, many considered "unemployable" due to racial and social backgrounds, Dr. Safar demonstrated his belief in a diverse workforce's ability to provide high-quality emergency medical care and mitigate racial and socioeconomic healthcare disparities.

Dr. Safar leveraged his influence, shattered barriers, and expanded boundaries. Soon after starting Freedom House, Dr. Safar recruited Dr. Nancy Caroline, a female physician with an interest in EMS, to serve as the Medical Director for the ambulance service. It was through this experience that Dr. Caroline got her first hands-on experience in EMS. The Freedom House ambulance service staff were trained in resuscitation – from the Father of CPR and critical care medicine. The Freedom House ambulance was one of the first pre-hospital emergency medical services in the United States with staff trained in Advanced Life Support emergency care.

Dr. Safar's vision for the Freedom House Ambulance Service was to provide rapid and effective prehospital care to underserved communities. The service not only provided emergency medical care to those who desperately needed it but also provided employment opportunities to many young African Americans who would otherwise have been unemployed. The ambulance service became a model for community-based EMS programs, demonstrating that a diverse workforce could provide high-quality emergency medical care while breaking down the socioeconomic and racial disparities in healthcare.

Multiple projects lead to multiple successes.
- Peter Safar, MD

Dr. Safar also believed that EMS practitioners should receive rigorous training and education to ensure competence and skill in providing emergency care. He helped establish the first formalized EMS training programs and was a vocal advocate for standardizing EMS education across the country. His work not only laid the foundation for modern EMS education programs and helped elevate the professionalism of EMS practitioners, but his work helped standardize EMS around the nation.

In May 1969, at the Airlie House Conference on Emergency Medical Services[48], Dr. Safar presented a paper entitled "Ambulance and Emergency Department Records". In this paper, he argued for the uniformity of ambulance report forms on a national scale to evaluate the public health aspects of emergency transportation. He also advocated for revisions to these forms for computerized bookkeeping and prospective studies, such as the evaluation of patient care quality. This proposal for a standardized patient care report form was an early conceptual precursor to what would, decades later, become the National EMS Information System (NEMSIS). In addition to his vision for NEMSIS, he also outlined the design of a new national certification organization for EMS personnel (established the following year as the National Registry of EMTs).

On September 30, 1974, Dr. Safar was appointed by President Gerald R. Ford[49] to be one of five public members on the Interagency Committee on Emergency Medical Services, established pursuant to the requirements of the 1973 EMS Act. Concurrently, the University of Pittsburgh received a grant from the U.S. Department of Transportation to create a national standardized curriculum for emergency medical services based on the Freedom House Ambulance Service training. While Dr. Safar oversaw the project, most of the project work was led by Dr. Caroline. The Department of Transportation adopted the curriculum in 1977 as the EMT-Paramedic National Standard Curriculum.

Apart from his foundational work in resuscitation science and the establishment of a model Paramedic service, Dr. Safar is also significantly responsible for the design of modern ambulances and chaired the Committee on EMS Taskforce on "Medical Requirements for Ambulance Design and Equipment."[50] Following a 1963 trip to the Soviet Union,[51] where he observed physician-staffed ambulances delivering intubation, defibrillation, medication, and infusion, Dr. Safar collaborated with his colleagues Jerry Esposito and Richard Brose to create a new ambulance design, including a rear-facing airway seat. Although they experimented with larger vehicles and vans, they ultimately proposed a custom-designed box that could be placed on a truck chassis,[52] known as a Type-1 Ambulance today.

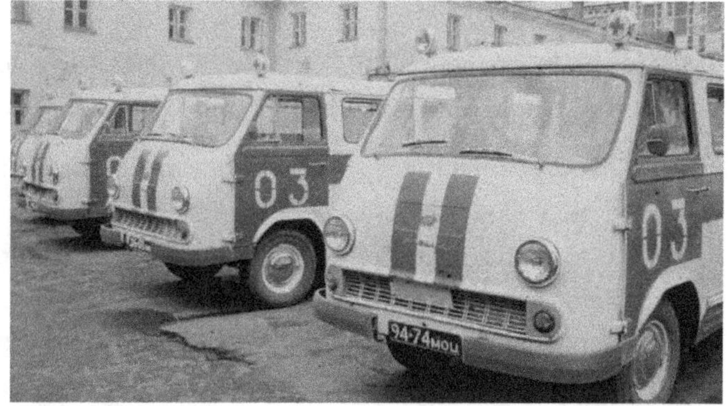

Figure 1Riga Autobus Factory (RAF) 977 Ambulance used in the Soviet Union (1960s)

Dr. Safar's ground-breaking contributions to EMS and resuscitation science have left an enduring impact on emergency medicine, and his innovative ideas, advocacy efforts, and educational contributions have shaped the modern landscape of EMS. His work has set a high bar for excellence in EMS care and has inspired future generations of EMS practitioners, educators, and researchers to continually advance the field of emergency medicine and improve patient outcomes.

Throughout his distinguished career, Dr. Safar received numerous awards and honors, including being nominated three times for the Nobel Prize in Medicine. He also received the Cross of Honor, Austria's highest civilian honor, for his contributions to the field of medicine. His influence in the medical community, both in the United States and globally, serves as a testament to his relentless efforts and lifelong dedication to improving patient care, championing equality, and advancing medical science.

Gratitude For Those Who Have Gone Before Us

The development of modern Emergency Medical Services in the United States stands as a testament to the unwavering dedication of numerous visionary individuals who significantly influenced emergency medical care. As explored in this chapter, these courageous and visionary leaders revolutionized pre-hospital care, laying the groundwork for the contemporary EMS system that has undoubtedly saved countless lives.

However, it is important to acknowledge that these individuals did not accomplish their feats alone. The rapid progression of EMS in the United States also owes its success to the untiring efforts of many unsung heroes who tirelessly established local ambulance services in their communities. These individuals, too, possessed visionary mindsets, and their hard work and commitment should serve as an inspiration to present-day EMS leaders. Without their invaluable contributions, the EMS system as it exists today would not have come into being.

Furthermore, it is crucial to recognize that failures also played a role in the evolution of the EMS system. Those who attempted innovative approaches and experienced setbacks provided valuable lessons about what did not work, ultimately guiding future endeavors toward success. It is important to remember that progress often stems from a process of trial and error.

As the legacy of the EMS pioneers is honored, it is essential to acknowledge that EMS remains a relatively young profession with countless opportunities for visionaries and innovators to make their mark. There are individuals today who continue to cast bold visions and advocate for continued advancements within the profession. These visionaries may present ideas that seem impossible to some, but it is important to seek out and encourage them. Supporting and nurturing the innovators and visionaries of today can foster a culture of continuous progress and drive further advancements in the field of EMS.

Looking forward, embracing the spirit of innovation, and actively seeking out those who are pushing the boundaries of what is possible in EMS becomes crucial. These individuals are instrumental in shaping the future of emergency medical care, and their ideas and advancements hold the potential to transform the profession in remarkable ways. Supporting and collaborating with these visionaries can collectively work towards achieving new heights of excellence in EMS and further improving patient care and outcomes.

Therefore, as gratitude is expressed for the contributions of past visionaries, it is equally important to encourage and uplift the innovators and visionaries of today. Their unwavering commitment and dedication are essential in driving the profession forward, ensuring that EMS continues to evolve, adapt, and deliver the highest standard of care to those in need.

3

Hollywood's Role In Designing the United States EMS System

"Movies can and do have a tremendous influence in shaping young lives in the realm of entertainment towards the ideals and objectives of normal adulthood."

THE POWER OF HOLLYWOOD IS INESCAPABLE. IT SHAPES OUR perceptions, influences our beliefs, and can ignite social change. Movies and television shows have played a crucial role in shaping the development of modern Emergency Medical Services. Popular media, including Hollywood and television shows like "Emergency!", established public perception of EMS and contributed to the need for standardized training and certification of EMS practitioners. The depiction of EMS as a heroic and essential part of the healthcare system in these shows helped generate public support for EMS and led to the creation of national standards for EMS training and certification. TV shows and movies have also played a vital role in public education, policy development, and system development. These shows raised awareness about the importance of emergency services, highlighted the challenges and dangers faced by EMS practitioners, and provided education on how to respond to emergencies and call 911 for help. Recently, shows like "Nightwatch" provided viewers with a glimpse into the personal stories, struggles, and triumphs of the EMS practitioners, helping to bridge the gap between EMS practitioners and the communities they serve. Overall, the impact of TV shows and movies on public perception of EMS and the critical role of EMS practitioners in saving lives and providing care during emergencies has been significant, leading to increased support for EMS agencies and improved outcomes for patients.

EMERGENCY! (1972-1979)

"Emergency!" was a popular TV drama that aired in 1972, featuring the fictional Los Angeles County Fire Department and its crew, including the characters of Paramedics Johnny Gage and Roy DeSoto, portrayed by Randolph Mantooth and Kevin Tighe. The show depicted the day-to-day work of paramedics responding to medical emergencies and providing pre-hospital care to patients. The characters of Gage and DeSoto are often credited with popularizing the role of paramedics and bringing awareness to the vital work they do.

The impact of "Emergency!" on the public perception of EMS and paramedicine was significant. The show helped raise public awareness about the role of paramedics and the importance of EMS in providing critical care in the field. As a result, the demand for local EMS agencies surged, and more individuals sought to become paramedics. The show also contributed to the professionalization of the EMS field, leading to advancements in training, education, and regulations for paramedics across the country.

Furthermore, both actors, Mantooth and Tighe, completed six months of paramedic training to accurately portray their roles on the show. This realistic portrayal helped to highlight the professionalism, competence, and dedication of paramedics and garnered respect for their work from the public. The show also depicted the physical, emotional, and mental demands placed on paramedics as they responded to high-stress situations, dealt with life-or-death decisions, and navigated the dynamics of working in a fast-paced, high-pressure environment.

Overall, "Emergency!" had a lasting impact on the public perception of EMS and paramedicine in the United States. It helped to generate interest and support for the advancement of EMS education, training, and regulation. As the show gained widespread recognition, it contributed to the increased recognition of paramedics as a distinct and essential part of the healthcare system, leading to improvements in the quality of care provided by EMS professionals and the development of standardized practices and protocols.

M*A*S*H (1972-1983)

MASH was a landmark television series that broke new ground in its exploration of the intersection of war and medicine. The show's depiction of medical professionals working in a Mobile Army Surgical Hospital (MASH) during the Korean War offered a unique insight into the challenges faced by those who provide emergency medical care in conflict zones. The show's portrayal of the intense pressure and chaos of working in such an environment resonated with audiences and helped to raise awareness about the critical importance of prompt emergency medical services.

Although the show was not explicitly focused on EMS, its influence on the development of EMS and emergency care in the United States cannot be understated. The show popularized the concepts of rapid access to organized trauma care and the pivotal role of specialized medical responders. The show's portrayal of emergency medicine as a vital and life-saving profession helped to create a greater sense of appreciation and support for the nationwide efforts to improve access to ambulances and establish an organized system for emergency care.

Perhaps one of the most significant contributions of MASH was establishing a foundation for former military medical personnel who had served during the Korean and Vietnam Wars to advance EMS and trauma care. These individuals played a pivotal role in establishing new training programs and research initiatives focused on enhancing the quality of care provided by emergency medical personnel. The show's depiction of the challenges and opportunities inherent in the practice of emergency medicine inspired many of these former military medical personnel to become leaders in the development of EMS and emergency care in the United States.

Overall, MASH had a profound influence on the way that Americans thought about emergency medical care. Its portrayal of medical professionals working under extreme conditions in a chaotic and high-pressure environment helped to raise awareness about the critical importance of accessing prompt emergency medical services. The show's impact on the development of EMS and emergency care in the United States cannot be overstated, and its legacy continues to be felt to this day.

MOTHER, JUGS & SPEED (1976)

"Mother, Jugs & Speed" is a 1976 comedy-drama film that provided a controversial representation of EMS in popular culture. Starring Bill Cosby as "Mother," Raquel Welch as "Jugs," and Harvey Keitel as "Speed," the movie follows the paramedic trio as they provide emergency medical care in Los Angeles. Although the film was a work of fiction, it helped raise public awareness about EMS.

The film had an impact on the public's perception of EMS, as it was one of the few mainstream films that depicted paramedics and their work during that period. It brought attention to the challenges faced by paramedics, including the physical demands of the job, quick decision-making, and the emotional toll of dealing with life-and-death situations. It also highlighted the camaraderie and teamwork among EMS practitioners, as well as their dedication to saving lives and providing care to those in need.

The film uniquely depicted the challenges and struggles of operating a private ambulance service in Los Angeles. The intense competition among private ambulance companies was highlighted, with each vying to be the first on the scene of an emergency to secure a patient and their business. The characters in the film represented different aspects of the private ambulance industry and the challenges they faced. "Mother" was the head of an established ambulance company, struggling to keep his business afloat amid increasing competition. "Jugs" was a recruit, struggling to prove herself and gain acceptance in a male-dominated field, while "Speed" was a reckless and unscrupulous ambulance driver who would do whatever it took to beat the competition.

The film depicted the dangerous and high-pressure nature of the private ambulance industry, with drivers often racing through traffic and disregarding traffic laws to reach emergency scenes first. It also highlighted the ethical dilemmas faced by private EMS agencies at the time, who were often torn between providing the best care for their patients and securing their business.

While the portrayal of EMS personnel as reckless and irresponsible does not reflect most real-life EMS professionals, "Mother, Jugs & Speed" inspired individuals to pursue careers in EMS and increased the demand for local EMS agencies.

RESCUE 9-1-1 (1989-1996)

Rescue 911 was a groundbreaking television show that aired from 1989 to 1996 and had a significant impact on both the public's perception of EMS and the connection between communities and EMS agencies. It was the first reality-based show to dramatize real-life emergency situations and the efforts of EMTs, paramedics, fire fighters, and police officers to rescue and provide care to individuals in crisis.

The show featured reenactments of actual 911 calls, along with interviews and commentary from the individuals involved in the emergencies, including the victims, their families, and the responding EMS practitioners. The episodes covered a wide range of emergencies, including medical emergencies, accidents, natural disasters, and other life-threatening situations.

"Rescue 911" was unique in that it brought real-life emergency situations into the homes of viewers, offering a compelling and often emotional portrayal of the work of EMS practitioners and other emergency responders. The show helped to raise awareness about the importance of emergency services, highlighted the challenges and dangers faced by EMS practitioners, and provided education on how to respond to emergencies and call 911 for help.

Moreover, the show played a vital role in connecting communities with EMS agencies. It helped increase public understanding of the critical importance of calling 911 during emergencies, which led to more timely responses and improved outcomes for patients. It also provided viewers with valuable information on how to recognize and respond to emergencies, which helped to prepare them for potential emergencies in their own lives.

Furthermore, "Rescue 911" helped to bridge the gap between EMS practitioners and the communities they served by fostering a sense of trust and understanding. By showcasing the human stories of EMS practitioners and the individuals they rescued, the show helped to humanize EMS practitioners and to showcase their dedication, professionalism, and compassion. This, in turn, helped to build stronger relationships between EMS practitioners and the communities they served, leading to increased support for EMS agencies and improved outcomes for patients.

NIGHTWATCH (2015-)

"Nightwatch" broke new ground by filming actual emergency calls inside ambulances during the night shift in New Orleans, Louisiana. The show offered viewers an intimate look into the challenges and experiences of EMS practitioners in one of the busiest and most diverse cities in the United States.

Through "Nightwatch," viewers gain insight into the daily lives of EMS practitioners as they respond to a wide range of emergencies, including medical calls, traumatic injuries, and critical incidents in the vibrant and dynamic city of New Orleans. The show captures the fast-paced and often unpredictable nature of EMS work in New Orleans, where providers face unique challenges, such as managing large crowds during special events and festivals, navigating through narrow streets and crowded areas, and responding to emergencies in diverse neighborhoods with varying socioeconomic conditions.

Moreover, "Nightwatch" highlights the impact of the city's rich cultural traditions, including its music, cuisine, and unique cultural celebrations, on the work of EMS practitioners. The show also emphasizes the human aspect of emergency services by revealing the personal stories, struggles, and triumphs of the EMS practitioners, as they balance their professional responsibilities with their personal lives and cope with the emotional toll of working in a high-stress and fast-paced environment.

In addition to its entertaining and informative look into the world of EMS in New Orleans, "Nightwatch" played a vital role in continuing the unique relationship between entertainment television and the development of EMS. The show highlighted the critical role of EMS practitioners in saving lives, providing care, and serving their communities during emergencies, while also humanizing their work. "Nightwatch" modernized and expanded the boundaries of the genre, providing a new and innovative format to raise public awareness about the importance of EMS agencies.

TELEVISION'S PORTRAYAL OF EMS PRACTITIONERS

The depiction of EMS practitioners in popular media, including television shows and movies, plays a pivotal role in shaping public perception and influencing the professionalization of the EMS field.

Popular media has often portrayed EMS practitioners as heroic, dedicated, and highly skilled professionals who play a vital role in saving lives and providing care during emergencies. Shows like "Emergency!" and "Nightwatch" have depicted paramedics and EMTs as compassionate, competent, and well-trained individuals who consistently prioritize patient care in high-stress situations. These positive portrayals have contributed to increased public awareness, confidence, and appreciation of the critical role that EMS practitioners play in the healthcare system, subsequently leading to advancements in training, education, and regulation within the field.

Moreover, such depictions have helped to humanize EMS practitioners, offering viewers a glimpse into the personal stories, struggles, and triumphs of the individuals who dedicate their lives to serving their communities. By showcasing the emotional, mental, and physical demands faced by EMS practitioners in the line of duty, popular media has fostered a greater understanding of the challenges they face, and the dedication required to excel in their profession.

While many portrayals of EMS practitioners in popular media have been positive, there have also been instances where they are depicted in a negative light. For example, the film Mother,

Jugs & Speed presented EMS practitioners as reckless, unethical, and driven by competition rather than patient care. Although the film was fictional and intended for entertainment purposes, it may have contributed to misperceptions about the professionalism and integrity of EMS practitioners among the public.

Similarly, some television shows and movies have exaggerated the drama and intensity of emergency situations to enhance entertainment value, potentially leading to unrealistic expectations about the capabilities and limitations of EMS practitioners. Such portrayals may inadvertently contribute to public confusion about the actual roles and responsibilities of EMS practitioners, as well as the nature of the work they perform. However, these shows often emphasize sensational emergency calls, such as the dramatic cardiac arrest patient that is revived, the thrilling rescue, the complex trauma patient, or the emergency childbirth, while neglecting to depict the more common, less dramatic, and sometimes routine patient encounters that EMS practitioners often face. The adrenaline-fueled portrayals of EMS practitioners in media have contributed to the recruitment of many individuals (including this author), but these portrayals can also lead to false expectations for newcomers to the profession. When new EMTs realize that many patient encounters are not as thrilling as those shown in Hollywood productions, they may experience frustration, disappointment, and, ultimately, leave the profession.

The portrayal of EMS practitioners in any type of popular media can significantly impact public perception and the professionalization of the EMS field. Positive portrayals help to generate interest and support for the advancement of EMS education, training, and regulation, leading to improvements in the quality of care provided by EMS professionals and the development of standardized practices and protocols.

Conversely, negative portrayals may undermine public trust and confidence in the EMS system, hindering the growth and development of the profession. It is therefore essential for popular media to strike a balance between entertainment and realism when depicting EMS practitioners, ensuring that the portrayals are accurate, nuanced, and respectful of the critical role they play in serving their communities and saving lives.

PUBLIC POLICY IMPLICATIONS

The representation of Emergency Medical Services in popular media has had a significant impact on public policy development, funding, and the establishment of national standards for EMS training and certification. The portrayal of EMS practitioners in television shows and movies has shaped public perception and understanding of the EMS profession, which, in turn, has influenced policy decisions at various levels of government.

One of the most notable examples of the influence of media representation on EMS policy development was the impact of the television show "Emergency!" on the professionalization of the EMS field. The show brought awareness to the importance of standardized training, education, and certification for paramedics, ultimately leading to advancements in EMS regulations across the United States. As a result of the show's widespread popularity, public demand for local EMS agencies surged, prompting policymakers to allocate funding and resources to develop and expand EMS systems in their communities.

The influence of popular media on EMS policy development is not limited to the United States. International audiences have also been exposed to American television shows and movies featuring EMS practitioners, which has contributed to the global growth and development of EMS systems. In many countries, these media portrayals have helped to create an understanding of the importance of a well-organized EMS system, leading to policy changes and the allocation of resources to improve pre-hospital care.

Additionally, the representation of EMS practitioners in television shows and movies has played a vital role in public education and awareness about the importance of emergency services. This increased awareness has led to policy changes aimed at improving access to emergency care, such as the widespread implementation of the 911 emergency call system and the establishment of national standards for EMS training and certification. These policy changes have helped to ensure that EMS practitioners are well-equipped and trained to provide high-quality care during emergencies.

Furthermore, the media's portrayal of EMS practitioners as dedicated, competent, and heroic professionals has generated public support for EMS agencies, which has translated into increased funding for EMS systems. Policymakers have recognized the critical role of EMS practitioners in saving lives and providing care during emergencies, leading to increased investment in EMS infrastructure, training, and equipment.

However, it is important to note that media representations of EMS practitioners are not always accurate or realistic, and there is a need for ongoing dialogue between the EMS community and the entertainment industry to ensure that portrayals are both engaging and informative. Inaccurate or overly dramatized depictions of EMS practitioners and their work may lead to unrealistic public expectations and misconceptions about the profession, which could have negative implications for policy development and funding.

The representation of EMS in popular media has significantly influenced public policy development, funding, and the establishment of national standards for EMS training and certification. The media's portrayal of EMS practitioners has shaped public perception and understanding of the profession, leading to increased support for EMS agencies and improvements in pre-hospital care. To ensure the continued positive impact of media representation on EMS policy, it is crucial for the EMS community and the entertainment industry to work together to create accurate and engaging portrayals of EMS practitioners and their work.

Public Health Education and Awareness

Popular media has played a critical role in educating the public about recognizing and responding to emergencies, as well as promoting public health initiatives related to emergency care. Television shows, movies, and news programs have used their platforms to inform audiences about the signs and symptoms of various medical emergencies, such as heart attacks, strokes, and respiratory distress, as well as the appropriate actions to take in these situations.

Moreover, popular media has been instrumental in promoting public health initiatives aimed at improving emergency care outcomes. Campaigns for bystander CPR, the use of automated external defibrillators (AEDs), Stop the Bleed campaigns, and the importance of calling 911 in emergency situations have been supported by media portrayals of EMS practitioners and their life-saving efforts. These portrayals have helped to increase public awareness and understanding of the crucial role of bystanders in the chain of survival, ultimately contributing to improved survival rates for out-of-hospital cardiac arrest and other time-sensitive emergencies.

Additionally, popular media has provided a platform for public health messages related to injury prevention, disaster preparedness, and mental health awareness. Television shows and movies often incorporate storylines that demonstrate the consequences of unsafe behaviors, such as distracted driving or substance abuse, thereby reinforcing the importance of prevention and personal responsibility in maintaining public health.

The Ongoing Influence of Popular Media on the Development of EMS

Despite the positive influence of popular media on public awareness and education regarding emergency care, there are ongoing challenges faced by EMS practitioners and the EMS system. These challenges include addressing misconceptions and unrealistic expectations about the capabilities and limitations of EMS practitioners, as well as the need for continued public support and funding to maintain and improve EMS agencies.

Popular media can play a role in addressing these challenges by providing more accurate and nuanced portrayals of EMS practitioners and their work. Collaborations between the EMS community and the entertainment industry can help to ensure that media representations are both engaging and informative, promoting public understanding and appreciation of the complexities and realities of emergency medical care.

In the future, popular media may continue to influence the development of EMS in the United States by exploring new and emerging trends in emergency care, such as the integration of telemedicine and other advanced technologies, as well as the expansion of community paramedicine programs. By showcasing these innovative approaches to emergency care, popular media can contribute to the ongoing evolution and improvement of EMS systems, helping to shape public opinion and policy development in support of high-quality, patient-centered emergency care.

In summary, popular media has played a significant role in raising awareness and educating the public about recognizing and responding to emergencies and promoting public health initiatives related to emergency care. Addressing the ongoing challenges faced by EMS practitioners and the EMS system requires continued collaboration between the entertainment industry and the EMS community to ensure accurate and engaging media portrayals. By doing so, popular media can continue to influence the development of EMS in the United States, fostering public support and driving policy changes that promote excellence in emergency care.

4

A GUIDING STAR (OF LIFE)

"The key is not to worry about being successful but to instead work toward being significant — and the success will naturally follow." - Wintley Phipps, as recounted by Oprah Winfrey

THE STAR OF LIFE IS A POWERFUL VISUAL REMINDER OF THE CRITICAL role that EMS practitioners play in saving lives and promoting public health. By serving as a unifying symbol for EMS professionals since the late 1960s, the Star of Life highlights the essential nature of the work and the significant impact EMS practitioners have on the well-being of individuals and communities they serve. The symbol has six blue, interlocking bars with a white "serpent" coiled around a staff in the center, symbolizing the rod of Asclepius, the Greek god of medicine and healing. The six points of the star correspond to the six essential components of the EMS system: detection, reporting, response, on-scene care, care in transit, and transfer to definitive care. Each point of the star represents a specific function in the EMS system, underscoring the importance of a coordinated approach to emergency medical care. The Star of Life is prominently displayed on almost every ambulance in the United States, incorporated into EMS patches and uniforms, and often seen on road signs to indicate the presence of emergency medical care nearby.

Editorials

Universal Medical Identification Symbol

This is the universal Emergency medical symbol devised by the American Medical Association.

The person who displays it carries information which should be known to anyone helping him during an accident or sudden illness.

First announced in June, 1963, this symbol is already in such general use that it is essential that it be recognized by all emergency personnel who care for the ill or injured. It means, "Look for medical information that can protect life." Failure to recognize this symbol and to heed its vital message could be disastrous.

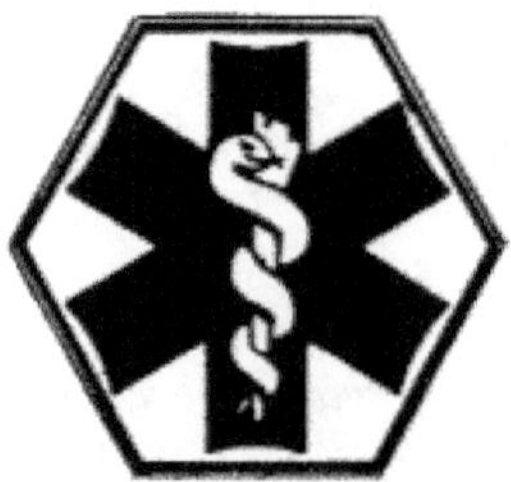

This symbol has been freely offered by the AMA to manufacturers and distributors of emergency medical signal devices and the publishers of medical identification cards. Thirty corporations and associations have adopted the universal symbol for use on their identifications and the number is increasing continuously. The AMA neither manufactures nor distributes signal devices.

Many signal devices of metal or plastic will bear this symbol on one side with a few words of vital information on the other. Other devices will have a pocket within which more detailed information can be found. Still others may consist of the symbol alone—a suggestion to look elsewhere in purse or pocket for important information or identification.

Fix this symbol in your memory—the star of life (or the asterisk of reference), bearing the snake entwined staff of Aesculapius, the mythical Roman god of medicine—taken from the seal of the American Medical Association, and all contained in a hexagon. This symbol may appear in any size or color. It is most likely to be found on the wrist or about the neck, though it may identify the presence of information in other locations.

Recognizing it as the universal symbol of emergency medical identification will help you to locate information that may protect life in an emergency.

A page from the 1964 Journal of the American Medical Association.

UNTANGLING THE HISTORY

The Star of Life has a rich, yet often misrepresented history. The original Star of Life was designed by the American Medical Association (AMA) in the early 1960s as the "Universal Medical Identification Symbol"[53] (also known as the "Universal Emergency Medical Identification Symbol"). The original intent was for this symbol to be freely available and printed on cards carried by persons with any medical conditions such as diabetes or epilepsy. This universal symbol would be easily recognized by the public and medical professionals during an emergency. The AMA did not trademark or copyright the symbol, but freely provided it to manufacturers and the public for use. The AMA widely promoted the use of this "Universal Medical Identification Symbol" in its journal (as seen in the image on the previous page) and in governmental publications.[54]

In 1964, the World Medical Association's Assembly in Helsinki, Finland, adopted the "Universal Emergency Medical Identification Symbol" for worldwide use, sponsored by the AMA. Shortly after, in March (1966), the "Universal Emergency Medical Identification Symbol" was being referenced as the "Star of Life" by the Federal Bureau of Investigation and others.[55]

In 1969, under the chairmanship of Irvin E. Henderson, MD, the AMA Commission on Emergency Medical Services encouraged the Department of Transportation to display the symbol on road signs to denote hospital Emergency Rooms. The next year, the AMA House of Delegates officially adopted the "Star of Life" design, which was the Universal Medical Identification Symbol without the surrounding hexagon.[56]

Simultaneously, President Lyndon Johnson's Committee on Highway Traffic Safety formed a Task Force tasked with establishing a national EMS certification agency.[57] The AMA led this Task Force, with many individuals who contributed to the creation and publication of the Universal Medical Identification symbol also appointed to the Task Force. The first meeting of this Task Force was on January 21, 1970, with additional representatives from the following organizations:

- Ambulance Association of America
- International Association of Fire Chiefs
- International Rescue and First Aid Association
- National Ambulance and Medical Services Association
- National Forest Service
- National Funeral Directors Association
- National Park Service
- National Safety Council
- National Ski Patrol

- American Heart Association
- International Association of Chiefs of Police

The Task Force moved quickly, and on June 4, 1970, the first meeting of the Board of Directors of the Registry of Emergency Medical Technicians (later renamed as the National Registry of Emergency Medical Technicians) was convened. Roddy A. Brandes, of the Ambulance Association of America, was elected the Board's first Chairman. However, this new national certification body for emergency medical services needed a logo, a unique symbol to unify the newest medical profession: a nationally standardized Emergency Medical Technician. Due to the close affiliation with the American Medical Association, the AMA transferred the Universal Medical Identification Symbol – a symbol already linked to emergency care - to the Registry of EMTs as a symbol to designate nationally certified EMS personnel. The symbol was incorporated into the Registry of EMTs branding and patches. In 1971, at 51 testing locations across the United States, 1,520 ambulance personnel took the first standardized national EMS certification examination. The successful candidates were presented with a patch that not only signified their newly demonstrated competence in Emergency Medical Services, but also indicated these personnel had a direct connection to the broader medical profession, the American Medical Association, and had met a unified national standard.

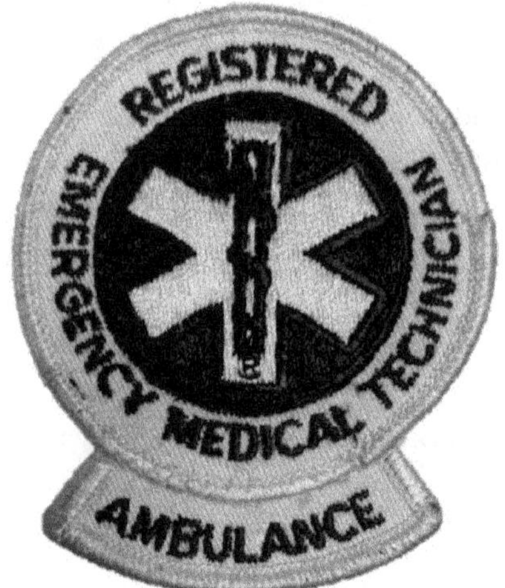

The 1971 Registry of EMTs National EMT-Ambulance Patch, featuring the Star of Life

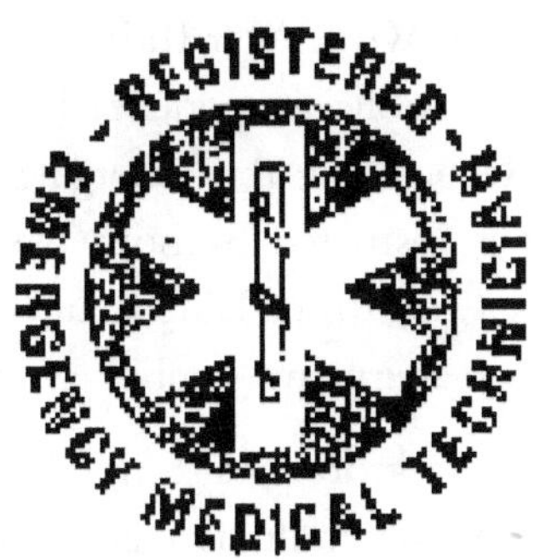

The original trademark of the Registry of Emergency Medical Technicians, incorporating the Star of Life.[58]

On April 12, 1973, the Registry of EMTs trademarked the Registered Emergency Medical Technician symbol that clearly incorporated the Star of Life. Honoring the work of the visionary physicians of the American Medical Association - that fought for a new medical profession and gifted the profession a unique symbol – the Star of Life has been incorporated into every National EMS Certification card and patch earned for over fifty years.

A Geneva Convention Violation?

It's 1972 and ambulance services are being established at a record pace in communities across the nation. Thousands of personnel are being trained as EMTs, and the nation is being entertained and educated by the new hit show, "Emergency!". However, there's a growing two-fold problem that is rapidly getting out of control: NHTSA's first attempt at a standardized symbol for the emerging profession was an Omaha Cross, which was an orange Greek Cross ✚ on a white background, and secondly many community ambulance services were using the actual Red Cross logo on ambulances.

First, NHTSA encountered serious issues with the Omaha Cross (the orange Greek Cross). In a 1974 highway safety manual, NHTSA acknowledged the error noting that,

> "a cross of reflectorized Omaha orange on a square background of reflectorized white might violate a Congressional grant to the Red Cross of 'the right to have and to use ... as an emblem and badge, a Greek Red Cross on a white background, as the same has been treated in the treaties of Geneva'...the orange cross specified by the National Highway Traffic Safety Administration (NHTSA) clearly is a 'colorable imitation' of the Geneva Red Cross".[59]

Secondly, as previously noted, many of the local ambulance service volunteers were veterans of the Korean War, the Vietnam War, or World War II. From the perspective and experience of these personnel, combined with the public's experience in the media, Red Cross logos were synonymous with ambulances. Recognizing this emerging concern that further use of the Omaha Cross or the Red Cross is restricted by both the U.S. Congress and the Geneva Convention, Dr. Dawson Mills, the Chief of the EMS Branch for the National Highway Traffic Safety Administration, had to find an alternative symbol for ambulances quickly.

Dr. Mills was very involved with the taskforce that formed the Registry of EMTs, so he raised this urgent concern to the organization's multidisciplinary board. Recognizing the Universal Medical Identification Symbol was quickly gaining recognition and acceptance, he requested permission to extend the use of the Star of Life symbol as the "national identifier for Emergency Medical Services" that would be used on all ambulances. (Subsequently, the federal ambulance standard was later known as a "Star of Life Ambulance".) The Registry's board agreed and approved this request, and Dr. J.D. Farrington, as Chair of the Board, memorialized this in a memo to Dr. Mills.

While the Registry of EMTs would continue to use the symbol, the Department of Transportation expanded the use of the blue 'Star of Life' and mandated its use on all ambulances purchased with federal funds. On September 26, 1972, the Office of the Secretary of Transportation issued a Memorandum adopting and recognizing the "Star of Life". By 1975, Leo R. Schwartz, the new Chief of the EMS Branch at NHTSA, modified the Star of Life by adding the six main tasks associated with EMS.

In 1974, the Department of Transportation noted[60],

> "It has been concluded by NHTSA that it is proper not to further interfere with the organizational identification provided by the Greek Red Cross. Rather, it is considered preferable to adopt a separate symbol which clearly and distinctively identifies the emergency care vehicle or ambulance within the total spectrum of the Emergency Medical Care system. The "Star of Life" has already been identified by the medical profession as a medical emergency symbol and its highway related use encouraged by the American Medical Association."

On February 1, 1977, the "Star of Life" was issued Registration Number 1058022 by the United States Patent and Trademark Office in the name of the Department of Transportation's National Highway Traffic Safety Administration.

The Star of Life holds immense significance within the EMS profession, serving as a powerful reminder of both its unity and the potential for history to fade into oblivion. It emerged as a unifying symbol, aiming to bring together a fragmented profession and instill public confidence by signifying that every ambulance, EMT, or Paramedic adorned with the Star of Life had successfully met the unified national standard. However, in a mere span of 50 years, the EMS profession forgot its roots and several iterations of fragmentation occurred. As EMS again undergoes a process of reunification, the Star of Life will hopefully symbolize integration and a renewed linkage with the healthcare system.

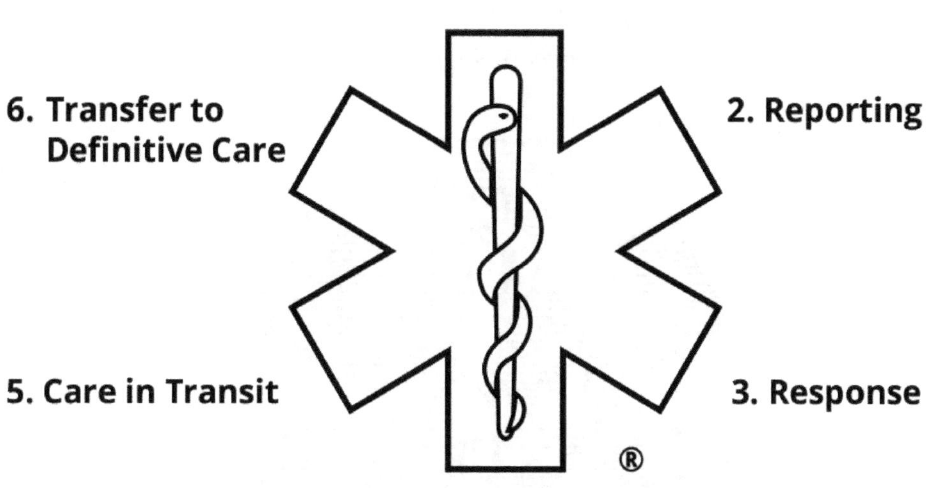
1. Detection
2. Reporting
3. Response
4. On Scene Care
5. Care in Transit
6. Transfer to Definitive Care
®

U.S. Cl: A,B **REG. No 1,058,022**

UNITED STATESPATENT OFFICE **Registered Feb. 1, 1977**

CERTIFICATION MARK

Principal Register

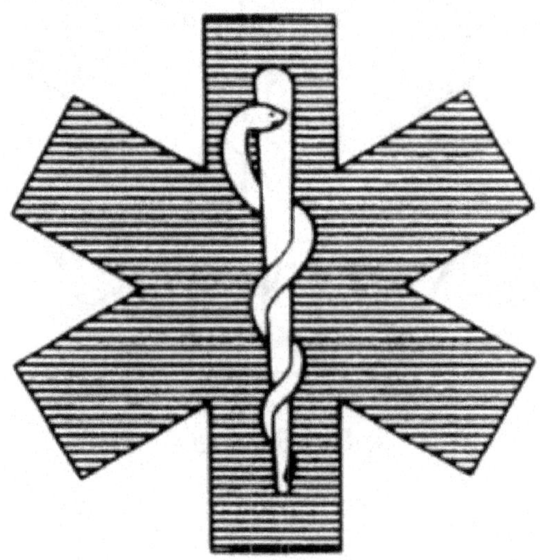

National Highway Traffic Safety Administration
United States Department of Transportation
400 7th Street SW
Washington, D.C. 20590

For: EMERGENCY MEDICAL CARE VEHICLES in CLASS A.
For: EMERGENCY MEDICAL CARE IN CLASS B.

First use in November, 1973; in commerce December 1973.
The drawing is lined for the color blue.

The certification mark is used by persons authorized by applicant to certify that emergency medical care vehicles meet U.S. Department of Transportation standards (Class A), the emergency medical care personnel operating the vehicle have been trained to meet U.S. Department of Transportation standards (Class B) or both.

Ser.No.33,491,filed Oct. 1, 1974

R.F. CISSEL, Examiner

5

FRACTURES & FRAGMENTATION

"Despite the obvious fact that a major portion of critically ill or injured patients enter the health care system through the hospital emergency department...no facet of medicine has been so widely ignored as Emergency Medical Services. For years EMS fell under the old canard, 'Everybody talks about it, but few do anything.' And even when they did, most approaches were both too little and poorly coordinated." [61]

- Robert E. Streicher, MD
Assistant Surgeon General & Director, Federal Health Programs
Health Services Administration 1974

THROUGHOUT THE 1960S AND 1970S, EMERGENCY MEDICAL SERVICES underwent a period of accelerated growth, garnering substantial public support and developmental advancements. However, the 1980s marked a significant transformation in the landscape of EMS due primarily to changes in federal funding, priorities, economics, and politics. The fragile and emerging EMS system survived, but the result was fragmentation. This chapter, titled "Fractures & Fragmentation," aims to explore the challenges that arose during this period, focusing on the impact of funding changes, the fragmentation of EMS systems, and the resulting inconsistencies in state requirements. An exploration of these issues will provide a more comprehensive understanding of the obstacles that hindered the progression of EMS, as well as the measures taken by various stakeholders to overcome these hurdles and enhance the quality of emergency medical services in the United States.

A PARADIGM SHIFT: THE BLOCK GRANTS OF 1980

The 1980s constituted a pivotal decade for Emergency Medical Services in the United States, characterized by substantial modifications in federal funding mechanisms, primarily through the introduction of block grants. This transformation elicited profound effects across EMS systems nationwide, influencing resource allocation, standardization, and ultimately, the efficacy of these systems.

Prior to 1980, the *Emergency Medical Services Systems Act* (EMS Act) of 1973[62] ensured dedicated federal funding for EMS systems. Notably, the EMS Act recognized the need and initial funding for the establishment of 300 defined and coordinated regional EMS systems across the United States. Nevertheless, by 1979, despite strong public favor and the infusion of substantial funds, the systematic implementation plan was faltering. On July 11, 1977, the Committee on Appropriations of the U.S. House of Representatives mandated an investigation. Select excerpts from the investigative report - which was presented to the Appropriations Committee in 1979, are included below:

> "[The Department of Health, Education and Welfare's] (DHEW) emergency medical services system development program has received nationwide support from State, local, and private organizations. It has resulted in improved emergency medical care in many sections of the country. Despite these successes, there are problems with the EMS systems development as there is a need for improved control over and evaluation of this program by HEW, and better coordination and cooperation at both the Federal and State levels... there has been a fragmented, uncoordinated departmental approach to implementing a viable, standardized EMS program…The investment by HEW and DOT in the Federal program to develop 300 EMS regions in the United States by 1985 could exceed $800 million…
>
> [Although the HEW Division of EMS] was delegated responsibility for administering the EMS program for HEW, no permanent positions have been budgeted for this purpose. Since FY 1975, requests for permanent staffing and additional personnel have been rejected by either the Secretary of DHEW or OMB…the Director of the Division of EMS traveled a total of 106 days during FY 1977 providing onsite technical assistance…
>
> **DOT Reluctant to Accept HEW Leadership Role in EMS**
>
> DOT and HEW conduct EMS programs under separate laws, DOT under the *Highway Safety Act* of 1966 and HEW under the *Emergency Medical Services Systems Act* of 1973, as amended.
>
> The DOT program emphasizes the prehospital functions of EMS, particularly as they relate to highway accident victims. The DHEW program includes the prehospital EMS functions and focuses on the development of comprehensive regional systems capable of providing the wide range of emergency medical care. The two programs have overlapping features and there is a need for better coordination.

> …DHEW and DOT have been trying to develop a Memorandum of Understanding clarifying their respective roles in EMS development. DHEW, as the lead agency for EMS, wants DOT's program to be coordinated with and approved by DHEW. DOT is reluctant to relinquish the leadership role derived from its earlier association with emergency medical care, established in the late 1960's and early 1970's, and actively resents having to coordinate any of its programs with DHEW[a]. Constant bickering between the two agencies has had an adverse effect on the national EMS program…
>
> **EMS is a State and Local Responsibility**
>
> Should Federal funding end, State support will be necessary to keep EMS systems intact. EMS regions are not political entities with direct taxing authority and must rely on the local governments participating in the system for financial and other support.
>
> The degree of support that the EMS regions might receive is unknown. In view of the competing demands for limited tax dollars, it appears doubtful, however, that adequate financial help will be forthcoming in many areas. As a consequence, the future of many in-place EMS systems will be in jeopardy, unless the States decide to actively support the program…
>
> **Uncoordinated EMS Programs Exist in Some States**
>
> In 9 of the 28 States in which EMS programs were reviewed by the Investigative Staff, two separate EMS programs were run at the State level, both funded through Federal grant programs. In these States, the Governor's Representative does not rely on the State EMS coordinator's assessment of EMS needs but instead makes an independent evaluation. This allows local governments which do not wish to be part of the regional EMS system to circumvent State and DHEW program requirements and still obtain Federal funding."[63]

Regrettably, the 1979 investigative report was not the sole indication of concerns. A prior 1976 report prepared by the Department of Health, Education, and Welfare, titled "Progress, But Problems in Developing Emergency Medical Services Systems" had already identified substantial challenges with implementing a national EMS system.[64] The cover of this congressional report read, "Development of regional emergency medical services systems on a self-sustaining basis depends on the willingness of local government and local providers, such as hospitals, to accept the regional system concept. So far, regional systems have not been able to gain the control and coordination necessary to achieve economic, effective, and efficient emergency medical services delivery called for by the *Emergency Medical Services Systems Act* of 1973."

---

[a] Following the investigation report, the Secretaries of the DOT and DHEW entered into an interagency MOU on October 26, 1978

Concurrently, as the investigative report brought to light significant challenges in the implementation of EMS Systems, Congress was confronted with mounting political and economic pressures. Notably, on November 4, 1979, Iranian students laid siege to the U.S. Embassy in Tehran, Iran, leading to the capture of more than 60 American hostages. This tense situation was further compounded in December by the Soviet Union's invasion of Afghanistan, which exacerbated Cold War tensions. These events unfolded against a backdrop of economic adversity, with the United States experiencing a surge in unemployment from 5.8 to 7.0 percent between 1979 and 1980, accompanied by an increase in inflation from 11.3 to 13.5 percent.[65]

REPORT TO THE CONGRESS

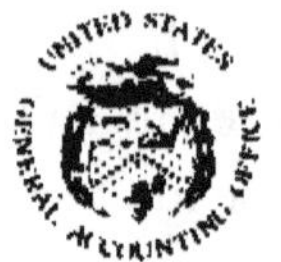

BY THE COMPTROLLER GENERAL OF THE UNITED STATES

Progress, But Problems In Developing Emergency Medical Services Systems

Health Services Administration
Department of Health, Education, and Welfare

Development of regional emergency medical services systems on a self-sustaining basis depends on the willingness of local government and local providers, such as hospitals, to accept the regional system concept.

So far, regional systems have not been able to gain the control and coordination necessary to achieve economic, effective, and efficient emergency medical services delivery called for by the Emergency Medical Services Systems Act of 1973.

Improvements have been made in the delivery of emergency medical services as a result of system developments encouraged and financed by the act. However, the regional concept is being compromised by virtue of the independence and differing priorities of local governments and providers.

HRD-76-150

JULY 13, 1976

As Congress grappled with challenging economic and geopolitical realities, EMS advocates made efforts to persuade Congress to maintain the plan. Unfortunately, the prophetic words of Sylvia Queen, Director of the Massachusetts Department of Health Office of EMS, in her 1980 written testimony to Congress, resonated deeply:

"Years of planning have been necessary in order to draw physicians, hospital personnel, emergency medical technicians, fire and police personnel and consumers together. All momentum will be lost if funds are not available with which to implement the planned systems. Federal support for this program was time-limited from its inception, and this we understood; however, to withdraw support from those regions which are at the very threshold of comprehensive implementation would be not only unjust but also counterproductive."
-Sylvia Queen, Director[66]

The convergence of these political and economic pressures, combined with the revelations of the congressional investigation report highlighting the faltering implementation of regional EMS systems, proved overwhelming. Despite public support for EMS, Congress reassessed the federal role in financing and developing EMS care systems. Consequently, in 1981, the *Omnibus Budget Reconciliation Act*[67] consolidated EMS funding into state-administered preventive health and health services block grants, effectively ending federal funding for the development of EMS. The Act also eliminated the designated lead federal agency for EMS System development, the Department of Health and Human Services (formerly HEW), Division of EMS. This pivotal shift had far-reaching implications, restricting funding specifically available for EMS systems, and significantly altering the federal leadership and coordination role in EMS system development. Federal responsibilities for EMS were divided among multiple agencies, including the EMS Division within the National Highway Traffic Safety Administration, EMS for Children and trauma systems development entities within the Health Resources and Services Administration (HRSA), and the Office of Rural Health Policy (ORHP).

Confronted with a new funding model, and fragmented federal support, the still-developing EMS systems and State EMS Offices struggled with substantial resource limitations. Although the block grant system provided states with more discretion in fund allocation, it also placed EMS in competition with other programs for a share of limited resources. This led to a noticeable reduction in funds available for infrastructure development, equipment upgrades, and training programs, all of which strained EMS systems' ability to maintain optimal care standards. Eloquently summarized by Dr. R. Adams Cowley, in his 1979 testimony before Congress:

> "In the political game of dividing the pie, you must convince the one with the knife that you deserve a fair share."
>
> - R. Adams Cowley, MD

Additionally, the introduction of block grants fostered further fragmentation and variability across EMS agencies in different states and jurisdictions. Without a dedicated federal funding stream and unified guidelines, the evolution and standardization of EMS systems were predominantly subjected to state-level decisions and preferences. This resulted in disparities in equipment, training protocols, and overall care quality, posing considerable challenges for the realization of a unified, nationwide EMS system.

Moreover, block grants intensified competition for limited funding. With numerous healthcare initiatives and social service programs vying for funding, EMS systems faced an uphill battle to secure essential resources for improvement and expansion. Consequently, many systems struggled to enhance infrastructure, modernize equipment, and invest in professional development opportunities.

The funding changes instigated by the emergence of block grants also impacted data collection and research within EMS. The scarcity of dedicated funding inevitably led to a reduction in resources set aside for data collection systems and EMS-related research. This compromised the ability to amass comprehensive data, conduct meaningful research, and implement evidence-based practices, thereby hindering EMS systems' capacity to optimize patient care and improve operational effectiveness.

By 1985, three significant observations became unmistakable: the predictions made by Sylvia Queen in 1980 had tragically materialized, leading to the loss of all momentum; Congress continued its dedication to block grants as a funding mechanism; and the cautionary words of Dr. R. Adams Cowley had also become an undeniable reality. Furthermore, it was evident that most states were not effectively utilizing block grant funding to develop their EMS systems.

In response to this reality, the National Association of State EMS Directors took decisive action by passing a resolution and delivering compelling congressional testimony, earnestly urging Congress to prioritize funding for EMS.

From the 1985 Congressional Record:

> **Statement of Paul B. Anderson, President, National Association of State Emergency Medical Services Directors**
>
> This testimony is offered on behalf of this national EMS association which has a variant serious concern relative to the continuation of comprehensive EMS systems programs in the United States in order to prevent death and disability thousands of times daily throughout the nation.

The National Association of State Emergency Medical Services Directors (NAEMSD) has approved the following resolution on the subject of the preventive health and health services block grant program:

WHEREAS, the delivery of Emergency Medical Services has been recognized as part of the healthcare delivery system, and

WHEREAS, Emergency Medical Service Systems funding was previously authorized and appropriated by Congress and administered by the federal Department of Health and Human Services, and

WHEREAS, the Congress currently provides EMS funding through the Preventive Health and Health Services Block Grant Program, and

WHEREAS, it is important not to dilute the funding initiative at the federal level,

NOW THEREFORE, BE IT RESOLVED THAT the National Association of State EMS Directors:

1) Supports the continuation of EMS funding at the federal level;

2) Recommends that this funding continue under the preventive health and health services block grant program at the Department of Health and Human Services

3) Feels that on both the state and the federal level greater emphasis be placed on the health services portion of the above named block grant; and

4) Recommends that the Department of Health and Human Services coordinate its activities relating to the EMS with the National Association of State EMS Directors.

The National Association of state EMS directors strongly believes that adequate funding for this block grant program is a necessity. The Congress is urged to continue this block grant program and to provide adequate funding for both the preventive and the health services aspect that must be addressed to serve the citizens of this nation.

The National Association of state EMS directors also believes that the flexibility of the block grant program must be maintained in order to permit states to use this funding in relation to the emergency medical services priorities that exist in each state now and in the future.

The subcommittee on labor, Health and Human Services, Education and related agencies is urged to act favorably to continue the Preventive Health and Health Services Block Grant Program and to ensure that adequate funding is provided in order that Emergency Medical Service Systems throughout the nation are kept viable to be able to reduce death and disability.[68]

FRAGMENTATION OF EMS SYSTEMS

The 1980s marked a challenging period for the United States' Emergency Medical Services system, with a significant rise in fragmentation due to the proliferation of EMS agencies, the evolution of personnel, and the fluctuations in federal funding. Predominantly spurred by abrupt changes in federal EMS leadership and funding structures, these shifts led to funding scarcity. The regional EMS systems and local ambulance services, established during the surge of the 1970s, were now lacking adequate funding and resources.

In the 1970s, a vigorous federal push for states and regions to develop EMS systems was visible. However, this momentum unexpectedly dwindled, leaving the relatively young and fragile regional and community EMS systems seemingly abandoned. Local community leaders had to innovate and find new mechanisms for sustainability as communities expected and heavily relied on ambulance services.

Simultaneously, the absence of robust state and national leadership amplified these challenges. Amidst this landscape, local EMS agencies, without clear guidance and faced with the conflicting federal directions from the Department of Transportation and the Department of Health, Education and Welfare (DHEW) in the late 1970s, found themselves independently navigating a multifaceted and complex terrain. This led to a patchwork of services with significant disparities in standards, quality, scope, and capabilities.

The 1978 congressional investigation report described the confusion and misalignment:

> "State EMS officials do not always have ready access to the Director of Division of EMS. Much of the program information is received thirdhand via the grapevine--by word of mouth...HEW regional offices were often not aware of program changes made by the Director of DEMS , and so the regional offices were unable to provide proper and timely guidance...".[69]

State EMS offices, after being somewhat abandoned by the strong (albeit conflicting at times) federal support of the 1970s, now lacked funding and resources. States were trying to manage the expanding number of EMS systems and community ambulance services and adjust to the new challenges. Amid the confusion, states began formulating their own regulations and certification prerequisites. Each state's choice—whether favoring DOT materials, DHEW materials, creating a hybrid, or producing unique materials—led to considerable inconsistencies among states. These inconsistencies complicated EMS professionals' attempts to transfer their licenses or certifications and led to confusion among EMS practitioners and the public.

The abrupt changes in federal support and priorities in the 1980s, including the prior conflicts between DHEW and DOT, had a lasting impact. Many of the states that had aligned more closely with DHEW guidance and materials opted to develop their own examinations and materials, rather than fully adopt the DOT-centric materials and the National Registry of EMTs. Established largely due to the *Highway Safety Act* of 1966, NREMT had a significant relationship with the DOT and its national standard curriculum.

This heightened fragmentation also led states to disregard model EMS legislation[70] and create their own rules, making it even more challenging to maintain a uniform standard of care nationwide. This discrepancy brought forth logistical challenges for EMS agencies operating across state boundaries, forcing them to navigate varying regulatory frameworks and distracted them from their primary focus—delivering high-quality patient care.

By the 1990s, this lack of uniformity culminated in more than 40 different variations of EMT certification,[71] each with distinct knowledge and skill requirements. This wide divergence obstructed the development of credentialing reciprocity agreements, impeded the standardization of the profession, and hindered EMS professionals seeking to transfer their certifications or licenses between states. The divergence from a nationally recognized exam also created misunderstanding between different EMS professional designations, thereby hampering efforts to standardize EMS practices and procedures, and negatively impacting EMS professionals' relationships with their peers in other medical fields.

Overall, the intensified fragmentation of EMS systems during the 1980s and the misalignment of state requirements presented substantial impediments to the advancement of emergency medical services in the United States. The federal initiatives and professional organizations worked relentlessly towards addressing these challenges, aiming to reorganize and consolidate EMS systems to improve the overall quality of EMS across the United States.

LASTING EFFECTS OF FRAGMENTATION ON EMS

In 1975, NHTSA commissioned a report to evaluate the development of EMS in the United States. While there were strides being made in theoretical development of a coordinated EMS system, the on-the-ground reality was different. The report cautioned:

There are numerous gaps and mismatches in the emergency medical care system that are associated with its fractionation ... Nowhere can there be said to exist a fully integrated system; the best examples merely have fewer discrete subsystems. In the worst instances all sub systems are autonomous--some privately owned, some public, and other simply independent non - profit...

Fractionation of the care system can at best only produce suboptimization of performance of both the units and total system, accompanied by waste of resources...Resource losses to the community or region also occur because a wide spectrum of response competences is not built up when there are many small units...

Utilization of personnel in short supply is difficult to maintain in fractionated subunits. Functions, duties, and activities cannot be reallocated, which contributes to under- or over - supply of needed competence. This further makes it difficult, if not impossible, to develop meaningful new occupations and careers to help with the manpower shortage.[72]

Though the issue of fragmentation was recognized within the EMS profession in the 1970s, developments in the 1980s further entrenched and amplified this challenge, which continues to shape the profession and impact the quality of care. Fragmentation emerged from numerous factors, such as misaligned state requirements, conflicting federal agencies, and community-driven EMS development. However, the ripple effects of fragmentation extended well beyond these issues, notably impinging on the operational efficiency, sustainability, and trajectory of EMS in the United States.

A major consequence was the inconsistency in patient care due to diverse training, certification, and professional standards across jurisdictions. With each state defining its own requirements, care quality offered by EMS professionals varied greatly. This inconsistency adversely affected patient outcomes, restricted interstate EMS personnel movement, and hindered the establishment of nationwide best practices for emergency medical care.

In 2009, the National Emergency Medical Services Advisory Council's Education/Workforce Committee found that:

> "The current lack of a standardized certification, licensure and credentialing of EMS personnel across the United States affects the performance of EMS systems as they cross jurisdictional and State lines in the execution of their duties. This impacts both routine emergency medical response and mutual aid support because of a disaster or mass casualty incident. This lack of standardization has implications on efficiency and effectiveness, compliance with States' statutes, workforce coordination and satisfaction, medical control, and EMS system human resource issues to name a few."[73]

Furthermore, fragmentation stifled the EMS field's growth and maturation. With EMS systems operating in silos, collaboration and knowledge exchange opportunities were diminished, which subsequently complicated the development of a cohesive professional identity and a unified set of best practices.

The fragmentation also contributed to an absence of a true unified national professional identity among EMS practitioners. Due to EMS systems' localized growth, EMS practitioners often felt a strong local allegiance but lacked a broader national EMS system understanding. This lack of a unified national identity has hindered EMS practitioners' ability to advocate for the profession at the federal level on matters such as insurance reimbursement and recognition of EMS as a highly specialized medical profession.

Allocation of resources and funding was another area affected by fragmentation. As communities established their own ambulance services, the thinly spread funding and competition for limited resources led to service delivery inefficiencies. These financial constraints hindered EMS agencies' ability to invest in essential equipment, training, and personnel, impacting the standard of care.

Fragmentation also erected significant barriers to integrating EMS agencies with other healthcare systems. The absence of coordination between EMS agencies and other medical providers made it difficult to provide seamless, patient-centered care. It also made it challenging to track patient outcomes and understand various EMS interventions' effectiveness over time.

The fragmented nature of EMS systems also led to a lack of mutual understanding and trust between EMS practitioners and other healthcare professionals. Variations in EMS practitioners' quality and scope of practice caused skepticism and confusion among other healthcare providers about EMS personnel's capabilities. This lack of understanding and trust complicated effective collaboration in managing patients' healthcare needs.

Moreover, consistent care protocols aligning with broader healthcare landscape best practices were challenging to develop due to fragmented EMS systems. The lack of unified standards led to diverse patient care approaches among EMS practitioners in different states and communities. These inconsistencies hindered the overall evaluation of EMS interventions' effectiveness and the development of evidence-based best practices which could be universally implemented.

Finally, fragmentation complicated the establishment of coordinated and efficient regional healthcare networks. With independent EMS agencies operating under varied state and local regulations, creating an organized system for optimal resource allocation became daunting. This challenge includes coordinating patient transport to the most appropriate healthcare facilities based on their needs and the capabilities of available hospitals.

Efforts to Address Fragmentation and Realign EMS Systems

Recognizing the challenges emerging from the fragmentation of U.S. Emergency Medical Services systems, a multitude of stakeholders – federal agencies, state governments, and professional organizations – continue efforts to address these issues and realign EMS systems. The goal continues to be a consistent, efficient, and patient-focused emergency medical care system nationwide.

In 1984, NHTSA entered into a collaborative agreement with the National Association of State EMS Directors (later, NASEMSO) to establish "reciprocity guidelines." In a congressional appropriations hearing, the NHTSA director described this

> "...as a means of encouraging States to adopt a uniform Emergency Medical Technician training program... while [States] had some form of Paramedic certification...it was not known whether the State certification program was based on NHTSA guidelines, or on individual State requirements."[74]

Following this, NHTSA inaugurated a technical assessment program for state EMS systems in 1988,[75] with the first assessment being conducted in Colorado. During these assessments, a team of subject matter experts evaluate the statewide EMS system on ten core components: regulation and policy, resource management, human resources and training, transportation, facilities, communications, public information and education, medical direction, trauma systems, and evaluation.

Another significant stride in the 1990s was the creation of new national guidance documents by the NHTSA Office of EMS and other stakeholders, such as the "*EMS Agenda for the Future: A Systems Approach*"[76] and the "*EMS Education Agenda for the Future: A Systems Approach*."[77] These documents provided a strategic vision for evolving and integrating EMS systems across the country, underscoring the need for enhanced coordination and communication amongst EMS agencies and the standardization of training, certification, and licensure procedures.

At the state level, efforts were made to align with this national guidance, with many states moving towards adopting the National Registry of EMTs exam as the standard for certification. This shift fostered a more uniform and rigorous testing process, thereby establishing consistent standards for EMS professionals, regardless of their practicing state.

In tandem, professional organizations such as the National Association of State EMS Officials (NASEMSO), the National Association of Emergency Medical Technicians (NAEMT), and the American College of Emergency Physicians (ACEP) played instrumental roles in realigning EMS systems. They developed and promoted best practices, advocated for the interests of EMS professionals at the state and federal levels, and encouraged collaboration and communication within the profession.

Integration of EMS with other healthcare systems also saw improvement with the development of electronic patient care reporting (ePCR) systems, like the National EMS Information System (NEMSIS), and the promotion of Health Information Exchanges (HIE). These efforts streamlined the transfer of essential patient information, enhancing the continuity of care.

Conceptualized in 2013, the EMS Compact standardizes certification and licensure processes across numerous states and provides a Privilege to Practice in multiple jurisdictions, based on one Home State EMS license. This strengthens the profession through uniform recognition of standards, improved workforce mobility, and increased EMS system efficiency. By 2023, 24 states enacted legislation supporting the EMS Compact. (Read more about the EMS Compact in Chapter 24.)

Today, all states recognize National EMS Certification as a pathway to state licensure (National EMS Certification is now mandatory in 48 states, read more in Chapter 18). This represents a significant achievement in creating a consistent standard of knowledge and competency for those entering the EMS profession after a fifty-year struggle. However, the pursuit of a fully integrated national identity for the profession is ongoing.

Stakeholders must persist in their collaborative efforts to promote uniform training, certification, and licensure standards nationwide. Coupled with stronger integration of EMS with other healthcare systems, these efforts can improve patient care and outcomes, support evidence-based best practices, and enable EMS professionals to efficiently advocate for their interests at the federal level. This unified approach will contribute to the progressive recognition of EMS as a specialized medical profession.

A Vision for Continued Unification

Despite significant strides in the past decade towards a nationwide, unified EMS system, substantial challenges persist. These have been exacerbated by the aftermath of the COVID-19[b] pandemic, which placed immense pressure on the broader healthcare sector, including EMS.

[b] SARS-CoV-2, Coronavirus disease of 2019

The crisis underscored and amplified existing difficulties, pushing EMS agencies to their limits. In the wake of this, the commitment to maintaining EMS as a service accessible to all communities requires renewed vigor towards a unified system approach.

Creating a unified EMS system is a complex task due to the unique nature of EMS agencies across different states. This fragmentation results from a confluence of factors such as diverse state and federal regulations, variations in service providers, funding and reimbursement challenges, and a lack of coordinated national oversight. However, the local pride that can contribute to fragmentation can also serve as a rallying force for unity. Like other healthcare professions like physicians, nurses, and physical therapists that uphold a nationally recognized identity, EMS professionals should prioritize establishing a unified national identity. This responsibility falls heavily upon local EMS leaders to nurture unity and collaboration on local, state, and national levels.

Federal and state agencies, professional organizations, and EMS stakeholders have acknowledged the challenges posed by fragmentation and have taken significant strides to address them. Initiatives such as the EMS Compact, the adoption of the NREMT National EMS Certification examination, and the ongoing development of national guidance documents have been instrumental in fostering a more uniform and efficient EMS system.

Nevertheless, it remains challenging to balance local needs and national standards. State-sponsored EMS legislation occasionally defaults to short-term solutions for local issues, at the cost of national standards and collective commitment to the EMS profession. This disheartening tendency, occasionally supported by local EMS practitioners, exacerbates fragmentation, and erodes the overall profession. When faced with legislation that threatens national standards, the EMS profession as a unified body must respond assertively, acknowledging the collective responsibility to address and resolve underlying challenges. This includes pushing elected officials to invest in education, allocating necessary resources, and tackling issues such as recruitment, retention, and certification. This unified stance not only safeguards the integrity of EMS as a profession but also upholds the quality of service provided to communities nationwide.

As the EMS landscape continues to evolve, it's vital to maintain collaborative efforts for consistency in training, certification, and licensure standards across the country. By fostering a stronger sense of unity and shared purpose within the profession, EMS professionals can better advocate for critical issues at the federal level, such as insurance reimbursement, workforce development, and the continued advancement of EMS as a specialized medical profession.

By channeling the local pride and commitment to excellence that has driven the evolution of EMS systems, stakeholders can collectively strive to create a more unified, efficient, and patient-centered system. This endeavor requires perseverance, collaboration, and an unwavering commitment to a unified systems approach. Although challenging, the ultimate reward will be a resilient and accessible EMS service available to all communities – a crucial component of our national healthcare infrastructure.

The MOU Between the DOT and HEW, 1978

The 1977 Congressional-led inquiry into the execution of the Emergency Medical Services System Act offered a harsh critique of the strife, rivalry, and dysfunction between the Department of Transportation and the Department of Health, Education and Welfare. Before the public release of the final report, these two federal agencies managed to establish a Memorandum of Understanding. Regrettably, this agreement did not last long, and it arrived too late to undo the effects of years of contradictory federal directives to States during the development of EMS systems.

**MEMORANDUM OF UNDERSTANDING
BETWEEN THE UNITED STATES DEPARTMENT OF TRANSPORTATION
AND THE
UNITED STATES DEPARTMENT OF HEALTH, EDUCATION, AND WELFARE
FOR PROCEDURES RELATING TO
EMERGENCY MEDICAL SERVICES SYSTEMS**

The Department of Transportation (DOT), under the Department of Transportation Act (49 U.S.C. 1651 et seq) and the Highway Safety Act of 1966 (23 U.S.C. 401 et seq) has authority to provide financial and technical assistance for the transportation phases of Emergency Medical Services. The Department of Health, Education, and Welfare (DHEW) is authorized to provide technical assistance and funds in the form of grants and contracts for Emergency Medical Services Systems under Title XII, Part A, of the Public Health Service Act (42 U.S.C. 300d et seq).

For the purpose of assuring a clear understanding by State, Regional, and local officials responsible for the implementation and administration of emergency medical services programs, it is essential that the primary areas of responsibility between DOT and DHEW be defined. Therefore, DOT and DHEW agree, pursuant to their respective statutory authorities, to the terms of this Memorandum. In carrying out this Memorandum, the goals of DOT and DHEW will be to develop, establish, and implement consistent and comprehensive national uniform standards, criteria, procedures, technical assistance, related requirements and to avoid duplication of effort.

Section 1206 of the Public Health Service Act identifies 15 components of an emergency medical services system. These component requirements are used in this document solely to delineate responsibilities of DOT and DHEW for the development of program standards and procedures.

A. <u>DOT RESPONSIBILITIES</u>

In coordination with DHEW, DOT will develop uniform standards and procedures for the transportation phases of emergency care and response as follows:

1. Manpower - EMS administrative personnel involved in the transportation phases of emergency medical services (EMS).

2. Training - First responders (fire, police, etc.) Emergency Medical Technicians - Ambulance and Paramedics, communications dispatchers, and system coordinators and administrators.

3. Communications - Telecommunications systems in areas of citizen access, central dispatch, ambulance to emergency department (ED), field resource management of EMS systems including utilization of basic and advanced telecommunications technology.

Attachment 6

4. Transportation - Ambulances and special transportation vehicles (air, surface, water) and equipment both carried and installed (extrication, communications, medical), including emergency and safety specifications.

5. Facilities - The transportation and care of emergency patients to the appropriately categorized and/or otherwise designated facilities.

6. Critical Care Units - Transportation and care to such designated units.

7. Public Safety Agencies - Integration and improved utilization of all personnel, facilities, and equipment.

8. Consumer Participation - The opportunity for private citizens to participate in making policy for the transportation phases of an EMS system.

9. Accessibility to Care - Transportation response and extra-hospital EMS care without prior inquiry as to patients' ability to pay.

10. Transfer of Patients - Inter-hospital transport and care of critical patients to advanced treatment centers.

11. Coordinated Medical Recordkeeping - Record systems utilized during the transportation phases (e.g., dispatcher and ambulance data forms and processing).

12. Consumer Information and Education - Education and training of private citizens along with dissemination of program information relating to training and educational concepts, principles, standards, and criteria for the transportation phases of EMS systems.

13. Review and Evaluation - Evaluation of the extent and quality of pre-hospital and inter-hospital emergency response and care services provided in the system's service area as it relates to emergency transportation.

14. Disaster Linkages - Coordination of pre-hospital and inter-hospital EMS transportation response and care services during mass casualties, natural disasters, or national emergencies.

15. Mutual Aid Agreements - Setting requirements for pre-hospital and inter-hospital EMS transportation response on a reciprocal basis.

B. DHEW RESPONSIBILITIES

DHEW will develop, in coordination with DOT, medical standards and procedures for initial, supportive and definitive care phases of EMS systems as follows:

1. Manpower - EMS personnel involved in all phases of EMS.

2. Training- First responders, private citizens, Emergency Medical Techinicians - Ambulance and Paramedics, communications, EMS hospital communicators, emergency nurses and physicians, EMS medical directors and system coordinators and administrators.

3. Communications - Telecommunications systems in areas of citizen access, central dispatch and field resource management of EMS systems. DHEW emphasis would be in the areas of medical communications and control for vehicle to hospital communications for both basic and advanced life support as well as hospital to hospital communications for advanced technology.

4. Transportation - Patient care standards for ambulances, special transportation vehicles (surface, air, water) to include equipment and treatment specifications.

5. Facilities - Development and implementation of regional hospital categorization programs.

6. Critical Care Units - Appropriate designation of critical care capability.

7. Public Safety Agencies - Integration and improved utilization of personnel, facilities, and equipment in day-to-day EMS and in major disaster operating procedures.

8. Consumer Participation - The opportunity for private citizens to participate in making policy for the EMS system.

9. Accessibility to Care - Care without prior inquiry as to ability of patient to pay.

10. Transfer of Patients - Inter-hospital transfer agreements for critical patients to advanced treatment centers in order to provide maximum follow-up care and rehabilitation.

11. Coordinated Medical Recordkeeping - Establishing and operating record systems utilized during transportation phases (e.g., dispatcher and ambulance data forms and processing) as well as in-hospital emergency and critical care treatment phases.

12. Consumer Information and Education - Education and training of private citizens along with dissemination of program information relating to training and educational concepts, principles, standards, and criteria for the EMS system.

13. Review and Evaluation - Evaluation of the extent and quality of regional emergency medical response and care services provided within the system's service areas.

14. Disaster Linkages - Coordination of EMS response and patient care during mass casualties, natural disasters, or national emergencies.

15. Mutual Aid Agreements - Setting requirements for pre-hospital, hospital, and inter-hospital emergency medical care on a reciprocal basis.

C. RESEARCH AND DEMONSTRATION

DOT and DHEW will pursue research and demonstration activities in support of their respective program responsibilities as defined above. Joint efforts are encouraged where possible.

D. FUNDING AND TECHNICAL ASSISTANCE

DOT may fund those activities pertaining to its responsibilities outlined above under both Section 402 and 403 of Title 23, U.S.C., Highway Safety Act of 1966. Under Section 402, it is recognized that in the apportionment of funds to the States for program implementation, DOT does not determine the priorities by which these funds will be applied to the transportation phases of the State's EMS system. Subject to applicable statutes and regulations and the availability of funds, DHEW may fund the full spectrum of eligible entities as defined in Section 1206 of the Public Health Service Act. When DHEW funds are expended for emergency ambulance vehicles and the training of Emergency Medical Technicians - Ambulance and Paramedics, DOT criteria as specified in EMS program regulations apply. DOT funds may be used to assist in the transportation phases of DHEW-funded projects. Both agencies will provide technical assistance as appropriate and as required in support of their program responsibilities.

E. INTERAGENCY COOPERATION

In addition to the statutory requirements pertaining to the Interagency Committee on Emergency Medical Services, DOT and DHEW will keep each other advised on a continuing basis and coordinate the development of standards within their respective responsibilities. With respect to communications systems, every attempt should be made to harmonize DOT-DHEW requirements to the maximum extent practicalbe.

F. EXCHANGE OF INFORMATION

Prior to the issuance of procedures, training manuals, regulations, funding or other information pertinent to the respective responsibilities, DOT and DHEW will exchange information, consult with, and assist each other within the areas of their special competence. Both Departments will actively maintain identified channels so as to share with each other, at both the central and regional office levels, all pertinent issuances to their respective staffs and clientele.

G. WORKING ARRANGEMENTS

DOT and DHEW will designate staff representatives and will establish joint working arrangements from time to time for the purpose of administering this Memorandum of Understanding. Pursuant to this Memorandum of Understanding, DOT and DHEW Regional Offices will promote coordination of DHEW-sponsored projects with DOT required State comprehensive EMS plans and programs through a mutually acceptable lead agency. These offices will also assist each other in the identification and application of all available resources to support EMS upgrading within the scope of such plans, programs and/or projects.

H. GENERAL

This agreement shall take effect upon the signing by authorized representatives of the respective Departments.

Nothing in this Memorandum of Understanding is intended to affect in any way the statutory authority of either Department.

For the Department of Transportation

Secretary

10/26/78
Date

For the Department of Health, Education, and Welfare

Secretary

10/26/78
Date

6

VOLUNTEERISM: THE ULTIMATE EMS SUBSIDY

"Volunteers do not necessarily have the time; they just have the heart."

VOLUNTEERISM PLAYED A CRUCIAL ROLE IN THE DEVELOPMENT OF emergency medical services across the United States. The reliance on volunteers in EMS is a unique aspect that sets it apart from other healthcare professions and most public safety fields. As EMS began to take shape in the mid-20th century, many communities turned to volunteers to provide emergency medical care due to limited financial resources and the absence of a well-established infrastructure for pre-hospital emergency care.

The volunteer model in EMS emerged out of necessity, with communities lacking sufficient funds and personnel to support a full-time, paid EMS workforce. Volunteers often came from diverse backgrounds, including veterans, local business owners, funeral home employees, and community members. For decades, these individuals stepped up to fill the gap in emergency medical services, providing essential care to their communities during emergencies.

Initially, the volunteer model proved to be an effective solution for providing emergency care in both urban and rural settings. In the early days of EMS, volunteers were trained in basic first aid, equipping them with the essential tools to respond to emergencies and save lives. The earliest volunteers often used their personal vehicles, such as station wagons or hearses, to transport patients to hospitals, improvising with the limited resources available to them at the time.

The importance of volunteerism in the early years of EMS cannot be overstated. Not only did these selfless individuals provide life-saving care, but they also played a key role in shaping the EMS profession as it evolved over time. Volunteers were instrumental in the development of EMS training and education programs, helping to establish the first EMT and paramedic courses across the country. Many volunteer EMS organizations also laid the groundwork for the development of more sophisticated EMS systems, with many eventually transitioning into full-time paid services.

Despite the invaluable contributions made by volunteers in the early years of EMS, the volunteer model also came with many challenges. As the demand for EMS increased and the complexity of pre-hospital care advanced, the limitations of a volunteer-based workforce became more apparent. While the role of volunteers will certainly continue in many communities for years to come, reliance on a volunteer-centric model is increasingly unsustainable for many communities.

Advantages and Challenges of a Volunteer-Based EMS Workforce

- **Cost-Effectiveness**: One of the most significant advantages of a volunteer-based EMS workforce is the cost savings for communities. With volunteers providing emergency medical services, communities benefit from *substantial* in-kind financial subsidies. For decades, this has allowed the communities to allocate financial resources to other essential services or infrastructure improvements while also having access to EMS.
- **Community Engagement**: Volunteer EMS professionals often have strong connections to their local communities, fostering a sense of ownership and responsibility for the well-being of their neighbors. This connection can lead to increased community support and trust in the EMS system.
- **Flexibility**: Volunteer EMS professionals can offer flexibility in staffing and scheduling, enabling EMS organizations to respond to fluctuating demand for services. This flexibility can help ensure that emergency medical care is available when needed, even during times of increased call volume or staffing shortages.

Challenges of a Volunteer-Based EMS Workforce

- **Recruitment and Retention**: Attracting and retaining volunteer EMS professionals is challenging, particularly as the demands and expectations placed on EMS personnel continue to grow. Balancing the demands of work, family, and volunteering is difficult, leading to high turnover rates among volunteer EMS practitioners.
- **Education, Training and Certification**: Ensuring that volunteer EMS professionals receive consistent, high-quality training and maintain necessary certifications is difficult. With limited resources and time, some volunteer organizations may struggle to provide the level of education and training required to maintain competency in the evolving field of EMS.

- **Sustainability**: As the demand for EMS agencies continues to rise, and the complexity of pre-hospital care increases, the sustainability of a volunteer-based EMS workforce is being called into question. As more communities face challenges in recruiting and retaining volunteers, the shift toward a paid EMS workforce is becoming increasingly necessary.

UNSUSTAINABLE EMPLOYER SUBSIDIES

In the early days of EMS volunteerism, it was common for the local EMS volunteers to work in small, community centric businesses. These community businesses were often very flexible and accommodating, supporting ambulance service volunteers' needs to quickly respond to emergency calls during working hours. Many of these same community businesses also acted as underwriters and supporters of the ambulance service financially. However, in recent decades, changing market dynamics, evolving employer-employee relationships, and the shift from local ownership to larger, more centralized businesses have contributed to the decline in employer support for volunteer EMS professionals. The decline in employer support for volunteer EMS professionals is attributed to several factors:

- **Changing Market Dynamics**: As markets have become more competitive and the economic landscape has evolved, businesses are under increasing pressure to maximize productivity, efficiency, and profit. As a result, many employers may no longer be able to afford the financial implications of allowing employees to remain on the clock while volunteering for EMS duties.
- **Evolving Employer-Employee Relationships**: The nature of work and employer-employee relationships has shifted significantly in recent decades. With the rise of the gig economy, remote work, and flexible work arrangements, the traditional model of employees being consistently available to volunteer for EMS duties has become less viable. Moreover, as the workforce becomes more diverse and the demands on employees' time increase, their ability to balance work, family, and volunteer commitments may be more challenging.
- **Shift from Local to Non-Local Ownership**: The transition from local business ownership to larger, more centralized corporations has also had an impact on employer support for volunteer EMS. Local business owners may have had a more direct connection to the community and a greater sense of responsibility for its well-being, making them more inclined to support volunteer EMS professionals. In contrast, non-local businesses may be less invested in the local community and less likely to prioritize supporting volunteer EMS personnel.

These factors have contributed to the decline in employer support for volunteer EMS professionals, further exacerbating the challenges faced by volunteer EMS organizations in recruiting and retaining qualified personnel. Additionally, the rising costs associated with transitioning from a volunteer-based workforce to a paid workforce have placed significant financial burdens on communities across the country. As the EMS profession continues to evolve and the role of volunteers becomes increasingly uncertain, it is essential for communities, policymakers, and EMS leaders to engage in ongoing discussions about the future of volunteerism in EMS and explore potential solutions to the challenges facing the profession today.

Difficult Transitions: Volunteer Model to a Paid Workforce

As the reliance on volunteer EMS professionals has become increasingly unsustainable, many communities have been forced to transition from a volunteer-based model to a paid EMS workforce. This shift brings with it numerous challenges and implications.

One of the most significant hurdles faced by communities transitioning to a paid EMS workforce is the increased financial burden. Employing full-time or part-time EMS practitioners requires funding for salaries, benefits, training, and equipment, which can strain community budgets. Additionally, the costs associated with recruiting, hiring, and retaining qualified EMS personnel can be substantial.

The transition to a paid EMS workforce often involves implementing a higher level of training (communities served by primary volunteers at the Basic Life Support level often desire paid personnel to provide Advanced Life Support). Implementing these higher standards is a challenge for communities that have traditionally relied on volunteer EMS personnel with varying levels of training and expertise.

Transitioning to a paid EMS workforce also requires communities to develop effective workforce management strategies, such as addressing issues related to scheduling, overtime, and employee retention. This is a complex and time-consuming process, particularly for communities that have limited experience in managing a paid EMS workforce.

The shift from a volunteer-based model to a paid EMS workforce can, in some communities, affect the relationships between EMS professionals and the communities they serve. When EMS personnel are volunteers, they often have very strong connections to the local community and a personal investment in its well-being. However, paid EMS practitioners are frequently not residents in the community and often commute (sometimes long distances) to the workplace. This may change the dynamics of these relationships and require additional efforts to maintain strong community ties.

As communities transition from volunteer EMS personnel to a paid workforce, it is essential to ensure a smooth handover of responsibilities to maintain continuity of care for patients. This may involve developing transition plans, providing training and support for new EMS professionals, and ensuring that the necessary resources and infrastructure are in place to support the new workforce model.

The transition from a volunteer-based EMS model to a paid EMS workforce presents numerous challenges for communities across the United States. To successfully navigate this shift, community leaders, EMS organizations, and policymakers must work together to address the financial, logistical, and relational implications of this change and develop strategies to ensure the continued delivery of high-quality emergency medical care to the communities they serve.

THE CRISIS: STRUGGLING TO TRANSITION A LABOR FORCE

As the volunteer-based EMS model becomes increasingly unsustainable, communities across the United States, particularly in rural and frontier areas, find themselves confronted with the task of addressing the challenge of transitioning from volunteers to paid labor. This crisis carries substantial implications for the delivery of emergency medical services and the wider healthcare system. Within this section, the focus will be on examining the fundamental issues and far-reaching impacts associated with this persistent crisis in these remote communities.

- **Financial Strain on Communities**: The most immediate and pressing concern for many rural and frontier communities is the financial strain associated with hiring paid EMS professionals. The cost of salaries, benefits, education, training, and equipment are frequently prohibitive for small or financially struggling communities, leaving them with difficult decisions about how to allocate limited resources. In some cases, communities may be forced to reduce other essential services to fund their EMS system, creating further challenges for residents.

- **EMS Service Gaps and Delays**: As rural and frontier communities struggle to replace volunteers with paid labor, there may be gaps in EMS service coverage and increased response times. These delays can have life-or-death consequences for patients in need of urgent medical attention, particularly in areas where access to emergency care is already limited due to geographical factors.

- **Recruitment and Retention Challenges**: Even when rural and frontier communities can allocate resources for paid EMS professionals, they frequently face difficulties in recruiting and retaining qualified personnel. The EMS profession is known for its demanding nature, with long hours, high-stress situations, and relatively low pay compared to other healthcare professions. Additionally, the remote locations of these communities may make it challenging to attract and retain talented EMS professionals, further exacerbating the crisis.

- **Impact on Quality of Care**: As rural and frontier communities struggle to replace volunteers with paid labor, the quality of EMS care provided may be at risk. With fewer personnel and increased pressure on existing staff, EMS professionals may experience burnout, leading to potential compromises in patient care. Additionally, as communities turn to hiring less experienced or underqualified personnel to fill staffing gaps, the overall quality of EMS care may suffer.

- **Ripple Effects on the Healthcare System**: The crisis faced by rural and frontier communities as they struggle to replace volunteers with paid EMS labor has broader implications for the healthcare system. Delays in emergency medical care can lead to increased pressure on hospital emergency departments, as well as increased costs associated with treating patients who have experienced delays in care.

To address the crisis faced by many rural and frontier communities as they struggle to replace volunteers with paid labor, it is essential for policymakers, EMS organizations, and community leaders to work together in developing sustainable solutions. This may involve exploring alternative funding mechanisms, developing innovative recruitment and retention strategies, and advocating for increased support and recognition for EMS professionals. By collaborating on these efforts, stakeholders can help ensure that these more remote communities continue to receive high-quality emergency medical care, even in the face of these mounting challenges.

THE PARADOX OF EMS IN RURAL AND FRONTIER COMMUNITIES

A paradox characterizes the Emergency Medical Services (EMS) environment in rural and frontier America. In these regions, the volume of medical emergencies is less due to lower population density. However, the remoteness and geographical challenges necessitate higher levels of expertise from EMS personnel. In contrast, the most qualified and experienced EMS professionals often find employment in urban settings where resources, salaries and support are more accessible.

This paradox presents significant challenges against the backdrop of volunteerism in rural and frontier communities. These areas, while transitioning from volunteers to paid personnel, must also ensure that their EMS professionals are equipped with the advanced expertise required to handle the unique challenges of their remote locations. This implies having not only the clinical skills necessary for extended transport times but also the ability to make critical decisions under resource constraints.

Retaining and recruiting proficient EMS professionals in rural and frontier communities is complex, often compounded by several factors:

- **Limited Resources**: Rural and frontier EMS agencies often have fewer resources, including lower salaries, less funding for equipment and training, and fewer opportunities for professional development, making it more challenging to attract and retain skilled EMS professionals.

- **Isolation**: The remote locations of these communities can make it difficult for EMS professionals to access education and training opportunities, as well as the support and networking opportunities available to their urban counterparts.

- **Competing Priorities**: The volunteer-based model in rural and frontier areas often means that EMS professionals must balance their responsibilities as EMTs or Paramedics with other work, family, or community commitments, which can limit their ability to focus on developing and maintaining their skills.

- **Lower Call Volume**: While the lower number of patient emergencies in rural and frontier areas might initially seem like a positive factor, it can contribute to a decreased exposure to clinical experiences, making it more difficult for EMS professionals to develop and maintain their skills and expertise.

Addressing the paradox of EMS in rural and frontier communities requires innovative solutions and collaboration among stakeholders. This may involve:

- Enhancing training and educational opportunities for rural and frontier EMS professionals, such as offering distance learning, telemedicine support, and targeted training programs that address the unique challenges of remote locations.
- Developing incentive programs and support structures to attract and retain skilled EMS professionals in rural and frontier communities, including competitive salaries, benefits, and opportunities for professional growth.
- Advocating for increased funding and resources for rural and frontier EMS agencies, to ensure that they have the tools and support necessary to deliver high-quality care.
- Promoting partnerships between rural and urban EMS agencies to facilitate knowledge sharing, training opportunities, and best-practice development tailored to the specific needs of rural and frontier areas.
- Examining the potential benefits of regionalization, mergers, consolidations, or other shared service models as sustainable options for lower-volume agencies.

The transition from volunteerism to a paid workforce has created a crisis in many rural and frontier communities, which are disproportionately affected by the challenges of replacing volunteers with paid labor. Moreover, it is vital that state and national EMS leaders and government officials collaborate with local communities, local government officials, and EMS leaders. Such collaboration is essential in assuring the reliability and sustainability of EMS across all communities. By addressing the paradox of EMS in rural and frontier America, stakeholders can help guarantee that these areas are served by knowledgeable, experienced, and skilled EMS professionals, thereby maintaining high-quality emergency medical care for all residents.

MEANINGFUL SUPPORT FOR VOLUNTEER SYSTEMS

Volunteer-based systems remain a vital pillar of the EMS workforce. In many communities across the nation, they serve as the indispensable backbone of EMS services and are projected to maintain this role in the foreseeable future. These systems are not only a testament to the spirit of service and community engagement, but they also provide essential emergency medical services in regions where access to full-time paid personnel may be challenging. As such, they will continue to be an integral part of the nation's EMS infrastructure, potentially for decades to come.

Considering the dependence on this model in numerous communities, states and jurisdictions bear a significant responsibility to provide meaningful support and incentives to volunteer EMS systems. Volunteer EMS clinicians balance the demands of their personal lives, regular jobs, and the crucial EMS roles they perform. The endurance and effectiveness of these volunteer systems depend largely on state and jurisdictional recognition and support.

Consequently, states and jurisdictions need to actively commit to supporting volunteer-based EMS systems. This includes enacting policies and launching programs aimed at attracting and retaining volunteer EMS professionals. Meaningful financial incentives, tax benefits, educational and training subsidies, as well as formal recognition programs, should be implemented at both state and local levels. States should offer volunteer-specific benefits, such as insurance or participation in a volunteer pension fund, as an example.

In addition, reducing the operational burdens for these volunteers is essential. This can involve helping with equipment and infrastructure costs, waiving state licensure fees, offering support for ongoing training and certification, and provisioning health and wellness resources. Investments in these areas not only validate and encourage the volunteers but also enhance the overall quality and resilience of the EMS system.

With volunteer-based systems continuing to play a critical role in many communities, the onus lies on the states and jurisdictions to provide the necessary incentives and support. By committing to such initiatives, they can help ensure the resilience, longevity, and efficacy of these systems, thereby securing an essential part of the nation's EMS provision. This robust support for volunteer systems embodies an investment in the nation's health security, community resilience, and the very essence of the EMS mission to serve.

7

EMS Data: The Most Powerful Healthcare Dataset

"Information is the oil of the 21st century, and analytics is the combustion engine."
- Peter Sondergaard

51,379,493

Structured Patient Care Records

13,946	**54**
EMS Agencies	States & Territories

2022 Data Submitted to the National EMS Information System

THE YEAR WAS 1969, A TIME OF SIGNIFICANT INNOVATION AND CHANGE in the United States. The National Aeronautics and Space Administration (NASA) was making final preparations for the Apollo 11 mission, while the Beatles had just played their last public performance in London, and Richard Nixon had been sworn in as the nation's 37th president. Amidst these events, the concept of computers was still new, with these machines being large, expensive, and reliant on punch cards for data input. Nevertheless, the Defense Advanced Research Projects Agency (DARPA) was already working to develop a computer network that could withstand a nuclear attack. It was in this context that Dr. Peter Safar, a world-renowned expert in resuscitation science and critical care medicine, attended the Airlie Conference in Warrenton, Virginia, to discuss Emergency Medical Services. At the conference, Dr. Safar presented a short paper titled "*Ambulance and Emergency Department Records*," which would ultimately lay the foundation for the modern National EMS Information System (NEMSIS).[78] Established in the late 1990s, NEMSIS has since become a valuable tool for EMS agencies, policymakers, researchers, and other stakeholders, enabling significant advancements in EMS data collection and reporting.[79]

The vision of Dr. Safar, clearly articulated in a few paragraphs, provides an insight into his brilliance. Not only does Dr. Safar recognize the need for standardization for patient care records, he also outlines:

- A national data standard for all EMS patient care reports
- The need to leverage computers to store and analyze EMS data
- The connection between EMS patient care records and public health
- The critical importance of communication and a direct handoff between EMS practitioners and the receiving physician
- The importance of structured quality assurance
- The need to legally preserve verbal orders between a base physician and the EMS Practitioner

Dr. Safar's vision for a standardized patient care report form for Emergency Medical Services came to fruition 21 years later with the establishment of the National EMS Information System. NEMSIS standardizes EMS data collection and reporting practices across the United States, and was developed collaboratively by EMS agencies, state EMS offices, and national EMS organizations such as the National Association of State EMS Officials (NASEMSO) and the National Highway Traffic Safety Administration (NHTSA). Since its inception, NEMSIS has undergone iterative development to evolve and adapt to changing EMS practices, technologies, and data needs.

As of 2022, the NEMSIS Public-Release Dataset (a subset of the National EMS database that is publicly available for researchers) contained 51,379,493 records from 13,946 EMS agencies representing 54 states and territories. The NEMSIS database provides a valuable resource for monitoring and improving EMS care, as well as for conducting research and informing policy decisions. Through standardizing EMS data collection and reporting practices, NEMSIS allows for consistent and reliable analysis of EMS systems nationwide. It also enables the tracking of performance measures and outcomes, which can be used to improve patient care and guide decision-making.

Dr. Safar's paper, as presented at the conference in 1969:

Ambulance and emergency department records

PETER SAFAR, M.D.

The forms used by police ambulance attendants in Pittsburgh were found to be inadequate for providing retrospective information about the patient's condition and treatment. Ambulance report forms should become uniform on a nationwide basis to permit evaluation of the public health aspects of emergency transportation. Unfortunately, national forms are not yet available. Therefore, three forms (Tables 1, 2, and 3, page 72) were designed for use, on a trial basis, by the mobile, ICU-type ambulance service which is based at the Pittsburgh Presbyterian-University Hospital. The attendant must fill out the short form (Table 1) for all calls by checking appropriate items. If a life-threatening condition exists, the long form (Table 2) is completed, and in cases of cardiac arrest the Cardiac Arrest form (Table 3) must be completed. After completing the long form, the attendant is debriefed by the supervising physician (ICU fellow) and the case is discussed at a weekly seminar for all attendants. After debriefing the attendant, the physician adds a short narrative report. The ambulance forms become part of the emergency room records and the patient's chart.

The forms should be changed as necessary for computerized bookkeeping and for prospective studies, such as evaluation of the quality of patient care. A record of vital signs proved useful for long trips, such as transfers of patients from rural to city hospitals.

Sound-recording events in the ambulance has been proposed. The practicality of continuous sound-recording in an ambulance is doubted because deciphering the tapes is difficult and time consuming. Such tapes yield less information than immediate debriefing. The dispatching center should record all verbal communication, including conversation in the center, over radio and telephone, and should note the time when these communications took place. Recording on video tape the treatment of patients in the ambulance and in the emergency room deserves consideration for the purpose of studying and supervising the procedures of patient care.

DR. SAFAR'S ORIGINAL PATIENT CARE REPORT DESIGN

Table 1

SHORT PATIENT CARE REPORT FORM
FOR AMBULANCE CREW

Complaint #________

Patient's Name____________________ Age____ Sex ____ Log #________

Ambulance dispatched to: ____________________ Date________

Ambulance attendants on run:

1. ________________ 3. ________________
2. ________________ 4. ________________

How was complaint received? ____________________

	TIME
Call received	___:___
Car Out	___:___
Arrive at scene	___:___
Leave scene	___:___
Arrive at hospital	___:___
Back in service	___:___

Before ambulance arrived, the patient received aid from:

- ☐ Nobody
- ☐ Public
- ☐ Lay bystander
- ☐ Employee
- ☐ Medically trained person
- ☐ Other________________

Aid consisted of: ________________

Upon observing the patient, the following were suspected or present:

☐ Airway problem		
☐ Respiratory distress		
☐ Chest pain	☐ Head injury	☐ Wound longer than 4 inches
☐ Shortness of breath	☐ Neck-back injury	☐ Deep tissue exposed
☐ Unconsciousness	☐ Chest injury	☐ Suspected fracture
☐ Heart Attack	☐ Abdominal injury	☐ Suspected internal hemorrhages
☐ Cardiac arrest	☐ Flowing bleeding	☐ Gunshot wounds
	☐ Spurting bleeding	☐ Stab wound

IF ANY OF THE ABOVE WERE PRESENT OR SUSPECTED, PLEASE USE LONG FORM.

When you arrived, how was the patient situated? (trapped in car, lying in bed, etc.)

What was the patient's condition (breathing, conscious, wounds, etc.)

What did you do for the patient?________________

Was the patient's condition on arrival at the hospital ☐ improved ☐ unchanged ☐ worsened ☐ don't know

Diagnosis at the hospital________________

Which hospital? ________________

Table 2

PATIENT CARE REPORT

Pt. Name ____________ LONG FORM ______ FHE Log # ______

A.A. Completing Form: AMBULANCE CREW

____

1. Were extrication methods needed?
   - ☐ YES ☐ NO ☐ DON'T KNOW

   A. Which type needed?
   - ☐ light (hand tools or hands alone)
   - ☐ medium (hand carried power tools)
   - ☐ heavy (power driven tools or power shovel)

   B. Was patient trapped?
   - ☐ in motor vehicle ☐ building wreckage
   - ☐ other______________

2. Status of Nervous System

   A. The patient was ☐ alert ☐ stuperous ☐ comatose ☐ don't know

   B. The pupils were:
   - ☐ small ☐ mid-dilated ☐ widely dilated ☐ don't know
   - ☐ equal ☐ right>left ☐ left>right ☐ don't know
   - ☐ reacting to light ☐ not reacting to light

   C. Did the patient move all extremities?
   - ☐ YES ☐ NO ☐ DON'T KNOW

   If not, which did he not move?

   - ☐ right arm ☐ left arm
   - ☐ right leg ☐ left leg

   D. Did the patient have sensation in all areas?
   - ☐ YES ☐ NO ☐ DON'T KNOW

   If not, where did he have no feeling?

   - ☐ right arm ☐ left arm
   - ☐ right leg ☐ left leg

Table 2—contd.

3. State of Respiratory System
   A. Was the airway obstructed when you arrived?
      ☐ YES ☐ NO ☐ DON'T KNOW
      If yes, which technique was used to open it?
      ☐ head tilt
      ☐ life saving grip
      ☐ oropharyngeal airway
      ☐ suctioning equipment
      ☐ wiping clean
      ☐ endotracheal tube
   B. Was oxygen given?
      ☐ YES ☐ NO ☐ DON'T KNOW
      If yes, which technique was used?
      ☐ plastic face mask
      ☐ elder valve
      ☐ cannula
      ☐ other
      ☐ Bag valve mask with
      ☐ oxygen delivery tube
      ☐ reservoir tube
   C. Was the patient given positive pressure ventilation?
      ☐ YES ☐ NO ☐ DON'T KNOW
      If yes, which technique was used?
      ☐ mouth to mouth
      ☐ mouth to S-tube
      ☐ bag valve mask
      ☐ other________
      Did the color improve?
      ☐ YES ☐ NO ☐ DON'T KNOW
      Did the chest rise with inflation?
      ☐ YES ☐ NO ☐ DON'T KNOW
4. State of Cardiovascular System
   A. Was the carotid pulse present?
      ☐ YES ☐ NO ☐ DON'T KNOW
   B. Was the radial pulse present?
      ☐ YES ☐ NO ☐ DON'T KNOW
      If yes, was the pulse rate
      ☐ >120 ☐ 80–120 ☐ <80
      Was the pulse regular?
      ☐ YES ☐ NO ☐ DON'T KNOW
   C. Color of skin and mucous membrane:
      ☐ normal
      ☐ flushed
      ☐ ashen (gray)
      ☐ pale
      ☐ cyanotic
      ☐ other ________

5. Were injuries present?
      ☐ YES ☐ NO ☐ DON'T KNOW
      If yes, complete the following:
   A. Areas injured:
      ☐ head
      ☐ face
      ☐ eye
      ☐ neck
      ☐ back
      ☐ chest
      ☐ pelvis
      ☐ upper extremity
      ☐ lower extremity
      ☐ general, multiple
      ☐ non-wound injury e.g. drowning, electrocution, etc.

TERRORISM AND EPCRS: THE INDIANAPOLIS-HAMILTON COUNTY PROJECT

In the wake of the 2001 terrorist attacks, the United States government acknowledged the necessity to enhance emergency response capabilities nationwide. Consequently, the Department of Homeland Security (DHS) was established in 2002 to orchestrate national security endeavors and allocate funding for homeland security initiatives. The Urban Areas Security Initiative (UASI), a program introduced by DHS, granted financial support to high-risk urban areas to improve their preparedness and response capacities. The Indianapolis-Hamilton County, Indiana, project was initiated in 2003. It aimed to expedite the adoption of electronic patient care records (ePCR) for emergency medical services in the greater Indianapolis area, create a mechanism for various independent EMS agencies to share data, and to perform near real-time syndromic surveillance of aggregate health data.

The ambitious Indianapolis-Hamilton County project sought to revolutionize ePCR utilization within EMS. Conceived a few months after the 2001 terrorist attacks, the project garnered funding from the Department of Homeland Security to establish a centralized ePCR system that would enhance patient care and facilitate large-scale EMS system research. Moreover, the project emphasized the potential role of EMS in national security.

Implementing this vision entailed transitioning over a thousand EMS practitioners from paper forms to computerized patient care reports, marking the first large-scale system transition of its kind in the EMS industry. This transition posed challenges, as EMS agencies were accustomed to paper reports and the technology to support the project's vision and scope was not yet sufficiently advanced. Rugged laptops were costly, cumbersome, and sluggish, while mobile packet data coverage was limited, and Wi-Fi was not widely available. Nevertheless, the project proved successful and illustrated the realm of possibilities.

The Indianapolis-Hamilton County project was the first multi-county, multi-system approach to adopt a centralized system for patient care reports, demonstrating its capacity to improve patient care and facilitate large-scale EMS system research. The project underscored the importance of collaboration and data-sharing among EMS practitioners, hospitals, public health departments, and law enforcement agencies.

One of the project's most notable achievements was the incorporation and development of syndromic surveillance capabilities within EMS. For the first time, EMS practitioners utilized near-real-time data for syndromic surveillance, allowing public health officials to promptly detect infectious disease outbreaks, which was crucial for addressing bioterrorism threats. The project paved the way for similar surveillance methods in other EMS systems and validated the significance of EMS data for national projects.

Furthermore, the Indianapolis-Hamilton County project shed light on EMS's emerging role in homeland security. Prior to the project, EMS was perceived as a provider of emergency medical care; however, the project revealed that EMS practitioners could play a critical role in detecting and responding to bioterrorism threats, thereby establishing EMS's unique position in national security.

The Indianapolis-Hamilton County project was a visionary endeavor that transformed ePCR usage in EMS. The project demonstrated that a centralized system for patient care reports could enhance patient care and enable large-scale EMS system research. Additionally, the project highlighted the value of collaboration and data-sharing among EMS practitioners, hospitals, public health departments, and law enforcement agencies. The project also set a precedent for other EMS agencies to transition to computerized ePCR and to use near-real-time data for syndromic surveillance. Ultimately, the project affirmed EMS's role in homeland security and showcased the critical role EMS practitioners could play in detecting and responding to bioterrorism threats.

Today, the use of near-real-time EMS data plays a crucial role in syndromic surveillance for public health and national security. While the ambitious vision of the Indianapolis-Hamilton County project in 2004 outpaced the technology available at the time, the theoretical framework has since been operationalized. The continuous evolution of technology has not only made the theory feasible but has also amplified its potential for real-world applications. This progression underscores the importance of forward-thinking initiatives in shaping the future trajectory of EMS, demonstrating how visionary ideas, when coupled with technological advancement, can revolutionize public health surveillance and security measures.

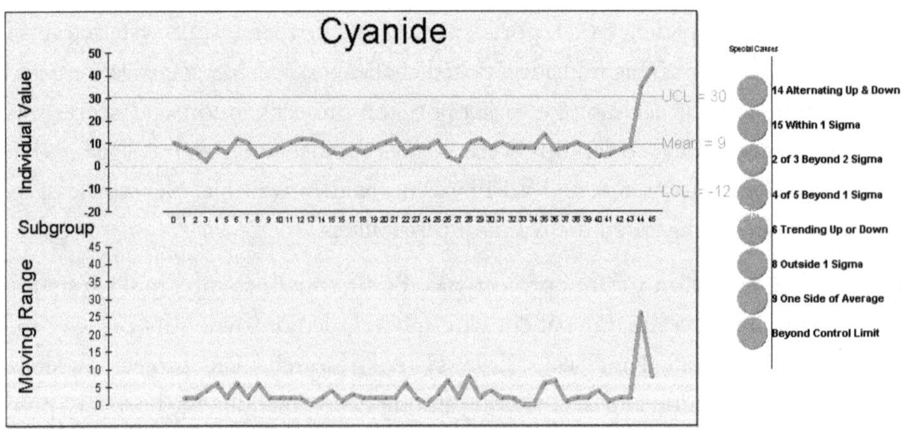

The first of its kind syndromic surveillance dashboard driven by near-real-time EMS data: Cyanide Monitoring Dashboard from the 2004 Pilot Project

Acknowledgements and Author's Disclaimer

The success of the Indianapolis-Hamilton County project is attributed to the hard work and dedication of its Project Steering Committee members. The committee comprised Steve Auch of the Indianapolis Fire Department, Tom Arkins of Wishard Hospital, Jeremy Pell of Warren Township Fire Department, Steve Davison of Fishers Fire Department, Tom Small of Carmel Fire Department, and Donnie Woodyard, Jr., of Riverview Hospital. (Participating in this group of visionaries and implementers was a tremendous honor for me.)

POWER OF EMS DATA IN PUBLIC HEALTH

In December, 2022, the Biden-Harris Administration demonstrated a significant public health application of NEMSIS data by launching a first-of-its-kind national data dashboard for non-fatal opioid overdoses. Developed in partnership between the White House Office of National Drug Control Policy (ONDCP) and the National Highway Traffic Safety Administration (NHTSA), the dashboard provides real-time, actionable information to first responders, clinicians, and policymakers to help save lives and direct resources to those most at risk.

This groundbreaking dashboard, which relies on the comprehensive data from the National EMS Information System (NEMSIS), helps to identify areas at the highest risk of overdoses and directs appropriate resources and support to address these issues before it's too late. The dashboard also enables service providers to connect people with life-saving treatment for substance use disorders.

The Nonfatal Opioid Overdose Dashboard represents a significant step in the Biden Administration's National Drug Control Strategy, which emphasizes the need to develop and strengthen the nation's data systems to reach people at risk of an overdose and expand access to treatment for substance use disorders and high-impact harm reduction interventions such as naloxone. By leveraging NEMSIS data, the dashboard provides unprecedented access to information for understanding and responding to the opioid overdose epidemic.

The dashboard allows for comparisons of jurisdiction and county-level data to national averages in four categories: population rate of nonfatal opioid overdose in a community, average number of naloxone administrations per patient, average EMS time in transit to reach an overdose patient, and the percentage of nonfatal opioid overdose patients who are not transported to a medical facility for further treatment. The dashboard is updated every Monday morning with a two-week lag and will continue to evolve to incorporate additional data and insights over time.

The launch of the Nonfatal Opioid Overdose Dashboard serves as a prime example of the valuable public health applications of NEMSIS data and highlights the importance of a standardized EMS data system in guiding evidence-based policies and interventions to save lives and address critical public health issues.

Dr. Peter Safar's visionary ideas in 1969 laid the groundwork for what would become the National EMS Information System (NEMSIS), paving the way for a new era of data-driven emergency medical services. His foresight to recognize the need for standardization, leveraging computers for data analysis, and the potential impact on public health demonstrated an extraordinary understanding of the future of EMS. Today, NEMSIS plays a crucial role in supporting research, informing policy decisions, and enhancing patient care, as exemplified by the recent launch of the Nonfatal Opioid Overdose Dashboard. Dr. Safar's groundbreaking vision has undoubtedly transformed the field of EMS, making it possible to respond more effectively to public health emergencies and improve the quality of care for millions of patients nationwide.

THE PIVOTAL ROLE OF NEMSIS DATA IN ADVANCING THE EMS SYSTEM

In the rapidly evolving healthcare sector, data-driven decision-making has become a cornerstone of efficient management and improved patient care. At the forefront of this movement in the EMS landscape is NEMSIS. By providing a wealth of standardized and comprehensive data, encompassing over 50 million annual EMS activations across the nation, NEMSIS has proven instrumental in shaping not just local EMS agencies but the broader national EMS system, state EMS offices, and related academic research.

The foremost benefit of NEMSIS lies in its facilitation of evidence-based policymaking. It offers a robust and standardized database that enables EMS agencies, policymakers, and researchers to derive actionable insights. This compilation of data—encompassing EMS responses, patient care, and health outcomes—allows strategic, evidence-based decision-making. Agencies can augment their performance, optimize resource distribution, and enhance patient care protocols using NEMSIS data. By identifying trends and patterns, they can predict demand, manage resources, and implement policies more effectively.

The ability to gauge performance against standardized benchmarks is another significant advantage conferred by NEMSIS. It empowers EMS agencies to evaluate their operations in relation to other agencies at local, state, and national scales. This comparative evaluation aids in pinpointing areas necessitating improvement, monitoring performance over time, and igniting quality enhancement initiatives. By having these metrics at their disposal, agencies can conduct a thorough and objective self-assessment, fostering a culture of continuous improvement.

NEMSIS also serves as a critical resource for research and program evaluation. Its rich data sets have enabled countless studies and evaluations, providing fresh insights, assessing the effectiveness of EMS interventions, and influencing EMS policies and practices. As such, it has become an invaluable tool for researchers and policymakers, enabling them to uncover EMS outcomes, identify trends, discern best practices, and utilize these findings in data-driven policymaking.

In terms of resource allocation, NEMSIS plays an indispensable role by offering data that reveals patterns and trends in EMS calls, response times, and patient profiles. EMS agencies, policymakers, and other key stakeholders leverage this data to identify high-demand areas for EMS agencies, optimize resource distribution, and enhance EMS system efficiency. As such, NEMSIS data has a direct impact on the quality of patient care, the efficiency of service provision, and the optimal utilization of scarce resources.

Public health monitoring is another arena in which NEMSIS data has been a game-changer. The granular view of EMS usage patterns, patient demographics, and health outcomes that NEMSIS provides has streamlined public health surveillance efforts. It has enabled the rapid identification of illness or injury trends, effective tracking of disease outbreaks, and robust support for comprehensive public health planning and responsive measures. This capacity not only strengthens the public health response but also aids in the proactive management of potential health crises.

The promotion of data system interoperability is another notable contribution of NEMSIS. By fostering standardized data elements, definitions, and reporting protocols, it has ensured seamless data sharing across different jurisdictions, states, and regions. This enhanced coordination, data exchange, and system integration have revolutionized information management within the EMS landscape.

Beyond these immediate applications, the national EMS data facilitated by NEMSIS has far-reaching implications for advancing research and enhancing patient care. Serving as the backbone of the National EMS Practice Analysis, it is also essential for effective scope of practice modeling and the formulation of evidence-based clinical guidelines. These functions demonstrate how NEMSIS not only improves immediate EMS operations but also significantly contributes to molding an efficient and impactful EMS system on a national scale.

The role of NEMSIS in the EMS landscape is as pivotal as it is diverse. From driving evidence-based policymaking to promoting interoperability, it has played a crucial part in streamlining operations, enhancing efficiency, and improving patient outcomes. Its significant contribution to research, both within individual EMS agencies and in the broader academic community, facilitates new insights, influences policies and practices, and drives continuous improvement.

Moreover, NEMSIS is pivotal in strategic resource allocation. The ability to identify patterns and trends, including high-demand areas for EMS agencies, means resources are directed where they are most needed, optimizing the overall EMS system's efficiency. As budgets in the healthcare sector continue to be stretched, having data to guide these important decisions is more crucial than ever.

Public health surveillance has also been considerably strengthened through the integration of NEMSIS data. With the ability to monitor trends in EMS utilization, patient demographics, and health outcomes, NEMSIS facilitates a rapid and effective response to public health emergencies. It allows health authorities to proactively track disease outbreaks and implement interventions, a function that has become particularly salient in the era of pandemic management.

The interoperability promoted by NEMSIS, through standardized data elements, definitions, and reporting protocols, is another testament to its significant impact on the EMS system. This functionality allows for more effective communication and data exchange among different jurisdictions, states, and regions, leading to more coordinated and integrated services. This seamless data sharing capability can accelerate the delivery of care, reduce duplication, and enhance the overall effectiveness of the EMS system.

Beyond its immediate applications, NEMSIS data is a foundational component of advancing research and patient care in the EMS field. Its use in the National EMS Practice Analysis is pivotal to understanding and advancing the profession, informing scope of practice, and developing evidence-based clinical guidelines. As such, NEMSIS not only enhances immediate EMS operations but also contributes substantially to shaping the future of an efficient, effective, and impactful EMS system on a national scale.

In a world that is increasingly driven by data, the significance of comprehensive, reliable, and accessible data cannot be emphasized enough. Within the realm of emergency medical services, the National Emergency Medical Services Information System (NEMSIS) assumes a crucial role in harnessing data to enhance systems, processes, and, ultimately, patient outcomes. As the full potential of NEMSIS continues to be unlocked, it will undeniably maintain its status as a significant catalyst for change, propelling continuous improvement and innovation in EMS delivery throughout the nation.

Author's Note:

In this era of digitization and data-centric decision making, it's important to note that the adoption of electronic Patient Care Reports should not overshadow the significance of detailed patient care narratives. EMS practitioners should understand and embrace the importance of maintaining a robust written narrative: it reduces liability by providing clear, comprehensive records of patient interactions; it optimizes reimbursement processes by accurately representing the services rendered; and most importantly, it facilitates continuity of care within the healthcare system by conveying valuable information for ongoing and future treatment plans. While embracing the benefits of structured data, we must also ensure that the art of narrative documentation remains a prominent component of our patient care strategies.

8

NATIONAL EMS INFLUENCERS

"Alone we can do so little, together we can do so much."
-Helen Keller

THE EVOLUTION OF THE NATIONAL EMERGENCY MEDICAL SERVICES system has largely been an organic process, leading to the establishment of a multifaceted array of national organizations and federal offices, each possessing distinctive roles, specializations, and stakeholders. Despite such diversity, a common thread unites these entities: the shared commitment to ensuring EMS practitioners render high-quality care to patients.

Over the years, through both formal and informal collaborations, numerous organizations have left an indelible mark on the EMS profession. Their combined efforts have significantly contributed to EMS progression, enhanced patient outcomes, and ensured that EMS practitioners are equipped with the requisite skills and knowledge to deliver quality care in emergency situations.

By fostering a cooperative environment, these groups have been able to streamline efforts and encourage the development of best practices and standardized procedures. Such sustained collaboration enhances the efficiency, effectiveness, and reliability of the EMS system, with far-reaching benefits for patients and the communities they serve. A brief overview of select national organizations is provided in this section.

List of Selected Organizations

AMERICAN AMBULANCE ASSOCIATION

The American Ambulance Association (AAA) was founded in 1979 and has a rich history of advocating for the interests of ambulance service providers and suppliers in the United States. The AAA was formed by a group of ambulance industry leaders who recognized the need for a unified voice to represent the unique challenges and needs of ambulance providers at the national level.

Since its inception, the AAA has been at the forefront of advocating for fair reimbursement policies for ambulance services. This includes advocating for adequate reimbursement rates from Medicare, Medicaid, and private insurers to ensure that ambulance providers can cover the costs of providing high-quality care to their patients. The AAA has also been instrumental in advocating for changes in reimbursement methodologies, such as the implementation of the Medicare ambulance fee schedule, which has helped standardize reimbursement rates across the country.

In addition to reimbursement advocacy, the AAA has been actively involved in promoting best practices in ambulance service delivery. The association has developed and promoted industry guidelines, standards, and educational resources on topics such as patient care, operations, safety, and quality improvement. The AAA has also been a strong advocate for the use of innovative models of care, such as community paramedicine and mobile integrated healthcare, which leverage the unique capabilities of ambulance providers to better meet the healthcare needs of their communities.

The AAA provides a wide range of resources and benefits to its members. This includes access to educational programs, industry research, networking opportunities, and tools for operational and financial management. The AAA also offers opportunities for engagement and collaboration among its members through committees, task forces, and special interest groups focused on various aspects of ambulance service delivery and management. These resources and benefits help members stay informed, enhance their operational capabilities, and improve the quality of care they provide to their communities.

Over the years, the AAA has achieved significant accomplishments in advancing the interests of the ambulance industry. For example, the AAA successfully advocated for changes in Medicare reimbursement policies, such as the extension of the temporary Medicare ambulance add-on payments, which have helped address reimbursement challenges faced by ambulance providers. The AAA has also been a vocal advocate for ambulance safety, working with federal agencies and industry partners to promote the adoption of safety standards and best practices. Furthermore, the AAA has played a key role in shaping federal regulations and policies related to ambulance services, including advocating for changes to the Medicare ambulance fee schedule and other regulatory issues that impact ambulance providers.

AMERICAN COLLEGE OF EMERGENCY PHYSICIANS

The American College of Emergency Physicians (ACEP) is a national medical specialty society that represents emergency medicine physicians in the United States. Founded in 1968, ACEP has become one of the leading organizations advocating for the specialty of emergency medicine, with a strong commitment to patient care and safety. ACEP members, including emergency physicians, residents, and medical students, provide high-quality emergency care to patients in need.

ACEP has a significant role in shaping and contributing to the national EMS system through its expertise in emergency medicine. One of its key roles is providing resources and guidelines for EMS practice, including evidence-based guidelines, protocols, and educational resources related to EMS care. These resources ensure that EMS practitioners are trained and equipped to provide high-quality care to patients in emergency situations.

Advocacy is also an important role of ACEP. The organization advocates for policies and regulations that support the practice of emergency medicine and EMS, including appropriate reimbursement for EMS agencies and state and federal policies that enhance the quality and safety of EMS care. ACEP also plays a role in EMS education and training, offering educational programs and resources for EMS practitioners, including continuing medical education (CME) opportunities, conferences, and online resources.

Furthermore, ACEP collaborates with other national organizations, such as the National Association of EMS Physicians (NAEMSP), the National Association of State EMS Officials (NASEMSO), and the National Highway Traffic Safety Administration Office of EMS (NHTSA EMS), to develop and implement best practices in EMS care. This collaboration helps to ensure a coordinated and cohesive approach to EMS care at the national level.

COMMISSION ON ACCREDITATION OF ALLIED HEALTH EDUCATION PROGRAMS

The Commission on Accreditation of Allied Health Education Programs (CAAHEP) and the Committee on Accreditation of Educational Programs for the Emergency Medical Services Professions (CoAEMSP) are the current reviewing entities responsible for accrediting paramedic programs. The accreditation process ensures that these programs meet or exceed national standards for quality and prepare students for the demands of the EMS profession.

In the early days of EMS education, the need for standardized accreditation of paramedic programs became apparent. The Council of Allied Health Education and Accreditation (CAHEA) and the Joint Review Committee for EMT-P recognized this need and began reviewing paramedic programs. These organizations later evolved into CAAHEP and CoAEMSP, respectively.

In 1980, the University of California, Los Angeles, (UCLA) and Eastern Kentucky University became the first institutions to have their paramedic programs reviewed under the new accreditation process. Other programs quickly followed suit, seeking validation through national accreditation.

Today, CAAHEP and CoAEMSP continue to work together to evaluate, reevaluate, and accredit paramedic programs across the United States. Their collaboration ensures that the programs maintain high standards of quality and remain aligned with the evolving needs of the EMS profession and the healthcare landscape. Accreditation by these organizations signifies professionalism, competency, and safety in EMS education, contributing to the overall integrity and effectiveness of the EMS system.

EMS FOR CHILDREN

The Emergency Medical Services for Children (EMSC) program was established in response to the need for specialized emergency care tailored to children, including infants, adolescents, and young adults up to 21 years of age.

The genesis of the EMSC program dates to the late 1970s, when the Hawaii Medical Association advocated for the development of EMS programs designed to reduce child morbidity and mortality. Further catalyzed by several significant incidents that underscored the inadequacies of emergency departments in treating children, Senators Daniel Inouye, Orrin Hatch, and Lowell Weicker initiated the creation of the EMSC program. Consequently, the *Emergency Medical Services for Children Act* (EMSC Act) was enacted by Congress in 1984, with reauthorizations in subsequent years.

The EMSC program, administered by the Health Resources and Services Administration's Maternal and Child Health Bureau, collaborates with various federal agencies, state and local partners, and national organizations. The program's primary objectives are:

- **Improving Pediatric Emergency Care:** The program aims to enhance EMS agencies, hospitals, and other emergency care providers' capacity to effectively manage pediatric emergencies. This is achieved through the promotion of pediatric-specific equipment, medications, protocols, and the training of EMS practitioners in safe and effective childcare during emergencies.

- **Enhancing EMS Systems for Children:** The EMSC program supports the development and improvement of EMS systems providing specialized care to children. It encourages the integration of pediatric care guidelines into EMS systems, improved communication among various stakeholders, and the consideration of children's unique needs in disaster and emergency preparedness planning.

- **Supporting Pediatric Research and Data Collection:** The program fosters research and data collection initiatives aimed at enriching the understanding of pediatric emergencies, their outcomes, and best practices. It accomplishes this by supporting research studies, data collection initiatives, and quality improvement efforts focusing on pediatric emergency care.

- **Providing Education and Training:** The EMSC program facilitates the enhancement of EMS practitioners, hospital staff, and other emergency care providers' knowledge and skills in managing pediatric emergencies. It does so by developing and disseminating pediatric-specific educational materials, offering training opportunities, and promoting ongoing professional development in pediatric emergency care.

- **Collaborating and Coordinating:** The program promotes partnerships and cooperation among federal agencies, state and local partners, and national organizations to advance pediatric emergency care.

The initial funding from the EMSC program supported four state demonstration projects, pioneering the development of strategies to address crucial pediatric emergency care issues. Over time, additional states received funding to devise other strategies and implement programs developed by earlier states. By the 1990s, all 50 states and the territories had received funding to improve and integrate EMSC into their existing EMS systems.

As the focus of EMS innovation shifted towards the prehospital care of children in many regions, there arose a need to make the innovative approaches and ideas more accessible. Thus, in 1991, two national resource centers were funded to provide technical assistance to states and manage the dissemination of EMSC information and products. By 1995, the EMSC National Resource Center in Washington, DC, emerged as the single national center. To address the critical need for research and lack of qualified individuals to conduct it, the National EMSC Data Analysis Resource Center (NEDARC) was established at the University of Utah School of Medicine. NEDARC's primary objective was to assist states in adopting common EMS data definitions and enhancing data collection and analysis nationwide.

The effectiveness of the EMSC program was validated by a comprehensive study conducted by the Institute of Medicine in the 1990s. This study uncovered significant deficiencies in pediatric emergency care and presented 22 recommendations for nationwide improvement. These insights convinced Congress of the necessity for additional resources, leading to an increase in funding for the EMSC program. This pivotal decision has strengthened the EMSC program's capacity to pursue its core objectives, thereby continuing its essential work of protecting and preserving the lives of children across the nation.

Federal Interagency Committee on Emergency Medical Services

The Federal Interagency Committee on Emergency Medical Services (FICEMS), established by congress in 2005,[80] fosters coordination, communication, and collaboration among various federal agencies involved in emergency medical services in the United States.[81] The committee, composed of representatives from agencies such as the Department of Transportation, Department of Homeland Security, Department of Health and Human Services, and Department of Defense, actively enhances the quality of care and services provided by EMS systems nationwide.

FICEMS serves as a dynamic forum for federal agencies to exchange information, share best practices, and coordinate efforts related to EMS. It actively promotes and supports the development and implementation of evidence-based standards, guidelines, and practices for EMS systems and providers. Additionally, FICEMS actively collaborates with state, local, and tribal partners, as well as EMS organizations, to ensure a well-coordinated and effective approach to EMS at all levels.

One of FICEMS' primary roles entails providing proactive leadership in advancing EMS policy and practice at the federal level. This proactive engagement includes spearheading initiatives related to EMS data collection, research, and evaluation, as well as workforce development and education. The committee actively offers guidance and support for emergency preparedness and response, actively engaging in planning, training, and coordination during various emergencies that may necessitate EMS involvement.

Moreover, FICEMS actively fosters partnerships and collaboration among federal agencies, state and local governments, and EMS organizations. It promotes information sharing, collaboration, and coordination among federal agencies while effectively aligning their efforts to achieve common goals and objectives related to EMS.

Throughout its existence, FICEMS has made significant and active contributions to the national EMS system through its collaborative efforts and proactive leadership. Notable examples include its active involvement in developing the National EMS Education Standards, which provide a fundamental basis for EMS education and training nationwide. FICEMS has also played an instrumental role in actively collecting EMS workforce data, conducting research and evaluation endeavors, facilitating emergency preparedness and response efforts, promoting collaboration and partnerships, as well as developing the comprehensive National EMS Scope of Practice Model. Through its proactive and multifaceted approach, FICEMS actively strives to enhance the quality of care and services delivered by EMS systems, actively benefiting patients and communities across the United States.

HEALTH RESOURCES AND SERVICES ADMINISTRATION

The Health Resources and Services Administration (HRSA) is a federal agency within the U.S. Department of Health and Human Services (HHS). HRSA's involvement in EMS is traced back to its establishment in 1982 through a departmental reorganization within HHS,[82] with the mission to improve health care access for underserved and vulnerable populations. In 1990, the *Trauma Care Systems Planning and Development Act*[83] established the Division of Trauma and Emergency Medical Systems within HRSA. Even though the division had limited funding and a brief existence, it signified a crucial revival of EMS under the authority of HHS.

HRSA's role in EMS includes:

- **Grant Funding**: HRSA provides funding through various grant programs to support the development, enhancement, and sustainability of EMS systems across the country. This includes funding for EMS workforce training and education, equipment and technology, community paramedicine programs, rural EMS initiatives, and other innovative projects aimed at improving EMS care and outcomes.

- **Technical Assistance and Guidance**: HRSA provides technical assistance, guidance, and resources to states, local governments, and other stakeholders to promote best practices in EMS. This includes developing and disseminating EMS-related guidelines, toolkits, and educational materials, as well as providing training and technical support to EMS agencies and personnel.

- **Data Collection and Research**: HRSA collects and analyzes data related to EMS systems, workforce, and patient outcomes to inform policy decisions, identify areas for improvement, and support evidence-based approaches in EMS. HRSA also conducts research and evaluation activities to advance the knowledge and understanding of EMS issues and best practices.

- **Collaboration and Coordination**: HRSA collaborates with other federal agencies, national EMS organizations, and state and local partners to promote coordination and integration of EMS agencies with other healthcare systems and public health initiatives. This includes working with agencies such as the National Highway Traffic Safety Administration (NHTSA) Office of EMS, Centers for Medicare & Medicaid Services (CMS), and the Federal Emergency Management Agency (FEMA) to align efforts and promote consistency in EMS policies and practices.

- **Workforce Development**: HRSA supports the development and training of the EMS workforce, including EMS practitioners, educators, and other EMS personnel. This includes funding initiatives to increase the number of qualified EMS professionals, enhance their skills and knowledge through continuing education and training programs, and promote workforce diversity and inclusivity.

International Association of Fire Chiefs

Founded in 1873, the International Association of Fire Chiefs (IAFC) is a professional association for fire chiefs and high-ranking fire service leaders. Throughout its history, the IAFC has been committed to the continuous improvement of fire services, including EMS. As EMS became an integral component of fire services, the IAFC expanded its focus to address the unique challenges and opportunities associated with EMS leadership.

The IAFC has long been a strong advocate for fire-based EMS systems, emphasizing their efficiency and effectiveness in delivering timely and high-quality pre-hospital care. The IAFC was part of the original Task Force charged with creating a national EMS certification organization in 1970. Since then, the IAFC has reiterated its support for the role of fire-based EMS through various resolutions (1975, 1980, and 1991). The organization has been instrumental in promoting the integration of EMS into the larger public safety framework, emphasizing the strategic positioning of the fire service as the first-line medical responder in nearly every community in the United States. In 2013, the IAFC was part of the committee that wrote the EMS Compact model legislation.

The IAFC's advocacy for fire-based EMS systems has been complemented by its contributions to EMS leadership in the following ways:

- **Development of educational programs and resources**: The IAFC has created and promoted numerous EMS-focused educational programs and resources aimed at enhancing the knowledge, skills, and abilities of EMS leaders.
- **Policy advocacy**: The IAFC has played a pivotal role in shaping national EMS policy through active engagement with legislators and regulatory agencies, ensuring that EMS remains a priority in public safety policymaking and funding decisions.
- **Collaboration and networking**: The IAFC facilitates collaboration and networking among EMS leaders across the country, fostering connections that have contributed to the sharing of knowledge, expertise, and best practices.
- **Research and innovation**: The IAFC supports research initiatives that advance EMS leadership, operations, and patient care, encouraging the dissemination of research findings to contribute to the ongoing evolution and improvement of EMS agencies.

The IAFC continues to play a vital role in EMS leadership by providing a platform for EMS leaders to collaborate, learn, and grow. As an advocate for fire-based EMS systems, the IAFC remains at the forefront of addressing emerging issues and fostering innovation in EMS. Through its various programs, initiatives, and advocacy efforts, the IAFC equips EMS leaders with the knowledge and tools necessary to excel in their roles and contribute to the ongoing development of the EMS field.

The International Association of Fire Chiefs is instrumental in shaping the landscape of EMS in the United States through its advocacy for fire-based EMS systems and its contributions to EMS leadership. By providing education, advocacy, and networking opportunities, the IAFC has helped to ensure that EMS remains a critical component of public safety and that EMS leaders are well-equipped to meet the challenges and opportunities of the evolving field.

INTERNATIONAL ASSOCIATION OF FIRE FIGHTERS

The International Association of Fire Fighters (IAFF) actively contributes to the development of Emergency Medical Services in the United States. Established in 1918, the IAFF, as the country's largest professional organization of fire fighters, recognizes the importance of EMS leadership within the fire service, playing a crucial role in shaping the evolution of EMS agencies.

The IAFF supports fire-based EMS systems, considering them the most efficient and effective method for delivering pre-hospital care. The organization promotes the role of fire-based EMS in public safety and actively participates in the development of national EMS policy. Moreover, the IAFF significantly contributes to EMS leadership through various initiatives:

- **Development of educational programs and resources**: The IAFF designs numerous EMS-focused educational programs and resources to enhance the knowledge, skills, and abilities of EMS leaders.
- **Policy advocacy**: The IAFF plays a crucial role in shaping national EMS policy, collaborating closely with legislators and regulatory agencies to ensure that EMS remains a priority in public safety policymaking and funding decisions.
- **Collaboration and networking**: The IAFF fosters collaboration and networking among EMS leaders nationwide, facilitating connections that contribute to the sharing of knowledge, expertise, and best practices.
- **Research and innovation**: The IAFF supports research initiatives advancing EMS leadership, operations, and patient care, promoting the dissemination of research findings to further the ongoing evolution and improvement of EMS agencies.
- **Health & Safety**: The IAFF supports the health & safety of fire and EMS personnel through initiatives such as peer support, behavioral health management, fitness, and nutrition and diet support.

Today, the IAFF Fire and EMS Operations/GIS Department provides comprehensive information on fire departments and fire-based EMS to assist in improving the working conditions of IAFF members. The Department promotes appropriate staffing and deployment for fire suppression and the effectiveness of fire-based emergency medical services systems by providing local affiliates with the tools necessary to develop, enhance, and protect their working conditions.

INTERNATIONAL BOARD OF SPECIALTY CERTIFICATIONS

The International Board of Specialty Certifications (IBSC), previously known as the Board for Critical Care Transport Paramedic Certification, is a professional organization that was established in 1997 and is dedicated to promoting and advancing specialty certifications in the field of emergency services. The IBSC provides certifications for emergency medical services professionals who seek to specialize and demonstrate their expertise in specific areas of practice.

The history of IBSC can be traced back to the recognition of the need for standardized, rigorous certifications that validate the knowledge and skills of EMS professionals in specialized fields. The organization was formed to develop and administer certification programs that assess the competency of EMS practitioners in various specialties, including flight paramedicine, tactical paramedicine, community paramedicine, and critical care paramedicine, among others. Since its inception, IBSC has become a globally recognized leader in specialty certifications for EMS professionals.

The role of IBSC is to establish and maintain standards for specialty certifications in EMS. The organization develops certification examinations that assess the knowledge, skills, and abilities of EMS practitioners in specific specialty areas. These examinations are based on comprehensive job analyses, which involve identifying the critical tasks and responsibilities of EMS professionals in each specialty field. IBSC also collaborates with subject matter experts, professional organizations, and stakeholders in the EMS community to ensure that its certification programs are relevant, valid, and reliable.

IBSC's certifications are designed to validate the expertise and competency of EMS professionals in their respective specialty fields. Achieving an IBSC certification demonstrates a high level of knowledge, skills, and commitment to the specialty practice. IBSC certifications are recognized nationally and internationally, and they serve as a benchmark for employers, patients, and peers to identify EMS professionals who have met rigorous standards of practice in their specialty field.

One of the significant accomplishments of IBSC is the development and maintenance of a robust portfolio of specialty certifications. The organization has developed certifications for various specialties in EMS, including Critical Care Paramedic (CCP-C), Tactical Paramedic (TP-C), Flight Paramedic (FP-C), Community Paramedic (CP-C), and Wilderness Paramedic (WP-C). These certifications have become widely recognized and respected in the EMS community and have helped elevate the standards of care in specialized areas of EMS practice.

IBSC has also played a significant role in promoting professional development and continuing education among EMS professionals. The organization provides resources, study materials, and practice exams to help candidates prepare for their certification examinations. IBSC also collaborates with other organizations and stakeholders in the EMS community to promote education, research, and innovation in specialty fields. Additionally, IBSC offers recertification programs that encourage EMS professionals to engage in ongoing learning and professional growth, ensuring that certified practitioners stay current with the latest developments in their specialty areas.

INTERSTATE COMMISSION FOR EMS PERSONNEL PRACTICE

The Interstate Commission for EMS Personnel Practice heralds an innovative era in national Emergency Medical Services leadership. Legislatively constituted and composed of state-appointed representatives from each EMS Compact member, the Commission holds authority over the governance of the Emergency Medical Services Compact. Its duties are diverse, extending from overseeing the Compact's implementation to regulating the cross-border practice of EMS personnel, while simultaneously promoting communication and collaboration among the member states.

Notably, the Commission functions as an official governmental body and, in essence, symbolizes a "super-state". This is a distinctive, unified voice of the 24 states (as of this writing) that have passed the Recognition of EMS Personnel Licensure Interstate Compact (REPLICA) legislation. The EMS Compact's main objective is to harmonize standards and practices pertaining to EMS personnel licensure while also overseeing the cross-state practice of EMS practitioners.

The Commission's distinguishing feature is not solely its mandate but extends to its reach and influence. As of the time of this publication, it represents over half a million EMS practitioners across the member states. These professionals now enjoy the privilege of practicing in multiple states, an important step in boosting professional mobility and ensuring consistent patient care across state boundaries.

In an era marked by growing challenges for EMS systems, the unified voice of the Commission stands as a collective reaffirmation of standardization in the profession, advocating powerfully for both the practitioners and the communities they serve. It bears testament to the potential of cooperative interstate governance, helping to shape the national EMS system's future by standardizing processes, boosting practitioner mobility, and guaranteeing high-quality emergency medical care for everyone.

For aspiring EMS managers and leaders, the Interstate Commission for EMS Personnel Practice shines as a beacon of unity and progress. Its work provides valuable insight into collective action's potential, and the important role innovative cross-jurisdictional solutions can play in shaping and managing EMS systems on a national level.

NATIONAL ASSOCIATION OF EMS EDUCATORS

The National Association of EMS Educators (NAEMSE) is a professional organization that was established in 1993 and serves as a leading advocate for EMS educators and the advancement of EMS education. NAEMSE is dedicated to promoting excellence in EMS education through professional development, collaboration, and advocacy.

NAEMSE's history is traced back to the recognition of the importance of high-quality EMS education in providing competent and skilled EMS practitioners. The organization was formed to provide a platform for EMS educators to collaborate, share best practices, and enhance the quality of EMS education. Since its inception, NAEMSE has grown into a prominent organization that represents the interests of EMS educators and plays a vital role in advancing EMS education.

One of the primary roles of NAEMSE is to provide professional development opportunities for EMS educators. The organization offers a variety of educational programs, workshops, and resources that focus on topics such as curriculum development, instructional design, assessment, and teaching methodologies. These educational opportunities help EMS educators enhance their knowledge and skills in delivering effective and evidence-based EMS education to their students.

NAEMSE also plays a crucial role in fostering collaboration and networking among EMS educators. The organization provides a platform for educators to connect, share ideas, and collaborate on initiatives that advance EMS education. NAEMSE hosts conferences, workshops, and online forums that facilitate networking and knowledge exchange among EMS educators from across the country. This collaborative approach helps promote consistency, standardization, and innovation in EMS education.

Another important role of NAEMSE is advocating for policies and standards that support EMS educators and the overall advancement of EMS education. The organization engages in legislative and regulatory advocacy efforts at the national and state levels, working to shape policies that promote high-quality EMS education, appropriate certification and licensure requirements, and favorable working conditions for EMS educators. NAEMSE also collaborates with other EMS organizations and stakeholders to advocate for issues that impact EMS education, such as accreditation, certification, and funding.

NAEMSE has achieved significant accomplishments in its mission to promote excellence in EMS education. The organization has been involved in the development of national EMS education standards, such as the National EMS Education Standards and the National EMS Scope of Practice Model, which serve as guidelines for EMS education programs across the country. NAEMSE has also been actively involved in curriculum development, instructional design, and assessment strategies to improve the quality of EMS education. Additionally, NAEMSE has been instrumental in advocating for EMS educators to have a strong voice in shaping EMS education policies and standards at the national and state levels.

National Association of EMS Physicians

The National Association of EMS Physicians (NAEMSP) is a professional organization that was founded in 1984 and serves as a leading advocate for the field of emergency medical services and the physicians who provide medical oversight and leadership in the EMS system. NAEMSP is dedicated to advancing EMS and improving the quality of prehospital care through education, research, and advocacy.

The organization was formed to provide a platform for EMS physicians to collaborate, share knowledge, and promote best practices in the field. Over the years, NAEMSP has grown into a prominent organization that represents the interests of EMS physicians and plays a vital role in advancing the field of EMS.

One of the primary roles of NAEMSP is to provide education and professional development opportunities for EMS physicians. The organization offers a variety of educational programs, conferences, and resources that focus on topics such as clinical practice guidelines, medical oversight, disaster preparedness, and leadership in EMS. These educational opportunities help EMS physicians stay updated with the latest evidence-based practices and enhance their knowledge and skills in providing high-quality care in the prehospital setting.

NAEMSP also plays a crucial role in promoting research and innovation in EMS. The organization supports and encourages research activities that contribute to the advancement of EMS knowledge and practice. NAEMSP's Research Committee provides guidance, resources, and support for EMS research initiatives, and the organization promotes the dissemination of research findings through its publications and conferences. This emphasis on research helps drive evidence-based decision making and fosters innovation in EMS care.

Another important role of NAEMSP is advocating for policies and regulations that support EMS physicians and the overall advancement of EMS. The organization engages in legislative and regulatory advocacy efforts at the national and state levels, working to shape policies that promote quality care, appropriate reimbursement for EMS agencies, and favorable working conditions for EMS physicians. NAEMSP also collaborates with other EMS organizations to advocate for issues that impact the entire EMS community, such as EMS workforce development, EMS system integration, and patient safety.

NAEMSP has achieved significant accomplishments in its mission to advance EMS and support EMS physicians. The organization has played a critical role in the development of clinical practice guidelines for EMS, providing evidence-based recommendations for prehospital care. NAEMSP has also been actively involved in disaster preparedness and response efforts, contributing to national guidelines, and coordinating resources for EMS physicians during disasters and emergencies. Additionally, NAEMSP has been instrumental in advocating for the inclusion of EMS physicians in federal initiatives, such as the Federal Interagency Committee on EMS (FICEMS), which helps shape national EMS policy.

NATIONAL ASSOCIATION OF EMERGENCY MEDICAL TECHNICIANS

The National Association of Emergency Medical Technicians (NAEMT) was founded in 1975 as a non-profit professional organization dedicated to representing and advocating for emergency medical services practitioners. At the time, the field of EMS was still in its early stages, and there was a lack of national coordination and representation for EMS practitioners.

The idea for the formation of the NAEMT originated from a group of EMS professionals who recognized the need for a separate national organization to represent the interests of EMS practitioners. One of the key figures in the formation of the organization was Rocco Morando, who was then the Executive Director of the National Registry of Emergency Medical Technicians(NREMT). Morando recognized the need for a professional organization that could advocate for the interests of EMS practitioners, that was distinctly separate from the National EMS Certification organization, and provide them with advocacy, educational, and professional development opportunities.

With the support of the NREMT and other EMS organizations, the NAEMT was established to provide a national voice for EMS practitioners. The organization quickly gained traction and membership, with thousands of EMS practitioners joining in its early years.

One of the primary objectives of the NAEMT was to promote EMS as a recognized profession. At the time of its formation, EMS was still considered a relatively new field, and there was little recognition or support for EMS practitioners. The NAEMT helped advance the recognition of EMS practitioners as healthcare professionals and promote the advancement of EMS practice. The organization has worked with federal and state agencies, EMS stakeholders, and other organizations to shape EMS policy and legislation, promote EMS research, and advocate for the advancement of EMS practice. It has also provided educational resources, programs, and certifications to support the ongoing professional development of EMS practitioners.

Today, the NAEMT is a leading national organization representing the professional interests of EMS practitioners. With over 75,000 members, the organization continues to advocate for the advancement of EMS practice, promote the safety and well-being of EMS practitioners, and provide educational resources and opportunities to support the ongoing professional development of EMS practitioners.

NATIONAL ASSOCIATION OF STATE EMS OFFICIALS

The National Association of State EMS Officials (NASEMSO) is a key organization that facilitates the exchange of information, encourages the application of best practices, and promotes policies that bolster the quality of Emergency Medical Services systems throughout the United States. The primary function of NASEMSO lies in coordinating state officials responsible for EMS oversight, offering an inclusive platform for these officials to engage in discussions, share information, and develop policies that improve national EMS systems. Tracing the origins of NASEMSO, the organization began as the Emergency Medical Services Administrators Association (EMSAA) in the late 1970s. Initially, it consisted of about 12 state EMS directors and another dozen or so city and county EMS directors. In 1980, the association redirected its focus towards state EMS administrators and renamed itself as the National Association of State Emergency Medical Services Directors (NASEMSD). Over subsequent decades, NASEMSD gradually expanded its membership to include other categories of state EMS office staff (including the National Council of State EMS Training Coordinators) and evolved into the present-day NASEMSO.

Throughout its existence, NASEMSO has significantly shaped the evolution and improvement of EMS systems across the country. The association has become an invaluable resource for states, facilitating the sharing of information and best practices, aiding collaboration in policy development, and championing EMS-related legislation and regulations.

A core function of NASEMSO is to foster communication and coordination among state EMS officials. Through a mix of regular meetings, conferences, and online forums, NASEMSO creates opportunities for EMS officials to discuss emerging issues, share successful strategies, and work together on initiatives to boost the performance of EMS systems. Additionally, NASEMSO acts as an intermediary between state EMS agencies and federal agencies like the National Highway Traffic Safety Administration (NHTSA) and others, advocating for policies and funding that underpin state-level EMS.

NASEMSO's historical timeline is marked by several significant achievements. One such milestone is the development and promotion of the *National EMS Scope of Practice Model*, which assists states in establishing consistent standards for EMS personnel and their scope of practice countrywide. NASEMSO has also contributed to the development of national patient care reporting standards, leading to an improvement in the quality of data gathered and reported by EMS agencies and promoting evidence-based decision making and patient care. Further, NASEMSO has been a potent advocate for legislative and regulatory changes that bolster EMS at both state and national levels. The organization has successfully championed for increased funding for EMS programs, supported legislation to advance EMS workforce development, and promoted policies that improve EMS system performance, such as the integration of telemedicine in EMS and disaster preparedness.

In recent years, NASEMSO has taken an active role in addressing emergent challenges in the EMS sphere, including the opioid epidemic, mental health and wellness of EMS personnel, and the integration of EMS into the wider healthcare system. As a leading voice in the field, NASEMSO continues to advocate for resources and support to tackle these critical issues and enhance the overall well-being of EMS practitioners.

NATIONAL EMS ADVISORY COUNCIL

The National Emergency Medical Services Advisory Council[84] (NEMSAC) is a federally established advisory committee that operates under the authority of Section 31108 of the *Moving Ahead for Progress in the 21st Century Act* of 2012. Its primary purpose is to provide recommendations, advice, and consultation to the U.S. Department of Transportation's National Highway Traffic Safety Administration (NHTSA) and the Federal Interagency Committee on Emergency Medical Services (FICEMS) on matters pertaining to Emergency Medical Services. NEMSAC acts as a liaison between the EMS community and federal agencies, ensuring effective communication, collaboration, and coordination in the development of national EMS policies and initiatives.

The authority of NEMSAC is derived from legislation, and it functions in accordance with the provisions of the *Federal Advisory Committee Act* (FACA), as amended. As a nationally recognized council of EMS representatives, NEMSAC serves as a forum for the exchange of information and perspectives from diverse stakeholders within the EMS community. This allows for the development, consideration, and communication of valuable insights and expertise in the field of EMS from an independent and knowledgeable standpoint.

NEMSAC's objectives and scope of activities encompass two main areas. Firstly, it provides advice and consultation to the Federal Interagency Committee on Emergency Medical Services (FICEMS) on EMS-related matters. FICEMS is a committee composed of representatives from various federal agencies involved in emergency medical services. By engaging with FICEMS, NEMSAC ensures that EMS issues are properly addressed and that the collective knowledge and experience of the EMS community are considered in federal decision-making processes.

Secondly, NEMSAC offers advice and consultation to the Secretary of Transportation on EMS issues that impact the Department of Transportation (DOT), specifically the National Highway Traffic Safety Administration's (NHTSA) Office of Emergency Medical Services (OEMS). As the federal agency responsible for promoting safe and efficient transportation systems, the DOT plays a crucial role in shaping EMS policies and regulations. NEMSAC's input and recommendations to the Secretary of Transportation ensure that EMS considerations are integrated into DOT initiatives, promoting the effective coordination and integration of EMS agencies within the broader transportation framework.

To fulfill its duties, NEMSAC is authorized to consider information and topics related to EMS issues presented by NHTSA OEMS. Based on this information, the council formulates recommendations and advice to be transmitted to the Secretary of Transportation and/or FICEMS through a designated federal officer (DFO). These recommendations and advice align with the guiding principles of EMS Agenda 2050, which include adaptability and innovation, equitable patient care, integration and technology, preparedness and education, professional safety, and sustainability and efficiency. By adhering to these principles, NEMSAC strives to ensure that its recommendations reflect the evolving needs and priorities of the EMS field.

Furthermore, NEMSAC is responsive to requests for consultation and advice from the Secretary of Transportation and/or FICEMS, demonstrating its commitment to addressing emerging issues and providing timely guidance on matters of national importance. The council prepares an annual report detailing its actions and recommendations, which is submitted to the Secretary of Transportation. Copies of the report are also shared with the Secretary of Health and Human Services, the Secretary of Homeland Security, and FICEMS, promoting transparency and accountability in the advisory process.

NEMSAC operates under the oversight of a designated federal officer (DFO), who facilitates its operations and acts as a point of contact between the council and the Secretary of Transportation. The DFO ensures effective communication and collaboration, supporting NEMSAC in fulfilling its responsibilities. By serving as a liaison between the EMS community and federal agencies, NEMSAC ensures that the perspectives, experiences, and expertise of EMS stakeholders are effectively communicated and incorporated into the development of national EMS policies and initiatives. The council's diverse composition and collaborative approach foster comprehensive discussions and enable a unified and strategic approach to addressing critical EMS issues.

NATIONAL EMS MANAGEMENT ASSOCIATION

The National EMS Management Association (NEMSMA) is a professional organization that represents EMS managers and leaders in the United States. NEMSMA is dedicated to promoting excellence in EMS leadership and management through networking, education, advocacy, and collaboration.

NEMSMA was founded in the late 1990s as an association of EMS quality professionals and has since expanded its mission to become a recognized authority on EMS leadership and management. Its members include EMS executives, managers, supervisors, and aspiring leaders who are involved in the administration, management, and leadership of paramedic services. NEMSMA uses the terms "paramedic" and "paramedic services" as it is applied in the broader international context to refer to all of EMS, and its related services.

The role of NEMSMA is to provide resources, support, and education to paramedic leaders, helping them enhance their leadership skills, stay updated on best practices, and navigate the ever-evolving landscape of administration and management. NEMSMA also serves as a platform for networking and collaboration among paramedic leaders, facilitating the exchange of ideas, experiences, and expertise.

Since 2016, NEMSMA has offered a voluntary professional certification program through its subsidiary, the American College of Paramedic Executives (ACPE) which offers a multi-step process to validate the skills of paramedic leaders at the supervisor, manager and executive level. NEMSMA strongly supports professionalization of the industry through formal education and each level of certification requires a college degree or equivalent experience. The ACPE credential recognizes EMS leadership education from a variety of sources and is not tied to a specific educational program. NEMSMA has also adapted the concepts of the law enforcement Field Training and Evaluation Program (FTEP) for use as an onboarding tool for EMS employers which is currently a popular educational offering. NEMSMA partners with the Pinnacle EMS Conference as their annual educational and networking event.

NEMSMA advocates for the development of paramedicine as a distinct profession and recognizes leadership as an important specialization within the profession. To support that development, NEMSMA launched the online *International Journal of Paramedicine* (IJOP) in 2023. The organization promotes the importance of effective leadership and management in driving high-quality EMS service delivery, advocating for policies and regulations that support the professional development. NEMSMA also collaborates with other EMS organizations and stakeholders to advance the interests of EMS organizations and ensure that the challenges of EMS leaders are addressed at the national level.

NHTSA Office of EMS

The National Highway Traffic Safety Administration (NHTSA) Office of EMS (OEMS) traces its roots back to the 1966 *Highway Safety Act.*[85] This act paved the way for a federal agency dedicated to enhancing highway safety across the United States and set the stage for the NHTSA's eventual role in leading EMS systems. Although individual states decided the specific structure and implementation of state highway safety programs, the Department of Transportation's (DOT) National Highway Safety Bureau, which later became the NHTSA, was granted the authority to oversee and regulate these efforts.

From the start, the Department of Transportation began to shape and progress EMS within the United States. Initially, the focus centered on building EMS systems adept at responding to motor vehicle accidents, delivering timely and appropriate care. To achieve this, the DOT spearheaded initiatives to establish national standards and education curriculums for EMS personnel, advocating for a systems approach at the state level.

As the EMS landscape evolved, so did the NHTSA's OEMS. It actively engaged in numerous initiatives aimed at enhancing EMS standards, guidelines, and practices. NHTSA has continuously offered an unwavering commitment to advancing the EMS profession, creating, and publishing pivotal documents that serve as the field's foundation. These include the original *National Standard Curriculum* in the 1970s, the *EMS Agenda for the Future*, the *EMS Education Agenda for the Future: A Systems Approach*, the *National EMS Scope of Practice Model*,[86] which provides guidance on the knowledge and skills required for different levels of EMS practitioners, and the *National EMS Education Standards*,[87] which detail the curriculum for EMS training programs.

Furthermore, the OEMS took a central role in funding and promoting EMS data collection and research. It embarked on studies and analyses on a wide array of EMS aspects, ranging from injury prevention, trauma care, and cardiac care to system performance. Such research informs policy decisions, program development, and resource allocation to enhance support for EMS systems and providers.

In addition to policy development and research, the OEMS has significantly contributed to EMS workforce development. It provided funding and resources for EMS workforce initiatives, such as recruitment and retention programs, EMS education scholarships, and professional development opportunities for EMS personnel.

The OEMS has also worked collaboratively with other federal agencies, state and local governments, and EMS organizations to establish national standards and guidelines for EMS systems and services. Furthermore, it made a significant impact on emergency preparedness and response, offering guidance and resources for EMS agencies during disasters and public health emergencies.

Since the 1966 *Highway Safety Act*, the Department of Transportation has invested hundreds of millions of dollars in the development of EMS systems, affirming its role as a consistent federal advocate for EMS.

NATIONAL REGISTRY OF EMERGENCY MEDICAL TECHNICIANS

The National Registry of Emergency Medical Technicians (NREMT) is an independent, non-profit organization dedicated to validating the proficiency of Emergency Medical Services (EMS) practitioners. On January 21, 1970, the NREMT was conceptualized by a Task Force comprising the National Academy of Sciences, the National Research Council, and the American Medical Association, in partnership with President Lyndon Johnson's Committee on Highway Traffic Safety. The objective was to consider the creation of a single national certification body for EMS.

By June 1970, the National Registry was officially established, fulfilling the mandate of President Johnson's committee. Acknowledging the importance of a unified national EMS standard, the American Medical Association granted the new entity their Universal Medical Identification Symbol, today known as the Star of Life, as its logo. This symbol also serves as the official designation for Nationally Certified EMS personnel. In 1971, the first NREMT-Ambulance exam was administered at 51 test sites nationwide to over 1,500 personnel, signifying the onset of official EMT certification. By 1974, the NREMT was calling for the development of national standards for Paramedics, and the following year, it advocated for the formal recognition of Paramedics as allied health professionals.

Currently, the NREMT's primary mission is to ensure a fair and unbiased assessment of EMS practitioners' knowledge and skills through the administration of legally defensible, objective examinations for National EMS Certifications. Moreover, the NREMT actively contributes to the unification and advancement of the EMS profession. Recognizing the necessity for an independent professional association, akin to the American Medical Association for physicians, the NREMT played a key role in the formation of the National Association of EMTs (NAEMT) in 1975, providing a collective voice for individual EMTs at a national level.

In addition to administering examinations and certifications, the NREMT also pioneers EMS research. Understanding the importance of robust research in the EMS field, the NREMT drives initiatives to improve the EMS workforce, elevate care quality, and evaluate the effectiveness of EMS systems. A noteworthy contribution in this area is the establishment of the EMS Research Doctorate Fellowship Program, aimed at promoting advanced research and nurturing future leaders and scholars in EMS.

Furthermore, the NREMT actively supported the creation and current operations of the National EMS Coordinated Database, the EMS Compact, and the National EMS Identification number. Through its commitment to certification excellence and collaborations with medical professionals, the NREMT reinforces the credibility and professionalism of the EMS profession. More details about the NREMT and National EMS Certification can be accessed in Chapter 18.

U.S. Fire Administration

The U.S. Fire Administration (USFA), an integral entity within the Federal Emergency Management Agency (FEMA), was established in 1974, in the aftermath of the 1973 National Commission on Fire Prevention and Control report entitled *America Burning.*[88] This pivotal report called attention to the extent of the national fire problem and urged immediate action to reduce the incidence and severity of fires across the country.

From the outset, the USFA was charged with a broad mission: to reduce loss of life and economic losses due to fire and related emergencies, through leadership, advocacy, coordination, and support. Over time, this mission has grown to incorporate responsibilities related to Emergency Medical Services.

Emergency Medical Services, a critical component of the overall health care system, is primarily involved in providing pre-hospital emergency care and transportation. EMS falls under the purview of the USFA because of the significant role the fire service plays in delivering emergency medical care. Most fire departments in the U.S., particularly in urban and suburban areas, provide some level of EMS. Indeed, for many departments, EMS calls constitute a large proportion of their overall responses.

The USFA recognizes the importance of this connection and, therefore, works diligently to support and enhance the provision of EMS through several mechanisms. Primarily, the USFA provides training, research, and data resources that allow fire-based EMS agencies to fulfill their crucial role effectively and efficiently.

The National Fire Academy (NFA), a part of the USFA, offers several educational programs specifically aimed at EMS. Courses such as *Emergency Medical Services Functions in the Incident Command System* and *Fire Service Emergency Medical Services Officer* are designed to enhance the knowledge and leadership skills of EMS professionals within the fire service. In addition, the NFA's EMS curriculum provides specific instruction in areas such as EMS operations at mass casualty incidents, quality management in EMS, and community risk reduction for the fire and EMS leader.

Moreover, the USFA conducts and disseminates research on a variety of EMS-related topics, offering valuable insights into the challenges and opportunities facing EMS today. This research helps shape national discussions about EMS and drives improvements in service delivery.

The USFA also provides important data resources, such as the National Fire Incident Reporting System (NFIRS). While primarily a tool for tracking fire incidents, NFIRS collects data on a wide variety of incidents to which the fire service responds, including EMS calls. This data aids in understanding the breadth and depth of the fire service's EMS activities, and can inform decision-making at local, state, and national levels.

The U.S. Fire Administration, since its inception, has evolved to acknowledge the expanding role of the fire service in delivering emergency medical services. Through education, research, and data provision, the USFA supports EMS within the fire service, enhancing the capabilities of these vital services and, ultimately, ensuring the health and safety of communities across the nation. For aspiring EMS leaders, managers, and state government officials, understanding the role and contributions of the USFA is an integral part of maximizing the effectiveness of EMS.

ADDITIONAL NATIONAL EMS ORGANIZATIONS:

There are many additional national organizations that have made significant contributions to the development of the U.S. Emergency Medical Services system. These organizations have significantly influenced EMS through advocacy, education, research, and the establishment of standards and guidelines, helping to shape the landscape of emergency medical care in the United States. It is essential to recognize that there are numerous organizations involved in this process, and the list provided in this section is by no means exhaustive. Nevertheless, it serves as an overview of some of the most influential organizations that have played a crucial role in the advancement of EMS across the nation.

- **American Academy of Pediatrics** (AAP): The AAP represents pediatricians and advocates for the health and well-being of children. They provide resources and guidelines for the pediatric care provided by EMS professionals.
- **American Association for the Surgery of Trauma** (AAST): The AAST promotes excellence in trauma care, research, and education, advocating for the development of trauma systems and the integration of EMS within these systems.
- **American Heart Association** (AHA): The AHA is dedicated to reducing death and disability from cardiovascular diseases and stroke. They develop evidence-based resuscitation guidelines and training programs for EMS practitioners, such as Basic Life Support (BLS) and Advanced Cardiac Life Support (ACLS).
- **American Paramedic Association** (APA)**:** The APA is a member-based organization advocating that the future of the discipline of paramedicine should be driven by its professional paramedic members. They are committed to professionalizing Paramedic practice across America and to ensuring the safety of the public served while promoting the advancement of the profession through autonomy and self-regulation.
- **American Trauma Society** (ATS): The ATS is dedicated to the prevention and treatment of trauma. They work to enhance trauma care through education, research, and advocacy, and support the development of trauma systems and EMS infrastructure.
- **Association of Air Medical Services** (AAMS): The AAMS is dedicated to the advancement of emergency air medical transport services, promoting safety, quality, and effectiveness of air medical and critical care transport through advocacy, education, and research.
- **Commission on Accreditation of Ambulance Services** (CAAS): The CAAS establishes standards for ambulance services and provides a voluntary accreditation process to ensure high-quality patient care and operational efficiency.

- **Council of State Governments** (CSG): The CSG is a nonpartisan organization that serves all three branches of state government. It fosters the exchange of insights and ideas to help state officials shape public policy, focusing on various issues, including public health and emergency services. The CSG has played a role in shaping EMS policy and regulations at the state level, which in turn influences the development and evolution of the U.S. EMS system.
- **Emergency Nurses Association** (ENA): The ENA represents emergency nurses and works to advance emergency nursing practice, advocating for high-quality patient care, and promoting professional development.
- **International Academies of Emergency Dispatch** (IAED): The IAED focuses on emergency dispatch services and provides training, certification, and accreditation programs for emergency dispatch professionals.
- **International Association of EMS Chiefs** (IAEMSC): The IAEMSC promotes leadership, cooperation, and information exchange among EMS chiefs and managers, fostering collaboration and growth in the EMS industry.
- **Association of Public-Safety Communications Officials (APCO International): APCO represents public safety communications professionals and works to promote best practices in emergency communications, advocating for efficient and effective emergency response systems.**
- **National Association of EMS Quality Professionals** (NAEMSQP): The NAEMSQP promotes best practices in EMS quality management and performance improvement, providing resources, networking opportunities, and professional development for EMS quality professionals.
- **National Association of Search and Rescue** (NASAR): NASAR is focused on search and rescue operations, providing education, training, and certification programs for search and rescue professionals, including those involved in wilderness EMS.
- **National Fire Protection Association** (NFPA): The NFPA develops and publishes standards and codes related to fire, rescue, electrical, and building safety, including standards for EMS systems and providers.
- **National Organization of State Offices of Rural Health** (NOSORH): The NOSORH enhances rural health care by supporting state offices of rural health and collaborating with federal and state partners to improve access to care, including EMS agencies, in rural areas.
- **National Volunteer Fire Council** (NVFC): The NVFC represents volunteer fire fighters, EMS practitioners, and rescue personnel, advocating for their interests and providing resources, training, and networking opportunities.

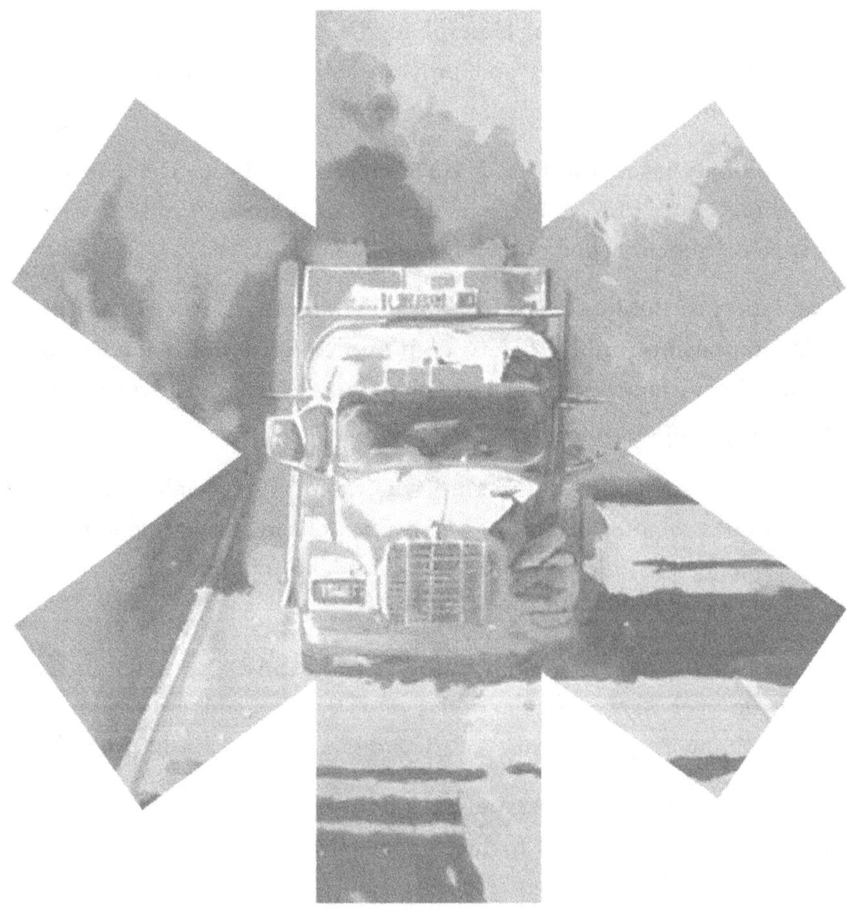

9

EMS WEEK

"We are a traveling nation and none of us knows when we might need help far from home. Let us affirm that the first year of this national legislation is only the beginning of our effort to improve this part of our total health care system so that no individual in this country will lack help when he needs it." – President Gerald R. Ford, Proclamation 4332, November 5, 1974

SINCE ITS INCEPTION IN 1974, EMS WEEK HAS STOOD AS AN ANNUAL tribute to the tireless efforts and unwavering dedication of Emergency Medical Services practitioners. Celebrated during the third week of May, this week underlines the pivotal role these professionals play in saving lives, preserving public health and safety, and supporting their communities.

The origins of EMS Week date back to 1974 when President Gerald Ford established the first "National Emergency Medical Services Week".[89] The goal was to recognize the vital work of EMS practitioners and raise public awareness about EMS. Today, EMS Week is celebrated annually with various events and activities that honor the achievements of EMS practitioners, highlight the importance of EMS in healthcare, and increase awareness of the challenges and issues faced by the EMS community.

One key aspect of EMS Week is the opportunity to express appreciation for the dedication, expertise, and sacrifices made by EMS practitioners, who serve on the frontlines of healthcare. Often risking personal safety and wellbeing to care for others, they contribute significantly to the well-being of individuals and communities. EMS Week helps raise awareness and inform the public about the importance of EMS. By showcasing the critical role EMS plays in responding to emergencies, providing medical care, and transporting patients to appropriate healthcare facilities, the national EMS week is often used to encourage individuals to learn basic life-saving skills like CPR and first aid, and to be prepared for emergencies.

Additionally, EMS Week facilitates collaboration and engagement between EMS agencies, policy makers, organizations, and communities. By fostering partnerships with healthcare professionals, public safety agencies, local governments, schools, businesses, and community organizations, EMS Week promotes community involvement and raises awareness of challenges and opportunities in the field of EMS.

> Through service, compassion, and dedication, EMS providers represent the very best of the American spirit. In the face of unprecedented challenges, their expertise, endurance, and hard work have been a literal lifeline for families in every community. Whether responding to the enormous suffering caused by COVID-19, the devastation of extreme climate events, or daily medical emergencies, EMS providers — many of whom are volunteers — prepare, sacrifice, and put others ahead of themselves. Not only do they assume the heightened risks associated with emergency care during a pandemic, but they also spend countless hours away from families and friends in order to serve their communities.
>
> -President Joseph R. Biden, Jr., May 14, 2021

EMS Week is also a platform for advocating policies and initiatives that support the EMS profession. This event allows EMS practitioners and organizations to address issues, challenges, and priorities within the EMS community, such as workforce development, funding, equipment and resource needs, and regulatory and legislative matters. Through these efforts, EMS Week promotes the interests and well-being of EMS practitioners and advances the EMS profession at local, state, and national levels.

Since the time President Ford was in office, Presidents and Governors have continued the tradition set by President Ford, issuing proclamations annually for EMS Week. The tradition of recognizing the breadth of services that EMS practitioners offer beyond emergency response, from disaster preparedness to public safety education, continues to grow. During this week, accolades are given to those who have shown outstanding service, providing a morale boost and acknowledgment of the unwavering dedication shown by the nation's EMS professionals.

Emergency Medical Services Week, 1974

A Proclamation

By the President of the United States of America

Each week more than a thousand Americans die as a result of accidents, heart attacks, and other medical crises because emergency medical assistance is not available.

For many years, physicians and health professionals have been urging improved national facilities for emergency medical care. Last year the Congress passed the "Emergency Medical Services Systems Act of 1973" to create a national thrust toward that goal.

Two Federal agencies, the Department of Health, Education, and Welfare and the Department of Transportation, are now working closely with States and communities to improve medical emergency services. Although many cities enjoy satisfactory services, the great majority of our communities, especially in rural areas, still require considerable improvement.

NOW, THEREFORE, I, GERALD R. FORD, President of the United States of America, do hereby designate the week beginning November 3, 1974, as Emergency Medical Services Week.

I call upon the Governors and mayors and all other State and local officials to assist hospital administrators and physicians, fire departments, and other public safety agencies in improving their emergency medical services.

I call upon Federal agencies, especially the two Departments mentioned above, to continue, with renewed vigor, their assistance to States and communities in accelerating their efforts to help those in need of emergency medical assistance.

And I call upon all our people to lend their support to these efforts. We are a traveling nation and none of us knows when we might need help far from home.

Let us affirm that the first year of this national legislation is only the beginning of our effort to improve this part of our total health care system so that no individual in this country will lack help when he needs it.

IN WITNESS WHEREOF, I have hereunto set my hand this fifth day of November, in the year of our Lord nineteen hundred seventy-four, and of the Independence of the United States of America the one hundred ninety-ninth.

Gerald R. Ford

The first presidential proclamation for EMS Week. (Digitized from Box 34 of the William J. Baroody Files at the Gerald R. Ford Presidential Library).

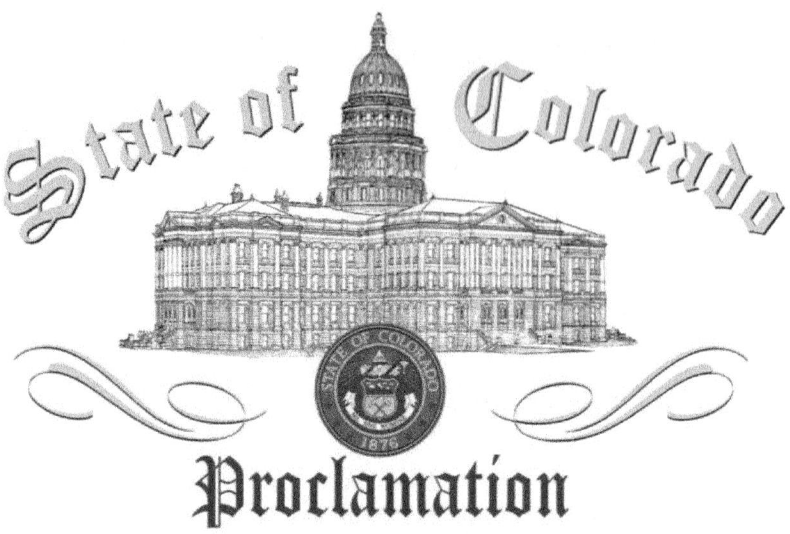

WHEREAS, the provision of emergency medical services is a vital public good; and

WHEREAS, each year, Colorado's emergency medical services provide vital care to those in need 24 hours a day, seven days a week; and

WHEREAS, access to quality emergency medical services dramatically improves the survival and recovery rate of those who experience sudden illness; and

WHEREAS, emergency medical services have grown to fill a gap by providing out of hospital care, including preventative medicine, follow-up care, and access to telemedicine; and

WHEREAS, the emergency medical services system consists of first responders, emergency medical technicians, paramedics, emergency medical dispatchers, firefighters, police officers, educators, administrators, pre-hospital nurses, emergency nurses, emergency physicians, trained members of the public, and other out of hospital medical care providers; and

WHEREAS, the members of emergency medical services teams, whether career or volunteer, engage in thousands of hours of specialized training and continuing education to enhance their lifesaving skills; and

WHEREAS, it is appropriate to recognize the value and the accomplishments of emergency medical services providers by designating Emergency Medical Services Week;

THEREFORE, I, Jared Polis, Governor of the State of Colorado, do hereby proclaim the period of time between May 21 and May 27, 2023, as

EMERGENCY MEDICAL SERVICES WEEK

in the State of Colorado.

GIVEN under my hand and the Executive Seal of the State of Colorado, this twenty-first day of May, 2023

Jared Polis
Governor

Since the 1970s, EMS Week has also been recognized with State Proclamations. This is an example of the 2023 proclamation issued by Colorado's Governor Jared Polis.

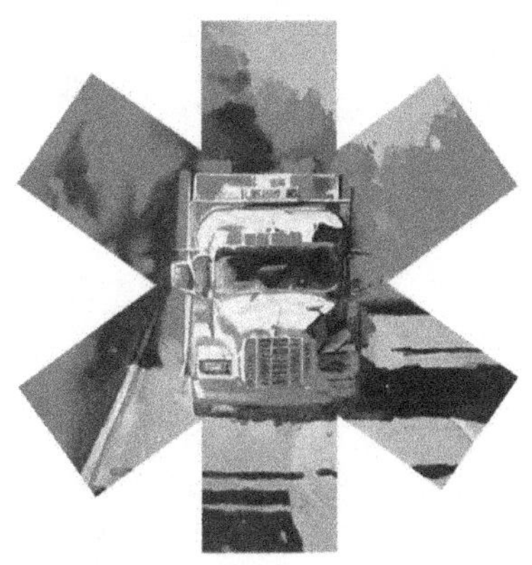

Section 2

EMS Systems & Operations

"All improvement happens project by project and in no other way."
-Joseph Juran

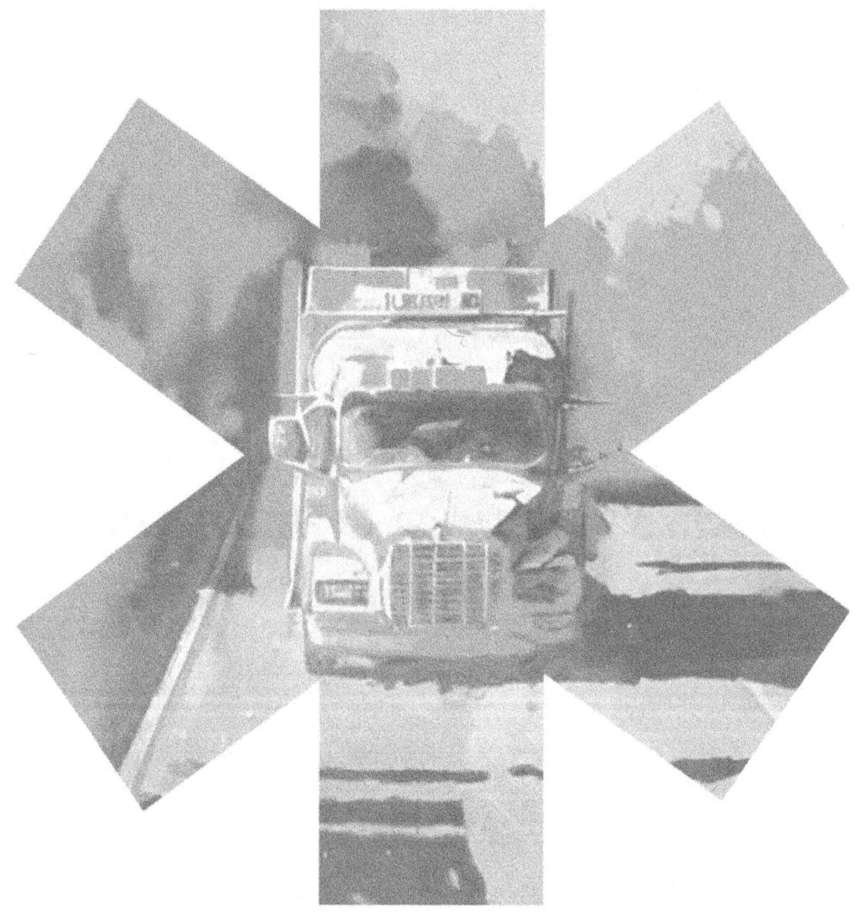

10

EMS Service Delivery Models

"If you've seen one EMS system, you've seen one EMS system."
- James O. Page

EMERGENCY MEDICAL SERVICE DELIVERY MODELS EXHIBIT A substantial degree of variation throughout the United States, with a diverse range of organizations and agencies undertaking the provision of these critical services. Each model possesses its unique set of characteristics, organizational structures, funding mechanisms, and operational frameworks, as well as a range of inherent advantages and challenges.

A comprehensive understanding of these various models is essential for all stakeholders involved in EMS provision, including policymakers, healthcare administrators, and emergency medical professionals, as it enables them to make well-informed decisions when determining the most suitable EMS delivery model to be implemented within their specific community or organization. By considering the unique needs, resources, and priorities of each community, stakeholders can better tailor their chosen EMS model to effectively address the community's specific requirements and enhance the overall quality of pre-hospital care, ultimately leading to improved patient outcomes and greater satisfaction for both patients and EMS practitioners.

PRIVATE FOR-PROFIT EMS

In the private for-profit EMS model, emergency medical services are operated by for-profit companies that are typically owned by individuals or corporations with the primary goal of generating profits. These companies may provide EMS services on a contract basis to municipalities, hospitals, or other entities, or they may operate as independent EMS providers. Revenue is generated through billing patients, insurance companies, and other payers.

Key Features and Considerations

Ownership	Private for-profit EMS companies are owned by individuals (sole proprietorships), groups of individuals (partnerships, LLPs, LLCs, etc.) or shareholders (either closely held or publicly traded). In some cases, corporations may hold memberships in LLPs or LLCs or possess shares. These shares could be closely held or publicly traded, depending on the structure and size of the organization.
Organizational Structure	These companies are organized as for-profit entities, often structured as corporations or limited liability companies (LLCs).
Funding Mechanisms	Revenue is generated through contract fees and fees charged for services rendered, including billing patients, insurance companies, and other payers.
Strengths	Private for-profit EMS companies may have flexibility in operations and decision-making and may be able to generate revenue and profits.
Weaknesses	Potential challenges associated with balancing fiduciary duty to shareholders and the commitment to delivering patient care, ensuring sufficient public accountability, managing potential conflicts of interest, and maintaining consistent quality of service.

PRIVATE NON-PROFIT EMS

In the private non-profit EMS model, emergency medical services are operated by non-profit organizations that are frequently community-based or regionally based. These organizations typically have a mission to provide EMS services to the community, and any revenue generated is typically reinvested into the organization to support its operations and goals. Private non-profit EMS organizations may be independent or may operate under contract with municipalities, hospitals, or other entities.

Key Features and Considerations

Ownership	Private non-profit EMS organizations are corporations formed for a charitable purpose and managed either by members of the corporation or by a board of directors. The assets of a non-profit corporation are held in trust for the benefit of the community served and as such are subject to ultimate oversight of the state's attorney general.
Organizational Structure	These organizations are organized as non-profit entities, such as corporations or charitable organizations.
Funding Mechanisms	Revenue is generated through fees charged for services rendered, donations, grants, and other sources, and is typically reinvested into the organization to support its operations.
Strengths	Private non-profit EMS organizations may have a community-oriented mission, focus on patient care over profits, and reinvest revenue into the organization to support operations and goals.
Weaknesses	Potential challenges include reliance on donations and grants, potential variability in service quality, and financial constraints.

Public EMS

In the public EMS model, emergency medical services are operated by government entities such as municipalities, counties, or other governmental organizations. Public EMS services may be funded via tax revenue or other government funding sources and are typically offered as a public service to the community.

Key Features and Considerations

Ownership	Public EMS services are owned by government entities, including municipalities, counties, or other governmental organizations.
Organizational Structure	These services are organized as part of the government, often as a department or division within the municipality or county.
Funding Mechanisms	Funding generally stems from tax revenue or other government funding sources supplemented by fees charged for services rendered, donations, grants, and other sources.
Strengths	Public EMS services are part of the governmental infrastructure and may provide services based on community needs. They may also have access to government resources and support and can provide consistent and reliable services to the community.
Weaknesses	Public EMS services often face challenges related to bureaucracy, budget constraints, and potential limitations in decision-making flexibility.

FIRE-BASED EMS

In the fire-based EMS model, emergency medical services are provided by fire departments, which often operate as part of municipal or county government entities. Fire-based EMS is typically integrated with firefighting services, with fire fighters frequently receiving EMS training. Fire departments may respond to both fire and EMS calls, delivering pre-hospital care and transportation to those requiring medical assistance.

Key Features and Considerations

Ownership	Fire-based EMS agencies are owned and operated by fire departments, which may be part of municipal or county government entities, further integrating them within the community. In some communities - even though they are closely aligned with the local governments they serve - fire departments may themselves be separate, non-governmental, nonprofit corporations.
Organizational Structure	These services are organized as part of the fire department, often as a dedicated division or unit within the department.
Funding Mechanisms	Funding for fire-based EMS agencies typically stems from tax revenue or other government funding sources, often supplemented by fees charged for services rendered, donations, grants, and other sources.
Strengths	Fire-based EMS agencies benefit from the existing infrastructure and resources of fire departments, including trained personnel, equipment, and facilities. Additionally, they may maintain a close relationship with the community and be able to respond quickly to emergencies.
Weaknesses	Fire-based EMS services may face challenges related to bureaucracy, budget constraints, and potential limitations in decision-making flexibility. In some fire departments, EMS is viewed as a secondary priority. In many agencies there is a potential conflict of interest between firefighting and EMS.

HOSPITAL-BASED EMS

In the hospital-based EMS model, EMS agencies are operated by hospitals or healthcare systems. These services extend the hospital's healthcare provisions by offering pre-hospital care and transportation, potentially integrating with the hospital's emergency department or other medical services.

Key Features and Considerations

Ownership	Under the hospital-based EMS model, services are owned and operated by hospitals or healthcare systems, positioning EMS as a crucial part of the larger healthcare network.
Organizational Structure	These services are typically organized within the hospital or healthcare system, often functioning as a distinct division or department.
Funding Mechanisms	Funding for hospital-based EMS agencies is primarily derived from the hospital or healthcare system's budget, often supplemented by fees charged for services rendered, donations, grants, and other sources.
Strengths	Hospital-based EMS agencies have the advantage of leveraging the resources and expertise of the hospital or healthcare system, including access to medical personnel, equipment, and facilities. Moreover, they may foster a close relationship with the hospital, enabling seamless care from pre-hospital to hospital-based care.
Weaknesses	Some challenges faced by this model include potential conflicts of interest between hospital and EMS priorities, limitations in serving the broader community beyond the hospital's catchment area, balancing the demands of internal (patient transfers) with external (911 emergency response), and potential resource constraints. In some hospital-based systems, EMS is perceived as a "loss leader." That is, while EMS agencies may not be profitable in themselves, they generate downstream revenues by securing hospital admissions that could otherwise be lost to competing facilities. As a result of this perspective, EMS may receive inadequate funding.

THIRD SERVICE EMS

The third service EMS model is characterized by EMS agencies provided by a standalone department within a city or county government. Like fire and police departments, these EMS agencies operate independently from other organizations such as fire departments, hospitals, or law enforcement agencies. Traditionally staffed with civilian employees, these EMS agencies are completely owned, financed, and operated within the local government structure.

Key Features and Considerations

Ownership	Third service EMS model agencies are owned by government entities, including municipalities, counties, or other governmental organizations.
Organizational Structure	These agencies are organized as autonomous EMS agencies, often possessing their own administrative structure and governance, which can streamline decision-making and foster innovation.
Funding Mechanisms	Financial support is generally derived from various sources, such as fees charged for services rendered, government funding, donations, and grants. This diversified funding approach can provide a more stable financial base for these agencies.
Strengths	A singular focus on EMS, enabling them to tailor their services to the community's specific needs. Furthermore, they may possess the flexibility to make decisions and implement changes independently, leading to a more agile and adaptive EMS service.
Weaknesses	While it's often believed that a separate department would offer EMS agencies equal attention, support, and stature given to police and fire departments, this is frequently not the case. Third-service EMS organizations often struggle for recognition and are valued less than their public safety counterparts. Cost containment may also be a significant challenge, as control of expenditures is typically dependent on the local government's budgetary and managerial processes.

PUBLIC UTILITY EMS

The public utility EMS model is built on the concept of delivering EMS services via a local governmental entity, such as a city, county, or district. This model is similar to other public utilities like water, gas, or electricity. Here, EMS agencies operate as a public service, but the provision of personnel, management, vehicles, and other resources is contracted out to a private ambulance company. This could either be a for-profit or non-profit entity. In this structure, the local government agency remains the provider of record and receives the revenue from fee-for-service billing. Meanwhile, the contracted services are paid based on an agreed-upon fee to the private provider.

Key Features and Considerations

Ownership	Public utility EMS agencies are owned and managed by a public utility entity, which could be a government agency or a separate organization.
Organizational Structure	Typically, these services are organized under the umbrella of a public utility organization, often as a division or department within the organization. This arrangement fosters integration with other public utility services and streamlines operations.
Funding Mechanisms	Financing is generally derived from the overall budget of the public utility organization, supplemented by patient billing, ensuring consistent financial support for EMS agencies.
Strengths	Ability to capitalize on the established infrastructure and resources of the public utility organization, benefiting from administrative support, financial stability, and access to equipment and facilities. This foundation can contribute to a more efficient and robust EMS service, better equipped to meet the needs of the community.
Weaknesses	Limitations in EMS expertise and training within the public utility organization could impact the quality of service. Conflicts of interest may arise between EMS priorities and other utility services, potentially compromising the allocation of resources and focus. Additionally, decision-making flexibility could be limited within the broader organizational structure, which may impede the ability to adapt and respond to the evolving demands of EMS agencies.

11

DISPARITIES IN ACCESS TO EMS

"Of all the forms of inequality, injustice in health care is the most shocking and inhumane."
– Dr. Martin Luther King, Jr.

IN A 1966 ADDRESS TO THE MEDICAL COMMITTEE FOR HUMAN RIGHTS, Dr. Martin Luther King Jr. asserted, “Of all the forms of inequality, injustice in health care is the most shocking and inhumane.” Regrettably, over half a century later, significant disparities and inequalities remain prevalent in access, quality, and provision of emergency medical services. These disparities are multifaceted and are influenced by various determinants such as geography, socioeconomic status, race/ethnicity, and insurance status.

As a relatively new healthcare model, EMS is just beginning to evaluate, research, understand, and address these disparities. It is crucial for EMS practitioners and policymakers to take steps to ensure that all individuals receive equal access to high-quality emergency medical care, regardless of their geography, socioeconomic status, background, or circumstances.

Some of the key issues related to EMS and ambulance access disparities in the United States include:

- **Geographic Disparities**: Regions such as rural areas, remote locations, and underserved urban areas often encounter obstacles in accessing EMS and ambulance services. In rural territories, substantial distances between healthcare facilities and residences can lead to prolonged response times and delayed delivery of timely care. The scarcity of EMS personnel, equipment, and infrastructure in these regions can also compromise the quality of care.

- **Socioeconomic Disparities**: Socioeconomic status can impede access to EMS and ambulance services. Lower-income communities may confront barriers due to financial constraints, lack of transportation, or insufficient health insurance coverage, potentially resulting in delayed or inadequate care and poorer health outcomes.

- **Racial/Ethnic Disparities**: Racial and ethnic disparities are also prevalent in access to EMS and ambulance services. Research indicates that communities of color, notably Black and Hispanic communities, often face challenges in procuring timely and quality health care[90]. Factors contributing to these disparities can include implicit bias, discrimination, language barriers, and mistrust of the healthcare system.

- **Insurance Disparities**: Health insurance coverage plays a role in accessing EMS and ambulance services. Individuals without health insurance or with inadequate insurance may face financial barriers to accessing EMS. Lack of insurance coverage can also result in increased out-of-pocket costs for ambulance transportation, which may deter individuals from seeking care.

- **Systemic Disparities**: Disparities in EMS and ambulance services are affected by systemic elements such as variations in EMS funding, resource allocation, and service delivery models across jurisdictions. Lack of standardization in EMS protocols, variability in ambulance response times, and differences in EMS practitioner qualifications and training can contribute to disparities in care.

- **Social Disparities**: Other social determinants of health can impact access to EMS agencies. Some social groups may face unique challenges in accessing EMS agencies, such as mobility limitations, lack of appropriate accommodations, discrimination, and stigma. These disparities can further exacerbate the existing inequities in access to EMS agencies and impact health outcomes for these populations.

- **Gender Disparities**: Studies continue to show that disparities exist in EMS access and treatment related to a patient's gender[91]. These disparities can be influenced by a variety of factors including societal biases, healthcare provider assumptions, and differences in presentation of symptoms. Addressing gender disparities in EMS requires increased awareness, education, and policy adjustments to ensure equitable care for all genders.

Addressing these disparities in EMS and ambulance access necessitates a comprehensive approach, encompassing policy changes, increased funding and resources, addressing social determinants of health, promoting diversity and inclusivity in the EMS workforce, and enhancing the coordination and standardization of EMS agencies across jurisdictions. Endeavors to ensure that all individuals, regardless of location, socioeconomic status, race/ethnicity, or insurance status, have equitable access to timely and high-quality EMS and ambulance services are vital for improving health outcomes and reducing health disparities in the United States.

Geographic Disparities

Geographic disparities in accessing EMS and ambulance services in the United States are often driven by the location and availability of healthcare facilities, infrastructure, and EMS resources. Rural areas, remote locations, and underserved urban areas face unique challenges in accessing EMS and ambulance services, which can result in delayed or inadequate care during emergencies.

One key factor contributing to geographic disparities is the distance between healthcare facilities and residences in rural areas. Rural communities often have limited access to nearby hospitals or healthcare facilities, resulting in longer response times and delays in receiving timely care. In emergencies such as heart attacks, strokes, or traumatic injuries, where time is critical, these delays can have serious consequences on patient outcomes.

Moreover, rural areas often face challenges in recruiting and retaining EMS personnel, resulting in a shortage of trained EMS practitioners. The cost of training, low population density, and remote locations can make it difficult to attract and retain qualified EMS professionals, leading to longer response times and reduced availability of EMS agencies.

Another issue is the lack of adequate infrastructure and resources in rural areas. Ambulance services require proper infrastructure such as roads, bridges, and communication networks to operate efficiently. However, rural areas may have poorly maintained roads, limited or no cell phone coverage, and challenges with communication infrastructure, making it difficult for ambulances to reach patients in a timely manner.

Addressing geographic disparities in access to EMS includes:

- **Expanding EMS resources in rural areas**: Increasing funding and resources for EMS agencies in rural areas, including hiring and training more EMS practitioners, improving ambulance fleet availability, and equipping ambulances with advanced medical equipment, can help improve access to care.
- **Telemedicine and tele-EMS**: Utilizing telemedicine and tele-EMS technologies can help bridge the gap in rural areas by enabling remote consultation with medical professionals and providing guidance to EMS practitioners in the field, especially in emergencies where access to specialized care is crucial.
- **Community paramedicine programs**: Community paramedicine programs, also known as mobile integrated healthcare, involve paramedics providing preventive and primary care services in underserved areas, including rural communities. These programs can help expand access to care, provide preventive services, reduce call volume, and stress on designated emergency resources, and address chronic health conditions in remote areas.
- **Improving infrastructure:** Investing in improving transportation infrastructure, such as roads, bridges, and communication networks, in rural areas can help ambulances reach patients more quickly and efficiently, reducing response times.

- **Coordination and integration of services**: Improving coordination and integration of EMS agencies with other healthcare providers, including hospitals and primary care clinics, can help ensure that patients in rural areas receive appropriate and timely care, including transport to appropriate healthcare facilities.
- **Targeted policies**: Implementing policies that specifically target geographic disparities, such as funding incentives for EMS practitioners to operate in underserved areas or expanding Medicaid coverage in states with high rural populations, can help improve access to EMS and ambulance services.
- **Community engagement**: Engaging local communities and understanding their unique needs and challenges can help in developing tailored solutions that are culturally appropriate and address the specific barriers to EMS and ambulance access in rural areas.

Addressing geographic disparities in access to EMS will require a multi-faceted approach that involves increasing resources, improving infrastructure, utilizing telemedicine and community paramedicine programs, promoting coordination and integration of services, implementing targeted policies, and engaging local communities. These efforts can help ensure that individuals in rural areas have equitable access to timely and quality EMS and ambulance services during emergencies.

Socioeconomic Disparities

Socioeconomic disparities also play a significant role in access to EMS and ambulance services in the United States. Disadvantaged communities, including those with lower incomes, limited education, and inadequate health insurance coverage, often face barriers in accessing timely and quality EMS care, resulting in disparities in care, quality, and outcomes.

One key factor contributing to socioeconomic disparities is the cost of EMS and ambulance services. EMS is expensive, and communities with lower incomes may face challenges in funding or sustaining the cost of services. This can result in delayed or deferred care during emergencies, leading to poorer health outcomes.

Moreover, individuals with lower incomes may face challenges in accessing transportation to healthcare facilities, including hospitals and clinics. Lack of reliable transportation options, including public transportation or access to private vehicles, can hinder their ability to access healthcare in a timely manner, resulting in delays in care and potentially worse outcomes. Often, EMS is the community safety net that provides treatment and transport for these individuals, and often these services are uncompensated.

Limited health literacy and education can also contribute to socioeconomic disparities in EMS and ambulance access. Individuals with lower levels of education may have limited understanding of the importance of EMS agencies, how to access them, and how to navigate the healthcare system. This can result in delays in seeking care or not utilizing EMS agencies appropriately, leading to disparities in care and outcomes.

Possible solutions to address socioeconomic disparities in EMS and ambulance access include:

- **Health insurance coverage**: Expanding access to health insurance coverage, particularly for low-income populations, can ensure that individuals have financial protection and can access EMS and ambulance services without incurring high out-of-pocket costs.
- **Transportation assistance programs**: Implementing transportation assistance programs, such as subsidized transportation options or partnerships with local transportation providers, can help overcome transportation barriers for individuals with limited access to reliable transportation, ensuring they can access non-emergency healthcare services in a timely manner.
- **Health literacy and education:** Implementing health literacy and education programs targeted at underserved communities can help improve their understanding of the importance of EMS agencies, how to access them, and how to navigate the healthcare system effectively.
- **Community outreach and engagement**: Engaging with underserved communities through community outreach programs, health fairs, and partnerships with community organizations can help raise awareness about EMS and ambulance services, build trust, and encourage utilization of these services.
- **Culturally competent care**: Providing culturally competent care that respects the diverse needs and beliefs of underserved communities can help build trust and encourage utilization of EMS and ambulance services.
- **Addressing social determinants of health**: Recognizing and addressing social determinants of health, such as poverty, housing instability, and food insecurity, that contribute to socioeconomic disparities in EMS and ambulance access can help improve access to care for vulnerable populations.

Addressing socioeconomic disparities in EMS access requires addressing the financial, transportation, health literacy, and cultural barriers that individuals from underserved communities may face. Implementing affordable pricing, expanding health insurance coverage, providing transportation assistance, promoting health literacy, engaging with communities, providing culturally competent care, and addressing social determinants of health can all contribute to reducing socioeconomic disparities and ensuring equitable access to EMS and ambulance services for all individuals, regardless of their socioeconomic status.

RACIAL/ETHNIC DISPARITIES

Racial and ethnic disparities in access to EMS and ambulance services are another significant issue in the United States. Studies have shown that individuals from racial and ethnic minority groups, including Black, Hispanic, Native American, and Asian communities, often face inequities in accessing timely and quality EMS care, resulting in disparities in care, quality, and outcomes. A 2013 retrospective analysis[92] of EMS patient care reports showed that African American blunt trauma patients were 50% less likely to be provided morphine for pain, compared with Caucasian patients.

One consideration is the under-representation of minorities in the EMS workforce. A peer-reviewed study published in the *Prehospital Emergency Care Journal* noted that only 5% of newly certified EMTs and 3% of paramedics identified as Black, and 13% of EMTs and 10% of paramedics identified as Hispanic. [93] Compared to the U.S. population racial/ethnic minorities and females continue to be underrepresented in the EMS profession.

Language barriers can also contribute to disparities in access to EMS and ambulance services for individuals with limited English proficiency (LEP). Language barriers can hinder communication with EMS practitioners, resulting in delayed or inadequate care, and can also lead to challenges in understanding how to access EMS agencies or navigate the healthcare system, resulting in disparities in care.

Geographic location and neighborhood characteristics can also intersect with racial and ethnic disparities in EMS and ambulance access. Studies have shown that racial and ethnic minority communities are more likely to be in areas with limited access to healthcare facilities, including hospitals and EMS stations. This can result in longer response times for EMS agencies, leading to delays in care and poorer outcomes for these communities.

Addressing racial and ethnic disparities in EMS requires a multifaceted approach, to include:

- **Language access services**: Implementing language access services, such as interpreter services or translated materials, can help overcome language barriers for individuals with LEP, ensuring that they can effectively communicate with EMS practitioners and access necessary care.

- **Community-based EMS programs**: Implementing community-based EMS programs that are tailored to the specific needs of racial and ethnic minority communities, including culturally competent care, language access, and community engagement, can help build trust and increase utilization of EMS and ambulance services in these communities.

- **Addressing structural racism**: Recognizing and addressing structural racism and bias within the healthcare system, including EMS and ambulance services, through policy changes, organizational culture shifts, and diversity, equity, and inclusion initiatives, can help reduce racial and ethnic disparities in care.

- **Improving geographic access**: Increasing access to healthcare facilities, including hospitals and EMS stations, in underserved racial and ethnic minority communities can help reduce response times and improve access to timely EMS and ambulance services.
- **Collaborations with community organizations**: Partnering with community organizations, such as local advocacy groups, faith-based organizations, and community health centers, can help facilitate outreach, education, and engagement efforts within racial and ethnic minority communities, promoting awareness and utilization of EMS and ambulance services.
- **Data collection and monitoring**: Collecting and analyzing data on EMS and ambulance utilization by race and ethnicity can help identify disparities and guide targeted interventions to address these disparities.

Addressing racial and ethnic disparities in EMS requires a multifaceted approach that addresses language barriers, geographic access, implicit bias, and community engagement. Strategies such as anti-racism training, language access services, community-based EMS programs, addressing structural racism, improving geographic access, collaborations with community organizations, and data collection and monitoring are potential solutions to promote equitable access to EMS and ambulance services for individuals from diverse racial and ethnic backgrounds.

However, implementing education and training programs to address these issues is costly and requires additional funding. Unfortunately, EMS systems often operate on significant budget deficits, and EMS practitioners may have to self-fund their education to enter a career with low wages. As a result, addressing racial and ethnic disparities in EMS and ambulance access is challenging due to competing financial barriers, ironically limiting progress towards equitable access.

INSURANCE DISPARITIES

Insurance disparities also contribute to inequities in access to EMS and ambulance services in the United States. Insurance status, including being uninsured or underinsured, can influence an individual's confidence and ability to access EMS in a timely and affordable manner, leading to disparities in care and outcomes.

Individuals who are uninsured or underinsured may face financial barriers to accessing EMS and ambulance services, including high out-of-pocket costs, co-pays, or deductibles. This can result in delayed or avoided utilization of EMS and ambulance services, leading to potential delays in care and poorer health outcomes.

Insurance disparities can also impact the type and quality of EMS and ambulance services available to individuals. Some insurance plans may have limitations or exclusions on coverage for certain EMS agencies or providers, resulting in disparities in the level of care received. For example, individuals with lower insurance coverage may face challenges related to interfacility transfers or access to specialized ambulances, leading to disparities in care quality.

Furthermore, insurance disparities can intersect with other disparities, such as socioeconomic and racial/ethnic disparities. Individuals from low-income communities, racial/ethnic minority communities, or communities with limited access to healthcare facilities may be more likely to be uninsured or underinsured, exacerbating existing disparities in EMS and ambulance access.

Possible solutions to address insurance disparities in EMS and ambulance access include:

- **Expanded insurance coverage:** Implementing policies to expand insurance coverage, such as Medicaid expansion, can help reduce the number of uninsured or underinsured individuals, increasing their ability to access EMS and ambulance services.
- **Financial assistance programs:** Establishing financial assistance programs, such as sliding scale fees or subsidies, can help individuals with limited insurance coverage afford EMS and ambulance services, reducing financial barriers to access.
- **Insurance policy reform:** Advocating for insurance policy reform to eliminate limitations or exclusions on coverage for EMS and ambulance services can ensure that individuals have comprehensive coverage for these essential services, regardless of their insurance status.
- **Information and education**: It is crucial to educate communities, policy makers, and other relevant stakeholders on the true cost associated with providing Emergency Medical Services in every community. This can help create informed policies, accurate budgets, and realistic expectations among the public.
- **Community outreach and education:** Conducting community outreach and education efforts to raise awareness about the importance of EMS and ambulance services, the availability of insurance coverage, and financial assistance programs can help individuals understand their options and navigate the insurance system effectively.
- **Collaboration with insurance providers:** Collaborating with insurance providers to promote equitable coverage of EMS and ambulance services, including addressing disparities in coverage limitations or exclusions, can help ensure that individuals have access to necessary care without financial hardships.
- **Advocacy and policy change:** Engaging in advocacy efforts to promote policy change at local, state, and national levels, such as advocating for equitable insurance coverage and reimbursement for EMS and ambulance services, can help address insurance disparities in EMS and ambulance access.

Insurance disparities are a significant barrier to equitable access to EMS and ambulance services in the United States. Expanded insurance coverage, financial assistance programs, insurance policy reform, community outreach and education, collaboration with insurance providers, and advocacy and policy change are potential strategies to reduce insurance disparities and promote equitable access to EMS and ambulance services for all individuals, regardless of their insurance status.

SYSTEMIC DISPARITIES

Systemic disparities, including structural and institutional factors, also contribute to inequities in access to emergency medical services and ambulance services in the United States. These disparities arise from various systemic issues that impact the availability, distribution, and quality of EMS and ambulance services, resulting in differential access and outcomes for different populations.

- **Resource allocation**: EMS and ambulance services may be disproportionately allocated to certain areas or populations, resulting in disparities in availability. For example, urban areas may have more EMS stations and ambulances compared to rural or remote areas, leading to longer response times and decreased access to timely care for individuals in those areas.

- **Funding and reimbursement**: Disparities in funding and reimbursement for EMS and ambulance services can affect the availability and quality of care. EMS agencies, particularly those serving low-income communities or areas with low population density, may struggle with limited funding, leading to inadequate staffing, equipment, and resources, which can impact the quality and timeliness of care.

- **Dispatch and triage protocols**: Dispatch and triage protocols used by EMS systems may inadvertently contribute to disparities. Implicit bias, cultural competency, and language barriers may affect decision-making in dispatching and triaging patients, leading to differential access to EMS and ambulance services based on factors such as race, ethnicity, or language proficiency.

- **Transportation barriers**: Systemic transportation barriers, such as lack of public transportation or limited availability of ambulance services in certain areas, can disproportionately impact individuals with limited mobility, those in low-income communities, or rural areas, resulting in disparities in access to EMS and ambulance services.

- **Health system fragmentation**: Fragmentation of the healthcare system, including lack of coordination and communication among different healthcare providers and agencies, can lead to delays and inefficiencies in EMS and ambulance services. This can disproportionately affect underserved populations who may face challenges in navigating the complex healthcare system.

- **Cultural competency and language barriers**: Systemic issues related to cultural competency and language barriers can impact the quality of care provided by EMS and ambulance services. Inadequate understanding of diverse cultural and linguistic needs of patients can result in miscommunication, misunderstandings, and suboptimal care, leading to disparities in care outcomes.

Addressing systemic disparities in EMS and ambulance access includes:

- **Equitable resource allocation**: Ensuring equitable distribution of EMS and ambulance resources, including personnel, equipment, and funding, to underserved areas and populations to reduce disparities in availability and response times.
- **Adequate funding and reimbursement**: Advocating for adequate funding and reimbursement for EMS agencies, particularly those serving low-income communities or rural areas, to ensure adequate staffing, equipment, and resources for providing high-quality care.
- **Culturally competent care:** Implementing culturally competent care protocols, including training in cultural competency and language proficiency for EMS practitioners, to improve communication, understanding, and trust between EMS practitioners and patients from diverse backgrounds.
- **Coordination and communication:** Enhancing coordination and communication among different healthcare providers and agencies involved in EMS and ambulance services to ensure seamless and efficient care delivery, particularly for underserved populations who may face challenges in navigating the healthcare system.
- **Transportation solutions**: Exploring and implementing transportation solutions, such as telehealth, community-based transportation options, or mobile integrated healthcare programs, to address transportation barriers and improve access to EMS and ambulance services for individuals in underserved areas.
- **Health policy and advocacy**: Engaging in health policy and advocacy efforts to address systemic issues related to EMS and ambulance services, such as advocating for changes in dispatch and triage protocols, reimbursement policies, and healthcare system integration to reduce disparities in access and outcomes.

Systemic disparities permeate various aspects of emergency medical services and ambulance care in the United States, including resource allocation, funding and reimbursement, dispatch, triage protocols, transportation barriers, health system fragmentation, and cultural competency and language barriers. These disparities contribute to inequitable access to emergency medical services, disproportionately affecting vulnerable populations such as those who are socioeconomically disadvantaged, racially/ethnically marginalized, or lacking insurance coverage. To address these systemic disparities, a comprehensive and multifaceted approach is necessary, encompassing policy changes, advocacy efforts, and cultural competency training for EMS practitioners, among other strategies.

Promoting equitable resource allocation involves ensuring that resources are distributed in a manner that addresses the needs of underserved communities and populations. Adequate funding is crucial for sustaining and expanding accessible emergency medical services and ambulance care. Additionally, cultural competency training for EMS practitioners enhances their ability to provide care that is sensitive to the diverse backgrounds and needs of patients.

Improving coordination and communication among healthcare providers is essential for delivering comprehensive and cohesive care. Addressing transportation barriers, such as limited access to ambulances or difficulties in reaching healthcare facilities, is vital for ensuring timely and appropriate care for all individuals. Advocacy efforts aimed at shaping health policies that prioritize equity and inclusivity can also drive meaningful change in the EMS landscape.

To reduce disparities, it is necessary to prioritize culturally competent care that respects the values, beliefs, and cultural practices of diverse patient populations. This involves fostering an inclusive and respectful environment within EMS organizations. By addressing these systemic factors, the goal is to create a more equitable and inclusive healthcare system that guarantees access to emergency medical services and ambulance care for all individuals in need, irrespective of their background or geographical location.

Recognizing the existence of systemic disparities and actively working to address them is paramount. By advocating for policy changes, promoting cultural competency, and ensuring equitable access to resources and care, we can strive towards a healthcare system that is truly equitable and provides fair access to emergency medical services and ambulance care, leading to improved healthcare outcomes for all individuals, regardless of their social, economic, racial/ethnic, or insurance status.

Social Disparities

Social disparities may hinder access to emergency medical services in some communities. Certain populations may face unique obstacles that impede their ability to obtain timely and appropriate EMS care, resulting in disparities in health outcomes.

- **Age**: Older adults may encounter obstacles accessing EMS agencies due to mobility restrictions, cognitive impairments, and other age-related factors. They may also have difficulty navigating the EMS system or communicating their needs to EMS practitioners, leading to delays or inadequate care.
- **Disability status:** Individuals with disabilities may encounter barriers when accessing EMS agencies, such as a lack of appropriate accommodations or equipment, transportation challenges, and communication difficulties. EMS practitioners may also require specialized training in caring for individuals with disabilities, including those with sensory impairments, cognitive disabilities, or mobility limitations.

These social disparities in access to EMS agencies can have significant consequences on health outcomes for these populations. Delayed or inadequate care can result in increased morbidity and mortality rates, decreased quality of life, and exacerbation of existing health conditions.

IMPACTS OF DISPARITIES AND INEQUITIES ON EMS ACCESS

Disparities and inequities in access to EMS agencies in the United States can have far-reaching and significant impacts. These disparities can result in differential health outcomes for different populations, exacerbating existing health disparities and contributing to health inequities. Some of the impacts of disparities in EMS access include:

- **Delayed or inadequate care**: Disparities in EMS access can result in delayed or inadequate care for individuals in need of emergency medical attention. This can lead to increased morbidity and mortality rates, as timely access to appropriate emergency care is crucial in many medical emergencies.
- **Health disparities**: Disparities in EMS access can contribute to existing health disparities, as certain populations may face greater challenges in accessing timely and appropriate emergency care. This can result in disproportionate health outcomes, with marginalized and underserved communities experiencing poorer health outcomes compared to more privileged populations.
- **Increased healthcare costs**: Disparities in EMS access can also result in increased healthcare costs for individuals and the healthcare system. Delayed or inadequate care can lead to increased hospitalizations, complications, and long-term health consequences, which can result in higher healthcare costs for individuals and an increased burden on the healthcare system.
- **Reduced quality of life:** A lack of equitable access to EMS agencies can negatively impact the quality of life for individuals who are unable to access timely and appropriate emergency care. This can result in prolonged pain and suffering, long-term disability, and reduced quality of life for affected individuals.
- **Disparities in outcomes for marginalized populations**: Disparities in EMS access can disproportionately impact marginalized populations, including racial/ethnic minorities, low-income individuals, individuals with disabilities, and older adults. These disparities can further contribute to social inequities and perpetuate health disparities among these vulnerable populations.
- **Economic and social consequences**: Disparities in EMS access can also have economic and social consequences, including lost productivity, increased healthcare costs, and strain on caregivers and families. These consequences can further exacerbate existing socioeconomic disparities and perpetuate cycles of poverty and health inequity.

To address disparities in EMS agencies, a comprehensive approach is necessary, involving data-driven strategies, cultural competency, community engagement, policy changes, and collaborations among various stakeholders. By implementing these strategies, EMS agencies can work towards overcoming disparities and ensuring equitable access to emergency care for all individuals, regardless of their social characteristics or identities.

OPPORTUNITIES TO ADDRESS DISPARITIES

To improve the equity of access to EMS agencies in the United States, a multifaceted approach is required that addresses disparities at various levels. Strategies to help overcome these disparities include:

- **Improve data collection and monitoring**: Collecting accurate and comprehensive data on EMS service utilization and outcomes, broken down by demographic characteristics, can help identify and monitor disparities. This can inform evidence-based interventions and policy changes to address disparities effectively.
- **Increase awareness and education**: Raising awareness among EMS practitioners and the broader healthcare community about disparities in access to EMS agencies is crucial. Education and training on cultural competence, implicit bias, and addressing social determinants of health can help EMS practitioners better understand and respond to the unique needs of diverse populations.
- **Enhance cultural competency and sensitivity**: Ensuring that EMS practitioners are culturally competent and sensitive to the needs of diverse populations is essential. This includes understanding diverse cultural practices, language barriers, and addressing biases to provide equitable care to all individuals regardless of their background or identity.
- **Improve outreach and community engagement**: Collaborating with community organizations, leaders, and advocates can help build trust and engagement with marginalized populations. Community outreach programs, health fairs, and community-based initiatives can increase awareness about EMS agencies, provide education, and facilitate access to care.
- **Increase resource allocation to underserved areas**: Ensuring adequate resources, including EMS personnel, equipment, and facilities, in underserved areas can help reduce geographic disparities. This may involve allocating more resources to rural and low-income areas and addressing workforce shortages through recruitment and retention efforts.
- **Implement policy changes**: Policy changes at the local, state, and federal levels can help address systemic disparities in EMS agencies. This may include improving reimbursement rates for EMS practitioners, promoting diversity and inclusion in EMS workforce, implementing policies to reduce discrimination and stigma, and addressing structural barriers that limit access to care.
- **Foster collaboration and coordination among healthcare stakeholders:** Collaboration among EMS practitioners, hospitals, community organizations, and other healthcare stakeholders can improve coordination and ensure a seamless continuum of care for underserved populations. This can include implementing referral systems, care coordination protocols, and shared decision-making processes.

- **Promote health equity in EMS leadership and governance**: Ensuring that EMS leadership and governance reflect the diversity of the communities they serve can help promote health equity. This may involve diversifying EMS leadership, involving community members in decision-making processes, and promoting inclusivity in EMS policies and practices.
- **Use technology and telehealth:** Leveraging technology, such as telehealth, can expand access to EMS agencies, especially in remote or underserved areas. Telehealth can provide triage, assessment, and consultation services remotely, improving access to timely and appropriate care.
- **Advocate for policy changes**: Engaging in advocacy efforts to address disparities in EMS agencies at the policy level can help create systemic changes. This may involve advocating for legislation, regulations, and funding to support initiatives aimed at reducing disparities in access to EMS agencies.
- **Improve diversity in the EMS workforce**: An EMS workforce that reflects the racial composition of the populations served influences reducing disparities in care for underserved populations. Focus on recruitment and educational opportunities among historically underrepresented populations.

Addressing disparities in EMS agencies is a complex and multifaceted challenge that requires a comprehensive approach. By implementing strategies such as data-driven interventions, cultural competency training, community engagement, policy changes, resource allocation, and collaborations among various stakeholders, EMS agencies can work towards overcoming disparities and ensuring equitable access to emergency care for all individuals, regardless of their social characteristics or identities. It is crucial to continue advocating for policy changes, promoting health equity in EMS leadership, and leveraging technology to expand access to EMS agencies. Ultimately, addressing disparities in EMS agencies is crucial to promoting health equity, reducing healthcare costs, and improving health outcomes for marginalized and underserved populations.

12

PHYSICIAN MEDICAL DIRECTION

"The art of medicine is long, and life is short." - Hippocrates

PHYSICIAN MEDICAL DIRECTION IN EMERGENCY MEDICAL SERVICES IS a vital element in improving prehospital care for critically ill and injured patients. In the 1960s, the concept of physician medical direction took shape, primarily driven by the need for enhanced care in the prehospital setting. Prior to this period, ambulances were primarily used for transportation purposes, with minimal medical interventions beyond basic first aid. However, with the recognition that early intervention and advanced medical techniques could significantly impact patient outcomes, innovative programs were established to train ambulance attendants in more advanced life support (ALS) techniques. These programs, spearheaded by physicians, paved the way for the development of physician medical direction and the integration of advanced care practices in the field of EMS.

PHYSICIAN DRIVEN FOUNDATIONS

In the late 1950s and early 1960s, a series of groundbreaking programs emerged to address the limitations of prehospital care at the time. For example, Dr. J.D. Farrington started training the Chicago Fire Department on the management of traumatic injuries in 1959. These programs sought to equip ambulance attendants with the necessary skills and knowledge to provide more advanced care to patients in need. Led by physicians who recognized the necessity of early interventions, these initiatives focused on training ambulance attendants in basic life support

(BLS) techniques such as cardiopulmonary resuscitation, the use of oxygen, splinting and bandaging.

The implementation of these early programs represented a significant shift in the approach to prehospital care. By training ambulance attendants in BLS, the aim was to provide immediate, life-saving interventions to patients before they reached the hospital. Recognizing the critical role that physicians played in shaping these programs, physician medical direction began to emerge as a fundamental aspect of EMS.

As these initial programs progressed, it became increasingly evident that more advanced care was necessary to further improve patient outcomes in the prehospital setting. In the late 1960s and early 1970s, pilot projects were established with the goal of training ambulance attendants as paramedics, introducing the concept of Advanced Life Support (ALS) . These projects aimed to provide paramedics with additional training in advanced procedures such as intravenous therapy, intubation, cardiac defibrillation, and medication administration.

The Freedom House Ambulance Service, established in Pittsburgh, Pennsylvania, in 1967 by Dr. Peter Safar and members of the African American community, was another notable pilot project. This service, operating under physician supervision, provided ALS care, including medication administration and advanced airway management. With a remarkable response time of under ten minutes, the Freedom House Ambulance Service achieved outstanding survival rates for patients experiencing cardiac arrest. This project demonstrated the effectiveness of physician medical direction in underserved communities and emphasized the importance of equitable access to high-quality prehospital care.

In Miami, Florida, the "Dade County Experiment" began in 1969. At a 1964 meeting of the International Rescue and First Aid Association, Dr. Eugene Nagel met rescue officers who told him that despite CPR, the patients were dying. While some hospitals were experimenting with physicians on ambulances, Nagel knew that was not a reasonable or sustainable model. He proposed a new model: training Miami-Dade fire fighters to deliver ALS care, including advanced airway management, IV therapy, and drug administration. The success of this project demonstrated that non-physicians could provide high quality advanced life support care in the prehospital setting.

Similarly, the "Paramedic Program" in Los Angeles, California, served as another pioneering model for EMS systems across the United States. This collaboration between the Los Angeles County Fire Department and the UCLA School of Medicine trained paramedics in ALS techniques, including advanced airway management, defibrillation, and drug administration. The success of the program further solidified the importance of physician medical direction in ensuring the delivery of high-quality care in the prehospital environment.

Seattle, Washington, introduced the "Medic One" program in 1974, emphasizing rapid response, advanced training, and close medical oversight. Under the guidance of a physician medical director, fire fighters were trained to provide ALS care. The program showcased a high success rate in resuscitating patients suffering from cardiac arrest, highlighting the impact of physician medical direction in improving outcomes for critical emergencies.

Other notable pilot projects of the 1970s, such as those in Columbus, Ohio, and Memphis, Tennessee, aimed to provide ALS care under the guidance of physician medical directors. These initiatives further contributed to the growing recognition of the critical role played by physicians in shaping and leading prehospital care.

The early paramedic pilot projects of the 1960s and 1970s showcased the immense potential of paramedics in improving patient outcomes in the prehospital setting. These pioneering initiatives paved the way for the establishment of physician medical direction as an essential component of modern EMS systems.

Today, physician medical directors are integral to EMS systems, providing oversight, guidance, and supervision to ensure that patients receive appropriate and high-quality medical care in the prehospital setting. They play a pivotal role in the development and implementation of evidence-based protocols, medical supervision and guidance for EMS practitioners, and ensuring that providers receive the necessary education and training. Physician medical directors also offer real-time clinical support to EMS practitioners, assisting in critical decision-making during complex patient care situations.

The concept of physician medical direction emerged in response to the need for improved prehospital care. The early paramedic pilot projects of the 1960s and 1970s, led by physicians, laid the foundation for the integration of advanced life support techniques into EMS systems. Physician medical directors are now an indispensable component of modern EMS systems, driving advancements in prehospital care and ensuring the delivery of safe, effective, and timely medical care to patients in need.

Role of Physician Medical Directors in Modern EMS

Physician medical directors play a crucial and multifaceted role in modern Emergency Medical Services. Their expertise and oversight are essential in ensuring the delivery of safe, effective, and timely medical care in the prehospital setting. This section explores the various responsibilities and contributions of physician medical directors in EMS, highlighting their impact on protocol development, medical oversight, education and training, clinical support, collaborative relationships, research and innovation, credentialing and evaluation, policy and advocacy, and disaster preparedness and response.

- **Protocol Development**: One of the key responsibilities of physician medical directors is the development and implementation of evidence-based protocols and guidelines for prehospital care. These protocols outline the appropriate care and treatment that EMS practitioners should provide to patients in various medical, traumatic, and behavioral emergencies. By establishing standardized protocols, medical directors ensure consistency in care delivery, promote best practices, and optimize patient outcomes.

- **Medical Oversight**: Medical directors provide ongoing supervision and guidance to EMS practitioners, ensuring that patient care meets established standards and protocols. They review patient care records, provide feedback to providers, and address any clinical concerns or questions. This continuous oversight ensures quality assurance for the EMS service and providers, identifies areas for training and improvement, and facilitates the provision of high-quality care in real-world scenarios.

- **Education and Training**: Physician medical directors are responsible for ensuring that EMS practitioners receive appropriate education and training to maintain their competency and skills. They are an essential leader in coordinating regular training sessions, workshops, and continuing education programs to update providers on the latest medical advancements, protocols, and guidelines. By promoting lifelong learning, medical directors enhance the knowledge and expertise of EMS practitioners, thereby improving patient care outcomes.

- **Clinical Support**: Physician medical directors provide vital clinical support to EMS practitioners in real-time. This support is in the form of phone consultations, online medical control, or on-scene assistance during complex patient care situations. Medical directors assist providers in making critical decisions related to medical interventions, transport decisions, and destination choices. Their timely and expert guidance enhances patient care quality and helps optimize outcomes.

- **Collaborative Relationships**: Medical directors work closely with EMS agencies, hospitals, and other healthcare providers to establish collaborative relationships and ensure seamless transitions of care. They participate in regional and state-level EMS committees, coordinate with local healthcare systems, and engage in multi-agency training exercises. By fostering collaborative relationships, medical directors facilitate care coordination, promote effective communication, and improve overall patient care continuity.

- **Research and Innovation**: Medical directors contribute to the advancement of prehospital care by promoting research efforts and implementing innovative care models within their EMS systems. They stay informed about the latest research, best practices, and technological developments in emergency medicine. By integrating research findings and innovative approaches into practice, medical directors improve patient outcomes and drive the evolution of EMS systems.

- **Credentialing and Evaluation**: Physician medical directors are responsible for the local credentialing and evaluation of the clinical proficiency of EMS practitioners within their agencies. Many are involved in the hiring process for new personnel, ensuring that providers meet the necessary licensure and certification requirements. Medical directors also conduct regular evaluations of provider performance and competency, ensuring that EMS personnel deliver care at the highest professional standards.

- **Policy and Advocacy**: Medical directors serve as advocates for their EMS agencies, promoting the importance of prehospital care and working to influence policy decisions that affect EMS systems. They may participate in legislative efforts, engage with community stakeholders, and represent the interests of their agencies at local, regional, and national levels. By advocating for EMS resources and policy changes, medical directors help shape the future of prehospital care delivery. Many medical directors are actively engaged with the National Association of EMS Physicians (NAEMSP), while medical directors involved in state regulatory leadership are members of the National Association of State EMS Officials (NASEMSO).
- **Disaster Preparedness and Response**: Medical directors play an essential role in disaster preparedness and response planning for their EMS agencies. They collaborate with other emergency response organizations, develop, and implement disaster response plans, and ensure that EMS practitioners are adequately trained and prepared to respond to large-scale emergencies and mass casualty incidents. Medical directors' expertise in coordinating resources, triaging patients, and managing complex medical scenarios during disasters is critical in ensuring an effective and efficient response.

The multifaceted responsibilities of physician medical directors highlight their pivotal role in shaping and leading EMS systems. Their expertise and oversight contribute to the development and maintenance of EMS protocols, quality improvement programs, and patient care standards. Through their involvement in protocol development, medical directors ensure that EMS practitioners adhere to evidence-based practices, promoting standardized and optimal care delivery.

BOARD CERTIFICATION FOR EMS PHYSICIANS

The development of EMS physician as a recognized subspecialty within the field of emergency medicine marks a significant advancement in prehospital care. The recognition of EMS physicians as a distinct subspecialty has brought formal recognition to their specialized training, expertise, and contributions to prehospital care. The emergence of professional organizations dedicated to advancing EMS played a crucial role in the recognition of EMS physician as a subspecialty. The American College of Emergency Physicians (ACEP) established an EMS Section within its section membership program, providing a platform for EMS physicians to collaborate, share knowledge, and advocate for the recognition of their unique expertise. This organizational support helped raise awareness about the specialized role of EMS physicians and their contributions to prehospital care.

To formalize the specialized training and expertise of EMS physicians, formal board certification followed. In 2010, following a joint effort by NAEMSP, ACEP, ABEM, and SAEM, the American Board of Medical Specialties (ABMS) formally recognized EMS as a physician subspecialty of emergency medicine.

In 2013, the American Board of Emergency Medicine (ABEM) administered the first EMS subspecialty certification examination, with eligibility built around completion of an accredited EMS fellowship. Board certification in EMS signifies advanced knowledge, expertise, and commitment to the field of EMS.

The path to becoming an EMS physician involves specialized training and education. Physicians typically complete a residency in emergency medicine and then pursue additional specialized training in EMS through a formal fellowship program. The fellowship program provides advanced training in the unique aspects of prehospital care, including medical oversight, field management, disaster and mass casualty management, and EMS system administration. This specialized training equips EMS physicians with the skills and knowledge necessary to excel in the dynamic and challenging prehospital environment.

Board Certified EMS physicians bring specialized medical expertise to the field, enabling them to provide comprehensive medical oversight and leadership. Their advanced knowledge and skills in critical care, resuscitation, trauma management, and disaster response enhance decision-making and improve patient outcomes.

One of the key contributions of EMS physicians is their involvement in the development and implementation of evidence-based protocols and guidelines for prehospital care. Drawing on their expertise, EMS physicians ensure that EMS practitioners adhere to standardized practices and deliver optimal care to patients in various medical, traumatic, and behavioral emergencies. This standardization promotes consistency and quality in prehospital care delivery, improving patient outcomes.

EMS physicians also play a crucial role in quality improvement programs and research efforts. Their involvement in these initiatives contributes to the ongoing advancement of prehospital care standards and practices. By participating in research studies, EMS physicians generate new knowledge and insights that can further enhance the care provided in the prehospital setting.

Moreover, EMS physicians serve as valuable liaisons between prehospital care and hospital-based medicine. Their involvement in collaborative relationships with EMS agencies, hospitals, and other healthcare providers helps facilitate seamless transitions of care and improve overall patient management. By advocating for adequate resources and policy changes, EMS physicians contribute to the improvement of EMS infrastructure and the delivery of high-quality care to patients in need.

The development of EMS as a recognized subspecialty has brought formal recognition to the specialized training, expertise, and contributions of EMS physicians to prehospital care. Through the establishment of professional organizations, certification programs, and specialized training, EMS physicians have gained recognition for their unique role in the field. Their advanced knowledge, leadership, and commitment to prehospital care have contributed to improved patient outcomes and the ongoing advancement of emergency medical services.

13

EMS SYSTEM FINANCE

"If providing ambulance services does not prove to be economically feasible, not only will there be poor service, but there may be none at all." (November 1975)[94]
- Howard Mitchell, MD, MPH[a]

ADDRESSING THE FINANCIAL ASPECTS OF EMERGENCY MEDICAL SERVICES systems in the United States is a multifaceted endeavor, engaging a variety of stakeholders and demanding astute decision-making. This issue, notably complex, has remained unresolved since the establishment of modern EMS in the United States. Sustainable and adequate funding for EMS agencies is a cornerstone to ensuring the continuity and quality of EMS services.

These agencies, however, face an uphill financial battle due to the escalating costs of equipment, education, training, and personnel, compounded by limitations on reimbursement from insurance providers. Rural EMS agencies confront a unique set of financial constraints, given their lower call volumes, extended response times, and elevated operational costs. This chapter delves into the nuanced landscape of EMS system financing in the United States, presenting the challenges and considerations involved in formulating a financially sustainable model for national EMS.

Despite the longstanding financial sustainability challenges, EMS has displayed an exceptional resilience not typically seen in other medical professions or public services, such as police departments or waste management services. To illustrate, community fundraising events, like bake sales, are a common source of funding for EMS, while they are virtually unheard of for

---

[a] Dr. Mitchell was the Chief of the Bureau of Occupational Health, State Department of Public Health, Berkeley, California.

fueling police cars or garbage trucks. This reflects the EMS's knack for leveraging public goodwill and ingenuity in their ongoing survival efforts.

This ability of the EMS to consistently devise immediate solutions to pressing problems is admirable. However, it also obfuscates the larger, systemic issue - the development of sustainable financial models for EMS. This urgent challenge, deferred for decades, is the root problem that needs addressing to secure the future of EMS agencies. For EMS managers, leaders, policy makers, and state officials, it's a crucial task that needs immediate attention and decisive action.

HISTORICAL ROOTS: A SYSTEM WITHOUT SUSTAINABLE FUNDING

The current financial struggles persisting within EMS agencies have significant historical underpinnings. Even as far back as 1975, publications highlighting the economics of rural ambulance services recognized "rising labor and equipment costs"[95] as a concern. Tracing back to the early evolution of EMS agencies, these financial difficulties have endured, becoming entangled with the nation's shifting healthcare financing terrain.

As covered in more detail in previous chapters, the genesis of modern EMS was a direct answer to the escalating number of automobile accidents. This rise necessitated immediate pre-hospital care, particularly in rural America. Initially, ambulance services were largely provided by funeral homes, volunteers, and fire departments, all of which generally lacked structured training, established physician oversight, or standards for equipment. However, the purpose of EMS quickly transitioned from focusing mainly on providing trauma care for rural automobile crash victims, to also addressing urban medical emergencies. Over time, the EMS system grew to include trained paramedics, specialized vehicles, and advanced life-support equipment. Yet, the financial infrastructure intended to underpin these expanding services struggled to align with the escalating demand and growing complexity of the care provided, perpetuating a struggle for financial stability.

A key historical factor contributing to underfunding was the *EMS Systems Act* of 1973. The Act outlined 15 EMS system components, from Regulation and Medical Direction to Patient Care and Public Education. However, it notably omitted a component for long-term, sustainable funding. Historical records suggest that while this issue was acknowledged, it was expected and assumed that state and local governments would eventually find a solution.

The 1976 DHEW report, *Progress, But Problems In Developing EMS Systems,* highlights the concern to Congress, but no solutions are offered:

> "Regional (EMS agencies) are having difficulty finding permanent financing for the administrative and operating costs…consequently, **when Federal funding stops, continuation of regional systems providing services will not be assured**."[96]

This disjointed structure of the EMS system in the United States further exacerbates the issue. Initially, ambulance services emerged as localized pilots to cater to specific community needs and services were provided by a diverse group of public and private organizations. This fragmentation has posed significant challenges in creating a unified funding model capable of serving all EMS practitioners' needs. Moreover, during the early days of EMS System development, the conflicting requirements (DOT vs DHEW) resulted in varied EMS system designs and implementations state-to-state.

The evolving landscape of healthcare financing in the United States has further contributed to the underfunding dilemma. The rise of managed care and a growing focus on cost containment have profoundly affected EMS agencies. Insurance providers' efforts to curb costs often result in limited reimbursements and stringent utilization management policies, frequently leading to insufficient compensation for EMS agencies. This, in turn, creates financial stress and, in certain instances, service closures.

Adding to these complexities, EMS agencies are grappling with escalating costs. Innovations in medical technology, rising pharmaceutical prices, and the increasing burden of regulatory requirements all contribute to augmented expenses. Concurrently, a persistent shortage of qualified EMS personnel exacerbates labor costs, as agencies vie for skilled workers. These mounting costs have outpaced the growth of funding sources, adding further strain to the financial viability of EMS agencies.

The persistence of outdated funding models also contributes to some EMS agencies' financial distress. For years, many agencies have heavily relied on local tax revenues and federal grants, which are subject to fluctuations and offer no guarantee of a stable funding base. The prevailing fee-for-service reimbursement model, typically seen as a transportation benefit rather than medical service, further complicates the issue by prioritizing high service volume over efficiency or care quality.

Traditional, transport-based reimbursement models also fall short as they link EMS care directly to ambulance transportation. This ties payment to transport, creating a systemic bias that "everyone gets transported" to an acute care hospital, when many patient conditions could be more effectively managed in other settings, such as at home, clinics, urgent care centers, outpatient mental health facilities, and others.

Recent years have seen external factors, such as the opioid crisis and the COVID-19 pandemic, magnify these financial challenges. These public health emergencies have heightened the demand for EMS agencies, straining resources and exacerbating many agencies' already fragile financial standing.

Further complicating matters, many EMS systems have recently grappled with prolonged Ambulance Patient Offload Times (APOT) at hospital emergency departments. These extended APOT present not only operational and clinical challenges but also pose significant financial issues for EMS systems. Extended APOT result in decreased unit hour utilization (UHU), inflated EMS staffing costs, and often lead to substantial response time penalties in many performance-based systems.

Moreover, the unintentional provision of "free" EMS labor, required to care for patients inside the hospital after ED arrival but before hospital staff assume direct care, in effect, amounts to a coerced subsidy in many systems from EMS agencies to hospitals. Current EMS reimbursement rates do not account for these additional costs, leading to significant financial sustainability concerns for many EMS systems across the nation.

The underfunding and financial instability in EMS agencies can be traced back to early development, inherent system fragmentation, an evolving healthcare financing landscape, and the continued reliance on antiquated funding models. It is imperative to address these historical factors and construct a sustainable financing model to ensure the delivery of quality care nationwide, honoring the original intent of the *EMS Systems Act* of 1973.

Challenges Facing EMS System Financing

EMS agencies face a considerable hurdle of funding limitations, highlighting the critical need for astute financial resource management. Many of these agencies find themselves maneuvering through a mosaic of funding avenues, ranging from local tax revenues and federal grants to insurance reimbursements. Regrettably, these sources often provide inconsistent, inadequate, and unpredictable funding. This unpredictability fosters financial instability and complicates the maintenance of essential personnel, equipment, and infrastructure.

The complexities of reimbursement rates intensify these difficulties. The variability in these rates adds another layer of complexity to procuring proper reimbursement for EMS agencies, potentially creating financial strain, and exposing funding deficits.

Another significant facet of the financial challenges facing EMS is the burden of uncompensated care. The requirement for ambulances to provide care, regardless of a patient's ability to pay, culminates in considerable uncompensated care costs. While ethically justifiable, these costs can place a disproportionate burden on EMS agencies, especially those serving vulnerable populations, potentially endangering their sustainability. Moreover, Medicaid, which covers a vast segment of America's economically disadvantaged population, reimburses ambulance services at rates significantly below the cost-of-service provision. In areas with high numbers of Medicaid beneficiaries, this situation amplifies the financial challenges for many EMS systems, frequently necessitating local subsidies to maintain their operation.

Recent data highlight the magnitude of these challenges. According to an April 2023 report by the Colorado Department of Public Health and Environment,[97] 50% of the 185 licensed ground ambulance agencies in Colorado answer fewer than 603 service calls annually. Similarly, a 2023 report from the State of Maine[98] showed that 77% of ground ambulance services responded to fewer than 1,000 calls per year.

Regardless of their call volume, EMS agencies must maintain the requisite staffing and equipment to ensure uninterrupted, 24/7 ambulance response. Services must be geographically dispersed to respond to calls promptly, leading to the so-called "cost of readiness." When using call volume as a metric to calculate the "cost-per-call," an EMS service with a low call volume will inherently bear a higher cost-per-call, as the fixed operational costs of an EMS service are distributed across fewer transported patients.

These challenges are especially pronounced in rural and remote areas, where factors such as low population density, extended response times, and transportation obstacles can heighten financial pressures. This amalgamation of complex challenges underscores the importance of crafting a sustainable financial model for EMS agencies, a task of paramount importance for EMS leaders, policymakers, and state officials.

Societal and Political Questions

Financing the EMS system transcends the quest for diversified funding sources, mandating the need to tackle pivotal societal and political matters. Communities are tasked with discerning the magnitude of EMS agencies they regard as indispensable and devising strategies to fund them. Such decisions might entail re-evaluating community priorities and weighing various factors, including the size of the community, population density, and availability of local resources.

At the state and national levels, discussions often pivot around the theme of equity. Questions emerge about whether rural communities should be afforded the same access to EMS as urban communities. Policymakers are thus charged with determining how communities will have reliable access to EMS, and deciding if the level of service should be Basic Life Support or Advanced Life Support. These deliberations shed light on the convoluted nature of EMS financing, underscoring the demand for a holistic strategy that considers a multitude of factors and engages all stakeholders.

One essential component of EMS system financing involves deciding the extent to which the government should underwrite EMS infrastructure. This involves considering factors such as the level of service offered, the financial prowess of local governments, and the potential for synergies among various levels of government. Policymakers face the delicate task of offsetting the advantages of increased government funding against competing public priorities and fiscal constraints.

One must note, however, that while the EMS industry acknowledges these complexities, there is often a lack of awareness and understanding among community members and elected officials. The assumption prevails that a call to 911 will promptly summon an ambulance complete with a team of professional paramedics. In many communities, despite years of financial constraints, this assumption holds true. Yet, this situation underscores the importance of enhancing awareness and fostering a deeper understanding of EMS financing challenges among all community stakeholders to ensure the long-term sustainability of these vital services.

Balancing the Scales: Subsidies and the EMS System

EMS agencies are an integral part of our nation's healthcare system. Yet, the financial models supporting them often fall short of meeting the true costs of providing these essential services. The discrepancy between an EMS service's cost-per-call and the reimbursement received must be bridged through various forms of subsidies. The current landscape of subsidies is diverse and complex, with no two EMS agencies in the United States adopting the exact same model. Subsidies may come from taxpayer support, municipal contributions, commercial payers, philanthropy, and grants. However, one of the most significant, yet often overlooked, subsidies that underpins EMS is the contribution of volunteer and underpaid labor.

A case in point is the State of Maine, where EMS agencies have long been built on the foundations of volunteerism and community service. While this spirit of community service remains vital, it is not a reliable solution to the central sustainability challenges facing the EMS system. A decline in volunteerism, coupled with a dependence on an underpaid workforce, hampers recruitment and retention. This situation necessitates a greater reliance on other subsidies, thereby increasing costs to local municipalities and taxpayers. Furthermore, the decline in volunteerism has shed light on the true cost of EMS, a revelation that has left many communities grappling with the reality of providing these services locally.

According to data from Maine, absent a subsidy, transporting EMS agencies cannot break even in the state, regardless of service mix. This scenario extends to the national EMS system, where all transporting EMS agencies are currently operating at a loss. A high-efficiency service, registering 1,800 transports per year, would need a subsidy of approximately $322 per transport to break even. Meanwhile, a more rural, low-volume service, with 300 transports per year, would require a subsidy of $2,030 per transport. Current subsidies, without additional state assistance, are insufficient to meet the existing need for transporting EMS agencies.

EMS, perceived as an essential public service, is situated at the intersection of public health care programs, health care providers, and the low-income, uninsured population with unmet medical needs – a triad often referred to as the healthcare safety net. Unfortunately, EMS is often excluded from this safety net due to the lack of effective federal and state leadership and sustainable funding strategies. The current system guarantees universal access to EMS without a universal funding system in place, delivering services regardless of the patient's insurance status or ability to pay.

EMS relies heavily on reimbursements from third-party payers, but these are usually contingent on patient transportation. This poses a significant challenge as nearly half of ambulance providers report that local or state government entities set the rates charged to patients. National estimates of the percentage of patients transported within each major healthcare payer category demonstrate the reliance on a wide array of payers and the challenges posed by uncompensated and undercompensated care.

The 2016 National EMS Advisory Council[99] estimates the current magnitude of uncompensated care delivered by the nation's ground ambulance services to be a staggering $2.9 billion annually. This stark reality poses a significant threat to the financial stability of the entire EMS safety net.

Thus, the systematic cost of providing emergency ambulance services in the U.S. overshadows currently available revenue. This imbalance is addressed in two ways: increasing reimbursement or subsidies or decreasing costs. Given the fixed costs required to provide a clinically acceptable level of service, cutting spending would result in a direct negative impact on the quality of care provided. Consequently, the focus must be on developing comprehensive and sustainable solutions that increase financial support to EMS systems without compromising the quality of care provided.

NEMSAC RECOMMENDATIONS

In 2016, the National EMS Advisory Council made a series of astute observations and recommendations, acknowledging the intersectional nature of EMS and suggesting how this should inform its funding. A summary of some of NEMSAC's recommendations and conclusions included:

- EMS operates at the confluence of healthcare, public health, public safety, and emergency medical preparedness systems. Yet, EMS funding is usually solely dependent on healthcare user fees, leading to chronic underfunding. Therefore, all these intersecting fields need to recognize the value which EMS contributes to their individual missions and assume responsibility to provide appropriate financial support.

- The public expectation is round-the-clock, high-quality EMS response. In many communities, EMS is the sole health care safety net service. Yet, most policymakers do not consider EMS as an essential service, contributing to chronic underfunding. Therefore, EMS should be recognized as an essential service, with all stakeholders working towards establishing sustainable funding mechanisms. (Note, by 2023, only 11 states had passed legislation designating EMS as an essential service, and few states had funded EMS as an essential service.)

- Emergency services must be available 24/7. However, ambulance reimbursement is curtailed by the healthcare system's medical necessity rules. Hence, ambulance response reimbursement should be based on the prudent layperson standard and not restricted or reduced based on retrospective medical necessity reviews.

- To fully realize improved patient outcomes, efficiencies, and patient satisfaction, EMS must be integrated into the broader health care system. Funding mechanisms should account for the crucial role of EMS in producing these benefits.

- As the community healthcare safety net, EMS provides services regardless of the patient's ability to pay. Federal regulations should not be used as a reason to reduce EMS reimbursement rates as any reduction in service could negatively impact patient outcomes.

- New service delivery models such as community paramedicine and mobile integrated healthcare have shown promising results. These models should be encouraged, funded, and expanded. A shared savings model could help fund these initiatives, assessing total downstream health care savings produced by these programs.

- The federal government should support local, state, and federal policy efforts to ensure the financial stability and improved performance of all EMS functions. The EMS industry should collaborate and adopt position statements regarding all the following:
    - Improved coordination among all EMS functions.

- Optimized economies of scale, system efficiencies, and standards of care through regionalized planning activities.
- Sponsor stakeholder processes to establish local EMS System performance standards.
- Ensuring commensurate government funding from each respective discipline.
- Rational reimbursement mechanisms for EMS response, care, and transport.
- State laws requiring reimbursement for emergency medical services to be remitted directly to EMS practitioners.

The NEMSAC recommendations, which follow similar logical conclusions that have been expressed for decades, outline a path whereby the EMS industry can strive for sustainable, fair, and comprehensive funding solutions. These steps will, in turn, fortify EMS agencies nationwide, ensuring they can continue to provide indispensable, life-saving services to communities across the country.

In addition to the NEMSAC recommendations, a crucial step in ensuring EMS system sustainability is to reengineer system design where possible. For instance, systems with extended Ambulance Patient Offload Times (APOT) can adopt approaches that reduce unnecessary Emergency Department (ED) transports, such as telehealth and treatment without transport. Even if payers do not separately cover these modalities, avoiding unsustainable costs associated with extended APOT could prove advantageous. Similarly, systems with high utilization for mental health or substance abuse patients could benefit from exploring transport to non-hospital destinations. This approach would give these patients access to healthcare and social services that can more effectively manage their conditions.

The economic sustainability of EMS systems directly correlates to how those systems are structured and the service modalities they provide. EMS systems are obligated to continuously assess their communities' needs and meet these needs through a variety of services and deployment models. Where regulatory barriers to these emerging models exist, regulatory authorities should work to incorporate flexibilities to allow local EMS systems to adapt and meet these evolving needs.

There are multiple strategies that should be employed to address the challenges facing EMS financing and ensure the sustainability of EMS systems. While some of these strategies will require significant investments, they are critical to maintaining the ability of EMS systems to provide lifesaving services to communities across the country. The goal should be to create a financially stable, resilient, and efficient EMS system that can adapt to changing community needs and healthcare landscapes.

14

ECONOMICS OF PROVIDING EMS

" The economic problems can be summarized briefly by noting that rural ambulance finances are hampered by there being too few patients or population at risk to support even one ambulance, and that urban ambulance finances are a problem frequently because there may be too many companies in competition to provide any single one with an adequate economic base of operation. Add to this the additional burden and economic waste inherent in excessively frequent turnover of personnel which is due primarily to very low wages, but which then leads to further costs for constant rehiring and retraining of ambulance personnel."

- Howard W. Mitchell, MD, as written in 1965 in the American Journal of Public Health [100]

THE ECONOMICS OF PROVIDING EMERGENCY MEDICAL SERVICES IN the United States is a long-standing, intricate problem that has perplexed EMS stakeholders since the dawn of the modern EMS model in the 1970s. Historically, funding and economic issues have often challenged EMS agencies, with the lack of comprehensive solutions persisting across decades. This predicament is acutely evident in seminal reports from the era, like the 1975 National Highway Traffic Safety Administration (NHTSA) commissioned report on the Economics of Rural EMS, which shockingly recounts that EMS was financially insolvent even when funeral homes were offering the services:

> "In 1969, 221 funeral home businesses provided ambulance service in Oklahoma; by 1973, the number had declined to 124, a 44 percent decrease. Faced with rising labor and equipment costs, funeral home operators chose to discontinue the service." [101]

Similarly, the 1976 Department of Health, Education, and Welfare (DHEW) report titled "*Progress, But Problems*" highlights persistent challenges associated with local governments funding EMS agencies. Despite the passage of time, many of the same unresolved issues continue to underscore the economics of EMS, making the following aspects crucial when analyzing the financial dimensions of providing these services:

- **Funding Sources:** Historically, EMS agencies have been financed through an amalgamation of sources, such as fees for ambulance transportation and services, taxes, grants, and donations. However, the sufficiency of these sources has remained a contentious issue, requiring ongoing evaluation and innovation in funding approaches.

- **Reimbursement Challenges:** These difficulties, which encompass low reimbursement rates from insurance providers and challenges in collecting fees from patients, were present in the early years of EMS and continue to pose financial challenges to EMS practitioners today.

- **Operational Costs:** The escalating costs associated with maintaining and operating ambulances, equipment, facilities, and personnel have been a longstanding concern for EMS agencies, exemplified by the declining number of funeral home businesses providing ambulance service in the 1970s.

- **Rural and Remote Challenges:** Geographic disparities have always posed unique challenges to EMS agencies, impacting both the economics and delivery of prehospital care. The struggle to find economic solutions for these areas continues to be a critical issue.

- **Volunteerism and Recruitment:** As with the 1970s, volunteer-based EMS agencies remain essential in many communities, but a decline in volunteerism due to various factors, such as demographic changes, increased training requirements, and time commitments, exacerbates the economic challenges of EMS agencies.

- **Economic Impact of EMS:** Despite the economic struggles, it's important to remember that EMS agencies have continually contributed to the economy, creating jobs, supporting local businesses, and providing vital healthcare services.

- **Technology and Innovation:** With the advent of new technologies and strategies over the years, the potential for improved patient outcomes and cost efficiencies has increased. However, the implementation of these advancements often requires substantial investment, presenting an economic conundrum.

- **Regulatory Environment:** EMS agencies continue to navigate a complex regulatory landscape, which can impact their economic sustainability. Policies related to licensing, certification, accreditation, reimbursement, and insurance coverage significantly influence the costs and financial viability of EMS agencies.

- **Emergency Preparedness:** EMS agencies' critical role in preparing for and responding to emergencies has always had significant economic implications, influencing the demand for services, necessitating additional training and equipment, and potentially disrupting funding and reimbursement.

Navigating the complex economics of providing Emergency Medical Services in the United States necessitates understanding a multitude of interconnected aspects, including funding sources, reimbursement issues, operational costs, geographic disparities, volunteerism, and regulatory frameworks. A thorough understanding of these components is vital for ensuring the sustainability and effectiveness of EMS agencies, as well as informing policy decisions regarding EMS funding, reimbursement, workforce development, and emergency preparedness. By recognizing and addressing these key factors, stakeholders can collaborate to devise and implement strategies that tackle the distinct economic challenges faced by EMS practitioners, and in doing so, support the continuous delivery of high-quality prehospital care to communities across the United States.

Financial Challenges and Strategies for EMS Sustainability

EMS agencies operating in both urban and rural settings encounter financial challenges that require strategies to ensure their sustainability. These challenges arise from the evolving landscape of EMS service provision, the impact of payer mix, and the imperative to strike a balance between cost management and delivering quality care.

Readiness Costs

Readiness costs are the expenses incurred by EMS organizations to ensure that they are prepared and equipped to respond to emergency calls and provide timely and effective care. These costs can include personnel salaries, training, equipment maintenance, vehicle depreciation, and other operational expenses.

Urban EMS organizations, with their high call volumes and dense populations, often face increased readiness costs due to the need for more personnel, vehicles, and equipment. In contrast, rural and frontier EMS organizations may have lower call volumes but face unique challenges, such as longer response times and limited access to resources.

Formula: Readiness Cost = Personnel Salaries + Training + Equipment Maintenance + Vehicle Depreciation + Other Operational Expenses

---

EMS organizations must carefully manage their readiness costs and seek additional sources of funding, such as government subsidies, grants, or community support, to ensure their financial sustainability. Strategies may differ between urban and rural settings, but the goal remains the same: to provide quality care while maintaining financial stability.

First Dollar Insurance Coverage and Payer Mix

First dollar insurance coverage is a type of insurance policy that provides the insured reimbursement for medical expenses from the first dollar spent, without any deductible or copayment requirements. This type of coverage can have a significant impact on EMS billing, as it may result in higher reimbursement rates and reduced financial burdens on patients.

The payer mix refers to the proportion of revenues from different sources, such as Medicare, Medicaid, private insurance, and self-pay patients. A diverse payer mix can help insulate EMS organizations from fluctuations in reimbursement rates or changes in policy. However, a payer mix heavily reliant on government payers, such as Medicare and Medicaid, may face financial challenges due to relatively low reimbursement rates and stringent regulations.

National EMS Payer Mix[102]	
Medicare	44%
Commercial / Private Insurance	21%
Private Pay	14%
Medicaid	14%
Other	7%

Formula: Payer Mix =
(Revenue from each Payer Source / Total Revenue) x 100%

EMS organizations in both urban and rural settings should be aware of the potential implications of shifts in insurance coverage and payer mix and develop strategies to adapt their billing practices accordingly.

Unit Hour Utilization

Unit Hour Utilization (UHU) is a performance metric commonly used in the EMS industry to measure the efficiency of resource utilization. UHU is calculated by dividing the total number of ambulance transports by the total number of unit hours (the time an ambulance is available for service).

Formula: UHU = Total Ambulance Transports / Total Unit Hours

While there is not a consensus on UHU thresholds, most agencies that respond to emergency calls target a UHU not exceeding 0.50 (50%). A higher UHU indicates a more efficient use of resources, as it implies that the EMS organization is maximizing the productivity of its personnel and vehicles. However, a higher UHU can also result in increased wear and tear on equipment, higher personnel stress levels, and potential compromises in patient care.

Urban EMS organizations, with their high call volumes and dense populations, may naturally have higher UHU values compared to rural and frontier EMS organizations, which may have lower call volumes but face unique challenges such as longer response times and limited resources.

EMS leaders should closely monitor their UHU and strive to strike a balance between efficiency and quality care. This may involve adjusting staffing levels, re-evaluating deployment strategies, or investing in technology to improve dispatch and response processes.

Cost Per Call

Cost per call is a financial metric used to evaluate the efficiency of EMS operations, calculated by dividing the total operational costs by the total number of calls responded to during a specific period. This metric can help EMS leaders identify areas of inefficiency and develop strategies to improve operational performance.

Formula: Cost Per Call =
Total Operational Costs / Total Number of Calls

By monitoring and optimizing their cost per call, EMS organizations can enhance their financial sustainability and ensure that they are providing value for the resources invested. This may involve streamlining operations, reducing waste, or implementing innovative service delivery models that better meet the needs of their communities.

Urban EMS organizations, with higher call volumes, naturally have a lower cost per call due to economies of scale. In contrast, rural and frontier EMS organizations, with lower call volumes, generally have a significantly higher cost per call due to the unique challenges they face, such as longer response times and limited access to resources.

EMS organizations in both urban and rural settings face numerous financial challenges that can impact their ability to provide quality care and maintain financial sustainability. By understanding these challenges and implementing targeted strategies to address them, EMS leaders and managers can ensure the long-term viability of their organizations, ultimately benefiting the communities they serve.

THE IMPACT OF PAYER MIX ON EMS REVENUE AND SUSTAINABILITY

The concept of payer mix, comprising the proportion of an EMS organization's revenue from different sources such as Medicare, Medicaid, commercial / private insurance, and self-pay patients, exerts a significant impact on EMS revenue and sustainability. This concept is especially critical as reimbursement rates and collection rates vary among these payer types.

In more urban settings, EMS organizations typically have a diverse payer mix, often with a higher proportion of patients covered by private insurance. This insurance often provides higher reimbursement rates than government-funded insurance programs like Medicare and Medicaid, contributing to the financial stability of these organizations. In contrast, rural and frontier EMS organizations may have a payer mix with a higher proportion of patients covered by government-funded insurance programs or who are uninsured. These payer sources usually provide lower reimbursement rates or have higher rates of nonpayment, which can create significant financial challenges for rural EMS organizations.

As per national estimates, the payer mix includes 44% of patients covered by Medicare, 14% by Medicaid, 14% as private pay, 21% by commercial/private insurance, and 7% from other categories.[103] These percentages highlight the varied payer mix and its implications for EMS organizations.

Given that Medicare ambulance reimbursement rates are, on average, 6% below the cost per transport, and Medicaid rates in roughly half of all states cover only half the cost of service, this poses significant challenges for EMS sustainability.[104] Further complicating matters, some state Medicaid rates are so low they cover only one-quarter the cost of service. Thus, payer mix composition directly influences the fiscal health of EMS organizations.

To mitigate the financial challenges associated with payer mix, aspiring EMS leaders and managers can employ strategies including:

- Advocacy efforts to influence reimbursement policies at the federal, state, and local levels, thereby improving reimbursement rates and collection rates for EMS agencies.
- Development of partnerships and collaborations with other healthcare providers, such as hospitals and primary care clinics, to establish integrated care models potentially resulting in more favorable payer mixes.
- Diversification of revenue sources by offering additional services or exploring alternative funding mechanisms, such as grants or community fundraising initiatives.
- Implementation of efficient billing and collection processes to maximize revenue from all payer sources, including ensuring accurate and timely documentation to support billing claims and pursuing collections from self-pay patients.
- Optimization of resource utilization and implementation of cost-saving measures to counterbalance the financial challenges associated with less favorable payer mixes.

Understanding the impact of payer mix on EMS revenue and sustainability is vital for EMS leaders and managers. Through the implementation of these strategies, EMS organizations can navigate payer mix challenges, enhancing their financial stability and sustaining their capacity to deliver high-quality care to their communities.

Readiness Costs and the Impact on EMS Economics

Readiness costs encapsulate the expenses borne by EMS organizations to maintain preparedness and agility in responding to emergency calls and delivering timely, effective care. The remit of these costs includes maintaining a fleet of ambulances, workforce staffing, training, and the necessary medical equipment and supplies. In the grand scheme of EMS operating expenses, readiness costs constitute a significant component, irrespective of the volume of calls or service demand.

The Economics of Readiness Costs

Readiness costs pose a substantial challenge for EMS organizations as these costs are incurred irrespective of call volume or the reimbursement received for the services provided. High readiness costs can exert significant financial strain on EMS organizations, especially those in rural and frontier areas where call volumes tend to be lower, and the per-service cost is often higher.

The financial landscape of EMS becomes increasingly complex when readiness costs must be balanced against other influential factors such as payer mix, reimbursement rates, and resource utilization. This balance is essential to maintaining the financial sustainability of EMS organizations and ensuring their capacity to provide high-quality care.

Adding a layer of complexity, financial modeling conducted independently in Maine and Colorado in 2023 concluded that nearly all EMS agencies are likely to operate at a financial deficit. This is largely because readiness costs surpass the revenue generated, highlighting the crucial need for subsidies in such circumstances.

Balance Billing and its Challenges in EMS

Balance billing refers to billing patients the difference between the provider's retail charge and the amount paid by the insurer. Though retail charges are typically well above the costs of providing services, the amounts paid by insurers are often well below the costs of providing services. The challenge with balance billing laws is finding an appropriate amount for insurers to pay to the providers of services that covers necessary costs but holds patients harmless for excessive balances. Thus far, law and policy have strongly favored insurers in this tug-of-war, leaving many providers with insurance payment amounts that are below the costs of providing the services.

Balance billing is a contentious issue, as it can place a significant financial burden on patients and may be perceived as unfair or inequitable. EMS organizations in both urban and rural settings must carefully consider the ethical and financial implications of balance billing and develop strategies to minimize the negative impact on patients while maintaining financial sustainability.

Formula: Balance Billing Amount =
Total Ambulance Charges - Insurance Coverage

Balance billing in EMS presents several challenges, which are categorized into the following areas:

- **Public perception**: The practice of balance billing may be perceived negatively by patients and the community. This perception can lead to dissatisfaction with the EMS organization and potential damage to its reputation. Many patients may not fully understand the costs associated with EMS agencies, which can further contribute to negative perceptions. Transparency and community education about the costs of EMS agencies can help mitigate these concerns.
- **Financial burden on patients**: Balance billing may place a significant financial burden on patients, particularly those who suffered a catastrophic event and/or with limited or no insurance coverage. This burden can lead to financial hardship for individuals and families and may even deter some individuals from seeking necessary medical care. EMS organizations should be mindful of the financial impact on patients and consider implementing payment plans or charity care policies to alleviate the burden for those in need.
- **Collection issues**: EMS organizations may face difficulties in collecting the outstanding balance from patients, leading to increased administrative costs and potential losses in revenue. Pursuing collections can strain the resources of EMS organizations and may require the assistance of third-party collection agencies, which can further contribute to negative public perception and reduce the net amount recovered. Implementing effective billing and collection strategies is essential for EMS organizations to recover their costs while minimizing the negative impact on patients and the community.
- **Legal and regulatory considerations**: Ground ambulance providers in certain states and jurisdictions already face restrictions or prohibitions on balance billing, constraining EMS organizations' ability to recoup their costs through this practice. Additionally, in 2022, Congress enacted the *No Surprises Act,* which prohibits balance billing by air ambulance services nationwide.[105] Some anticipate this Act may be amended in the future to extend the same prohibition to ground ambulance services. Regulatory restrictions on balance billing can vary, and EMS organizations must ensure compliance with applicable laws and regulations. Advocacy efforts to influence regulatory policies may be necessary to ensure that EMS organizations can recover their costs and maintain financial sustainability.

THE IMPORTANCE OF BALANCE BILLING IN THE ABSENCE OF OTHER FUNDING

Despite the challenges associated with balance billing, it may be a necessary practice for EMS organizations that lack alternative funding sources, such as tax revenue, donations, grants, or community fundraising. Balance billing can help EMS organizations recover the costs of providing services, ensuring their financial sustainability and their ability to continue providing essential emergency care to the community.

In both urban and rural settings, the financial viability of EMS organizations is heavily dependent on their ability to recover costs through billing practices. In high-volume urban areas, EMS organizations face challenges related to high demand, payer mix, and varying insurance coverage levels. These challenges can result in a higher reliance on balance billing to recover costs and maintain operational efficiency. In contrast, low-volume rural and frontier areas may face challenges related to lower call volumes, higher per-call costs, and limited access to alternative funding sources. For these EMS organizations, balance billing may be an even more critical factor in ensuring financial sustainability.

To strike the right balance between the financial needs of EMS organizations and the potential burden on patients, it is essential for EMS leaders and managers to develop transparent billing practices and policies. This can include:

- **Clearly communicating the costs of services to patients and the community**: Educating the public about the costs involved in providing EMS services can help improve understanding and acceptance of balance billing practices.
- **Implementing payment plans or charity care policies**: Offering flexible payment options or financial assistance for those in need can help alleviate the financial burden on patients and ensure access to necessary medical care.
- **Developing effective billing and collection strategies**: Employing efficient billing processes and collection strategies can minimize administrative costs and maximize revenue recovery, while maintaining a positive relationship with the community.
- **Advocating for regulatory policies that support EMS organizations**: Engaging in advocacy efforts to influence regulatory policies can help ensure that EMS organizations can recover their costs through balance billing and maintain financial sustainability.

Balance billing is a complex and often contentious issue in the EMS industry. However, it is a crucial aspect of the financial sustainability of EMS organizations, particularly in the absence of alternative funding sources. By understanding the challenges and implications of balance billing, EMS leaders and managers can develop effective strategies to recover costs while minimizing the impact on patients and the community. This delicate balance is essential for the continued provision of high-quality emergency medical care and the overall viability of EMS organizations.

Cost Per Call and Unit Hour Utilization: Urban vs. Rural Considerations

The concepts of cost per call and unit hour utilization are essential in evaluating the performance and financial sustainability of EMS organizations. Understanding the differences between high-volume urban ambulance services and low-volume rural and frontier ambulance services in relation to these metrics is crucial for EMS leaders and managers.

Cost per call refers to the average cost incurred by an EMS organization for each emergency call responded to. It considers various expenses such as personnel salaries, equipment maintenance, vehicle fuel, and administrative costs. For high-volume urban ambulance services, the cost per call may be influenced by factors like population density, call volume, and the availability of resources. In contrast, low-volume rural and frontier ambulance services often face unique challenges, such as longer response distances, limited call volume, and resource scarcity, which can impact their cost per call.

Unit hour utilization measures the productive utilization of EMS resources by assessing the percentage of time an ambulance is actively engaged in responding to calls. High-volume urban ambulance services tend to have higher unit hour utilization due to the higher demand and call volume. In comparison, low-volume rural and frontier ambulance services may experience lower unit hour utilization due to longer response times and fewer calls.

Monitoring and analyzing these metrics are vital for EMS leaders and managers in different settings. By tracking cost per call, EMS organizations can evaluate the efficiency of their operations and identify areas where cost-saving measures could be implemented. For high-volume urban ambulance services, managing the cost per call becomes crucial in balancing the high demand and available resources. In the case of low-volume rural and frontier ambulance services, understanding the factors contributing to the cost per call can help in making informed decisions about resource allocation and optimizing service delivery.

Similarly, assessing unit hour utilization allows EMS leaders and managers to determine the effectiveness of resource deployment. By monitoring the percentage of time ambulances are actively engaged in responding to calls, organizations can identify underutilized resources and explore strategies to improve efficiency. For high-volume urban ambulance services, maximizing unit hour utilization can help ensure that resources are effectively utilized to meet the high call volume. In contrast, low-volume rural and frontier ambulance services may need to consider alternative strategies to maintain a reasonable level of unit hour utilization given the lower call volume.

Understanding the concepts of cost per call and unit hour utilization is vital for EMS leaders and managers as these metrics provide valuable insights into the operational efficiency and financial sustainability of their organizations. Monitoring and analyzing these metrics in different settings, considering the differences between high-volume urban ambulance services and low-volume rural and frontier ambulance services, allow for optimal resource allocation and service delivery. By effectively managing these metrics, EMS organizations can strive for operational excellence, financial sustainability, and the provision of high-quality emergency medical services to their communities.

Cost per call is a key metric used to measure the expenses associated with providing EMS services on a per-call basis. It is calculated using the following formula:

Cost per Call = Total Operational Costs / Number of Calls Handled

---

Operational costs can include personnel salaries, equipment, supplies, vehicle maintenance, and administrative expenses, among others. By calculating the cost per call, EMS leaders and managers can evaluate the efficiency of their service delivery and identify areas for improvement or cost-saving measures.

Unit Hour Utilization: Definition and Calculation

Unit hour utilization (UHU) is a measure of the productivity of EMS resources, specifically ambulance units. UHU is calculated using the following formula:

UHU = Number of Transports or Calls / Number of Unit Hours Available

---

A higher UHU indicates more efficient utilization of resources, while a lower UHU may suggest underutilized resources or inefficiencies in service delivery. Monitoring and analyzing UHU can help EMS leaders and managers optimize resource allocation, scheduling, and deployment strategies to improve overall operational efficiency.

Urban vs. Rural EMS: Cost Per Call and UHU Considerations

High-volume urban ambulance services and low-volume rural and frontier ambulance services face unique challenges and considerations when it comes to cost per call and UHU metrics.

Urban EMS organizations are likely to have more resources and a higher number of calls, which may result in a lower cost per call. However, urban EMS organizations may also face challenges related to high demand, congestion, and longer transport times, which can affect UHU and overall efficiency. Strategies to improve dispatch and response times, such as dynamic deployment or traffic management systems, can help urban EMS organizations optimize their UHU and cost per call metrics.

In contrast, rural and frontier EMS organizations may face challenges related to lower call volumes, higher per-call costs, and limited access to resources. In these settings, it may be more difficult to achieve optimal UHU and cost per call metrics due to the inherent challenges associated with rural service delivery. Rural EMS organizations should focus on strategies that maximize resource utilization, such as collaboration with neighboring agencies, shared resources, or regionalized dispatch centers, to improve their UHU and cost per call metrics.

EMS Subsidies and Alternative Funding Sources

EMS should be recognized and funded as an essential governmental service, given its critical role in providing emergency medical care to communities. However, many EMS leaders and managers face significant financial challenges in sustaining their services, especially in low-volume rural and frontier ambulance settings. To ensure the long-term viability of their organizations, EMS leaders must explore diverse funding streams and secure alternative sources of financial support. This involves identifying and pursuing options such as tax revenue, donations, grants, and community fundraisers. By actively pursuing these funding opportunities, EMS leaders can alleviate financial constraints and maintain the delivery of high-quality emergency medical services to their communities. It is important for EMS leaders to continue seeking sustainable models for funding and to advocate for the recognition of EMS as an essential service deserving of stable and adequate funding.

The Necessity of Subsidies and Alternative Funding Sources

EMS organizations often face significant financial pressures due to factors such as payer mix, insurance coverage limitations, and the high costs associated with maintaining a state of readiness. In the absence of adequate funding, EMS organizations may struggle to provide high-quality emergency medical services to their communities. Subsidies and alternative funding sources can help bridge the gap between operational expenses and revenue generated through billing, ensuring that EMS organizations can continue to deliver essential services without compromising their financial stability.

A crucial aspect of EMS economics is the dependence on subsidies to bridge the gap between an EMS service's cost-per-call and the reimbursement they receive in the United States. Subsidies can take various forms, and each EMS service in the country utilizes a unique combination of these financial supports. Commonly used subsidies include taxpayer support, municipal contributions, commercial payers, philanthropy, and grants. Importantly, one of the most significant subsidies underwriting rural and frontier EMS agencies in the United States is volunteer and underpaid labor.

Historically, EMS in the United States has relied on and valued the role of volunteerism in developing locally based EMS agencies. While volunteerism continues to play a role in EMS, it is increasingly acknowledged that this reliance is not a sustainable long-term solution to the system's financial challenges. Declining volunteerism, combined with an underpaid workforce that affects recruitment and retention, has led to an increased reliance on other subsidies, resulting in higher costs to local municipalities and taxpayers. Moreover, the decline in volunteerism has exposed the true cost of EMS, which has come as a shock to many communities struggling to provide local EMS agencies.

The State of Maine's 2022 Blue Ribbon Commission concluded that:

> Absent a subsidy, transporting EMS services cannot break even in the State, regardless of service mix, and all transporting EMS services are currently operating at a loss. As demonstrated in the previous chart, to break even, a high-efficiency (1,800 transports per year) service would need a subsidy of approximately $322 per transport; for a more rural, low-volume service (300 transports per year), a subsidy of $2,030 per transport is needed. Relying on current subsidies without additional State assistance is insufficient to meet the existing need for transporting EMS services and, as the commission heard throughout its work, all EMS services in Maine are currently operating at a loss.[106]

Subsidies and alternative funding sources are crucial in sustaining EMS organizations by bridging the gap between operational expenses and revenue. While volunteerism has historically played a significant role, it is not a sustainable long-term solution. Recognizing the financial challenges faced by EMS organizations, it is essential to explore diverse funding options and advocate for adequate subsidies to ensure the provision of high-quality emergency medical services to communities without compromising financial stability.

Tax Revenue as a Funding Source

One common source of funding for EMS organizations is tax revenue. Local or regional governments may allocate a portion of property, sales, or other taxes to support EMS agencies. This funding source can provide a stable and predictable revenue stream for EMS organizations, allowing them to plan and budget more effectively. EMS leaders and managers should work closely with government officials and policymakers to advocate for the inclusion of EMS agencies in local or regional tax allocations.

Donations and Grants

EMS organizations can also benefit from donations and grants from various sources, such as individuals, corporations, and foundations. These funding sources can provide crucial financial support for EMS organizations, particularly those operating in rural and frontier settings with limited access to other revenue streams. EMS leaders and managers should actively seek out potential donors and grant opportunities, as well as establish and maintain relationships with these funding sources to secure ongoing support.

Community Fundraisers and Support

Finally, EMS organizations may turn to their local communities for financial assistance through fundraisers and other community-based initiatives. Examples of such efforts include bake sales, charity events, or crowdfunding campaigns. These initiatives not only provide essential financial support for EMS organizations but also serve to engage and educate the community about the importance of EMS agencies and the challenges faced by EMS practitioners. EMS leaders and managers should collaborate with community partners and stakeholders to develop and implement creative and effective fundraising initiatives.

COST CONTAINMENT AND EFFICIENCY STRATEGIES FOR EMS ORGANIZATIONS

Cost containment and efficiency are critical considerations for EMS leaders and managers in optimizing resource utilization, reducing expenses, and maintaining high-quality services. Implementing these strategies is essential for both high-volume urban and low-volume rural and frontier ambulance services to address financial challenges and ensure the long-term sustainability of their organizations.

Efficient Resource Allocation and Utilization

One critical aspect of cost containment is the efficient allocation and utilization of resources. EMS leaders and managers should regularly evaluate their organization's resource allocation to ensure that staff, equipment, and facilities are being utilized effectively. This process may involve assessing the distribution of ambulances and personnel across different service areas, determining the optimal number of units and staff required for each shift, and identifying opportunities to streamline operations.

Implementing Technology Solutions

The integration of technology solutions can also contribute to cost containment and improved efficiency. Examples include adopting electronic patient care reporting (ePCR) systems, utilizing GPS and dispatch software to optimize response times, and employing telemedicine technology to reduce unnecessary transports. These technologies can help EMS organizations to streamline operations, enhance data collection and analysis, and improve overall patient care.

Training and Education

Investing in the ongoing training and education of EMS personnel is essential for maintaining a high standard of care while also containing costs. EMS personnel that are properly educated and trained can make more informed decisions about patient care, potentially reducing the need for costly interventions and transports. Furthermore, ongoing professional development helps to foster a culture of continuous improvement, leading to more efficient and effective EMS agencies.

Performance Measurement and Quality Improvement

EMS organizations should establish and maintain a robust performance measurement and quality improvement system. This system should include the regular collection, analysis, and reporting of performance data, as well as the identification and implementation of targeted quality improvement initiatives. By continuously monitoring and evaluating their performance, EMS organizations can identify opportunities for cost savings, service enhancements, and improved patient outcomes.

Collaboration and Partnerships

Finally, EMS organizations should explore opportunities for collaboration and partnership with other healthcare providers, government agencies, and community organizations. These partnerships can lead to more coordinated and efficient service delivery, shared resources, and potential cost savings. Examples of collaborative initiatives include integrated healthcare networks, joint purchasing agreements, and coordinated response plans with neighboring EMS agencies.

15

FUNDAMENTALS OF INSURANCE & BILLING

Healthcare is an essential safeguard of human life and dignity,
and there is a social and moral obligation to ensure it is available and accessible to all.
- Donnie Woodyard, Jr

THE EFFICIENT AND ACCURATE MANAGEMENT OF INSURANCE AND billing processes is essential for the financial sustainability of emergency medical services organizations. EMS leaders and managers must navigate a complex landscape of reimbursement policies, payer requirements, and regulatory changes to ensure their organizations receive appropriate compensation for the services they provide. This chapter aims to provide a comprehensive overview of the fundamentals of insurance and billing in the EMS context, with a particular focus on the needs and challenges faced by rising EMS leaders and managers.

By understanding the fundamentals of insurance and billing, EMS leaders and managers will be better equipped to address the financial challenges facing their organizations and advocate for policy changes that support the evolving needs of EMS care.

NAVIGATING MEDICARE AND MEDICAID REIMBURSEMENT

MEDICARE is a federal health insurance program that primarily serves individuals aged 65 and older, as well as certain younger individuals with disabilities. Medicare Part B specifically covers medically necessary ambulance services, both for emergency and non-emergency situations. However, to qualify for reimbursement, EMS practitioners must adhere to stringent documentation requirements that detail the medical necessity of the provided services.

It is crucial for EMS leaders and managers to understand the Medicare coverage criteria and billing guidelines to ensure proper reimbursement. Key aspects include:

- **Ground and air ambulance services**: Medicare covers both ground and air ambulance services, depending on the patient's medical condition and transportation needs. Reimbursement rates may differ based on the mode of transportation.
- **Service levels**: Medicare distinguishes between Basic Life Support (BLS) and Advanced Life Support (ALS) services, with separate reimbursement rates for each. Furthermore, ALS services include ALS-Level 1, ALS-Level 2, and Specialty Care Transport (SCT), each with specific documentation, staffing, and procedures performed requirements. Accurate documentation of the service level provided is essential for proper billing.
- **Medical necessity**: To qualify for reimbursement, ambulance transportation must be medically necessary, meaning it is the only safe and appropriate means of transportation given the patient's medical condition.

MEDICAID is a joint federal and state program which provides healthcare coverage to low-income individuals and families. Like Medicare, Medicaid covers emergency medical transportation, including ambulance services, for eligible beneficiaries. However, each state administers its own Medicaid program and sets its own coverage guidelines and reimbursement rates, which can result in considerable variation across states.

EMS leaders and managers should familiarize themselves with their respective state's Medicaid policies and procedures, focusing on the following:

- **Eligibility requirements**: States may impose specific eligibility criteria for beneficiaries to qualify for ambulance service coverage, such as medical necessity or prior authorization requirements.
- **Reimbursement rate**s: Medicaid reimbursement rates for ambulance services vary by state and are often lower than Medicare or private insurance rates. Understanding these rates is essential for accurate financial planning.
- **Documentation and billing**: Proper documentation and adherence to state-specific billing guidelines are crucial for ensuring timely and accurate reimbursement from Medicaid.

By gaining a thorough understanding of the nuances of Medicare and Medicaid reimbursement, EMS leaders and managers can better navigate the financial aspects of providing emergency medical services, ensuring the sustainability and success of their organizations.

MANAGING INSURANCE AND SELF-PAY REIMBURSEMENTS

Commercial / Private insurance companies offer a wide range of health insurance plans, with varying coverage for ambulance services. EMS leaders and managers must be adept at understanding and navigating these diverse policies to ensure appropriate reimbursement. Key aspects to consider when working with private insurance companies include:

- **Contract negotiation**: Establishing contracts with private insurance companies can help secure more predictable reimbursement rates and streamline the billing process. EMS organizations should carefully review contract terms and negotiate favorable conditions.
- **Verification of benefits**: Prior to providing services, EMS organizations should verify a patient's insurance coverage, including any applicable copays, deductibles, or coinsurance, to ensure accurate billing and minimize potential disputes.
- **Preauthorization requirements:** Some insurance plans may require preauthorization for non-emergency ambulance services. EMS practitioners should be familiar with these requirements to avoid denied claims or delayed reimbursement.

Handling Self-Pay Patient Billing

Self-pay patients, who lack insurance coverage or have insurance policies that do not cover ambulance services, present unique challenges for EMS organizations. Managing self-pay billing effectively requires balancing the need for financial sustainability with the ethical obligation to provide care regardless of a patient's ability to pay. To achieve this balance, EMS leaders and managers should consider the following strategies:

- **Clear communication**: Transparently communicate the cost of services to self-pay patients, ensuring they are aware of their financial responsibilities.
- **Payment plans and financial assistance**: Offer flexible payment plans or financial assistance programs to self-pay patients who may be struggling to pay their EMS bills. This approach can help mitigate the risk of nonpayment and maintain a positive relationship with the community.
- **Collection efforts**: While pursuing unpaid bills is often necessary for financial sustainability, EMS organizations should approach collections with sensitivity, considering the potential impact on patient relationships and community goodwill while concurrently providing education on the true costs associated with providing EMS.

By effectively managing private insurance and self-pay reimbursements, EMS leaders and managers can enhance their organizations' financial stability and ensure the continued provision of high-quality emergency medical services.

Implementing Best Practices in EMS Billing and Documentation

Proper documentation is critical for maximizing reimbursement from all payer sources. Incomplete or inaccurate documentation can lead to denied claims, delayed payments, or reduced reimbursement rates. To promote accurate and complete documentation, EMS leaders and managers should:

- **Develop clear documentation guidelines**: Establish standardized protocols for documenting patient care, ensuring that all required information is consistently recorded.
- **Train and educate staff:** Provide ongoing training and education for EMS personnel on documentation best practices, emphasizing the importance of accurate and complete records for billing purposes.
- **Implement quality assurance processes**: Regularly review patient care reports for completeness and accuracy, identifying areas for improvement and providing feedback to EMS personnel.

Streamlining the Billing Process

An efficient billing process can help expedite reimbursement, minimize errors, and reduce administrative burdens. To optimize their billing processes, EMS leaders and managers should:

- **Invest in billing software**: Implement a robust EMS billing software system that can help automate and streamline various aspects of the billing process, such as claim submission, payment tracking, and reporting.
- **Centralize billing functions**: Designate a dedicated billing department or staff member to manage all billing functions, ensuring a consistent and efficient approach.
- **Stay current with billing regulations**: Regularly review and update billing policies and procedures to remain compliant with evolving regulations and payer requirements.

Managing Billing Compliance and Audits

Compliance with billing regulations is essential to avoid potential penalties, fines, or loss of reimbursement. To promote billing compliance and successfully navigate audits, EMS leaders and managers should:

- **Develop a compliance program**: Establish a formal compliance program that outlines policies and procedures for detecting, preventing, and correcting billing errors or misconduct.
- **Conduct internal audits**: Periodically perform internal audits to assess compliance with billing regulations and identify areas for improvement.
- **Respond to external audits**: When facing an external audit, cooperate with the auditing entity, provide requested documentation, and promptly address any identified issues.

By implementing best practices in billing and documentation, EMS leaders and managers can not only maximize reimbursement but also reduce the risk of noncompliance, ultimately contributing to the financial stability and success of their organizations.

Medicare and Medicaid Fraud

Fraudulent activities involving Medicare and Medicaid reimbursement in the EMS sector can occur both accidentally and intentionally. These activities can lead to significant financial and legal repercussions for EMS organizations, including fines, penalties, and loss of reimbursement. EMS leaders and managers must be vigilant in preventing and addressing potential fraud to protect their organizations and maintain the trust of their communities. Examples of fraudulent activities in EMS include:

- **Upcoding**: Billing for a higher level of service than what was provided, such as billing for an Advanced Life Support (ALS) service when only Basic Life Support (BLS) was rendered.
- **Billing for medically unnecessary services**: Submitting claims for ambulance services that do not meet the medical necessity criteria established by Medicare or Medicaid.
- **Falsifying documentation**: This refers to the alteration or creation of fraudulent patient care reports, medical records, or billing documents to validate deceitful claims or deliberately providing partial documentation — the omission of certain information — that could potentially impact billing negatively.

The Impact of Licensing Issues on EMS Billing

Every year, EMS organizations lose significant revenue due to EMS personnel failing to maintain proper licenses. EMS agencies are not permitted to bill for services rendered by crew members who are not properly licensed and in good standing. Consequently, organizations may have to forego or refund significant sums of money.

Combating Fraud and Ensuring Compliance

To mitigate the risks associated with Medicare and Medicaid fraud and licensing issues, EMS leaders and managers should adopt a proactive approach, implementing the following strategies:

- **Develop a robust compliance program**: Establish a comprehensive compliance program that includes policies and procedures for detecting, preventing, and correcting fraudulent activities and licensing violations.
- **Monitor licensing status**: Managers should never rely on paper records for license verification, but rather use primary source verification for EMS personnel licenses. This includes directly searching the database records for the state EMS licensing system, or the EMS Compact's National EMS Coordinated Database. While it is rare, paper license records have been altered and if not recognized, the employer is at significant risk.

Finally, regularly track the licensing status of EMS personnel, ensuring that all staff maintain current and valid licenses. Implement processes to promptly address any lapses in licensing.

- **Conduct internal audits and reviews**: Perform periodic audits and reviews of billing practices and documentation to detect potential fraud or licensing issues. Provide timely feedback and corrective action when necessary.
- **Foster a culture of integrity and accountability**: Encourage open communication and reporting of potential fraud or licensing concerns, promoting a culture where staff feel empowered to report issues without fear of retaliation.
- **Provide ongoing education and training**: Offer regular training sessions for EMS personnel on billing compliance, fraud prevention, and the importance of maintaining proper licenses.

By actively addressing the challenges posed by Medicare and Medicaid fraud and licensing issues, EMS leaders and managers can safeguard their organizations' financial stability and reputation, ultimately ensuring the continued provision of high-quality emergency medical services.

Reimbursement for Specialized EMS Agencies

As the healthcare landscape continues to evolve, EMS organizations are increasingly incorporating specialized services, such as community paramedicine, mobile integrated health, and telemedicine, into their care models. These innovative services often require unique billing and reimbursement strategies, making it essential for EMS leaders and managers to understand the specific considerations involved.

Billing Considerations for Specialized EMS Agencies

Specialized EMS agencies often do not fit neatly into traditional billing categories, necessitating the development of new billing approaches. Key considerations for billing specialized services include:

- **Identifying appropriate billing codes**: EMS organizations must determine the correct billing codes for specialized services, which may differ from those used for traditional ambulance services. This may involve using new or modified Current Procedural Terminology (CPT) codes or Healthcare Common Procedure Coding System (HCPCS) codes.
- **Ensuring proper documentation**: Specialized services may require different documentation standards to demonstrate medical necessity and support billing claims. EMS leaders and managers should establish clear documentation guidelines and provide training to personnel involved in these services.
- **Collaborating with payers**: EMS organizations should actively engage with Medicare, Medicaid, and private insurance companies to advocate for coverage and

reimbursement of specialized services. This may involve negotiating contracts or working with payers to establish new reimbursement policies.

VALUE-BASED REIMBURSEMENT MODELS

As the healthcare system shifts towards value-based reimbursement models, specialized EMS agencies will likely become increasingly important in demonstrating the value and impact of EMS care. These services often focus on preventive care, population health, and care coordination, aligning with the goals of value-based care models. EMS organizations should consider:

- **Developing quality metrics**: Identify and track relevant performance metrics for specialized services, such as patient outcomes, cost savings, or patient satisfaction, to demonstrate the value of these services to payers and stakeholders.
- **Participating in value-based payment programs**: Explore opportunities to participate in value-based payment programs or pilot projects, such as bundled payment initiatives or pay-for-performance models, which can provide additional reimbursement for specialized services.
- **Building partnerships with healthcare providers**: Collaborate with hospitals, primary care providers, and other healthcare organizations to develop integrated care models that leverage specialized EMS agencies to improve patient outcomes and reduce healthcare costs.

Maximizing Reimbursement for Specialized EMS Agencies

To optimize reimbursement for specialized services, EMS leaders and managers should:

- **Stay informed of policy changes**: Monitor changes in Medicare, Medicaid, and private insurance reimbursement policies related to specialized services, and adjust billing practices accordingly.
- **Pursue alternative funding sources**: Seek grants or other funding opportunities that support the development and implementation of specialized EMS agencies, such as federal or state programs, private foundations, or corporate sponsorships.
- **Advocate for policy change**: Engage in advocacy efforts to promote policy changes that support reimbursement for specialized services, working with professional associations, legislative representatives, and other stakeholders.

By understanding and addressing the unique billing and reimbursement considerations for specialized EMS agencies, leaders and managers can help ensure the financial viability and success of these innovative care models within their organizations.

Common Challenges in EMS Billing

EMS billing presents several unique challenges that must be navigated by EMS leaders and managers to ensure appropriate reimbursement for their services. Key challenges include the perception of ambulance billing as a transportation benefit rather than a medical benefit, the growing emphasis on treatment in place programs, and the often-complex nature of EMS billing.

Ambulance Billing as a Transportation Benefit

Traditionally, ambulance services have been billed as a transportation benefit, rather than a medical benefit, which can limit the reimbursement available for EMS care. This perception can impact EMS organizations in several ways:

- **Limited coverage for medical services**: Insurance payers may not fully cover the cost of medical care provided by EMS personnel during transport, as reimbursement is primarily focused on the transportation component.
- **Difficulty in demonstrating medical necessity**: EMS organizations may struggle to justify the medical necessity of ambulance transports, particularly when patients could potentially be transported by other means.

The Growing Emphasis on Treatment in Place Programs

As EMS organizations increasingly focus on treatment in place programs, billing for these services can pose new challenges:

- **Lack of reimbursement for non-transport care**: Many insurance payers, including Medicare and Medicaid, do not currently provide reimbursement for treatment in place services when a patient is not transported. This can create a financial barrier for EMS organizations looking to expand these programs.
- **Demonstrating the value of treatment in place services**: EMS leaders and managers must effectively communicate the benefits of treatment in place programs, such as improved patient outcomes and reduced healthcare costs, to payers and stakeholders to advocate for policy changes that support reimbursement for these services.

The Complex Nature of EMS Billing

EMS billing involves a myriad of complexities that can create challenges for EMS organizations:

- **Varying payer requirements**: Navigating the diverse billing requirements and reimbursement policies of Medicare, Medicaid, and private insurance companies is time-consuming and resource-intensive for EMS leaders and managers.
- **Ensuring accurate documentation**: Proper documentation is crucial for successful billing but is challenging to maintain given the dynamic nature of EMS care and the variety of payer requirements.

- **Managing denials and appeals**: Denied claims and the appeals process are a significant administrative burden for EMS organizations, potentially resulting in higher administrative costs, and delayed or reduced reimbursement.

By recognizing and addressing these common challenges in EMS billing, leaders and managers can develop strategies to overcome these obstacles and improve the financial sustainability of their organizations.

COVID-19 AND THE NEED FOR PERMANENT CHANGE

During the COVID-19 pandemic, the Centers for Medicare & Medicaid Services (CMS) implemented a waiver to provide reimbursement for EMS treatment in place services. However, when the COVID-19 public health emergency (PHE) ended, this crucial waiver was also terminated. This section will discuss the details of the waiver program, its importance, and the need for it to be reconsidered as a permanent change in EMS billing and reimbursement.

The COVID-19 Treatment in Place Waiver Program

Medicare is the dominant payer of ground ambulance services, and therefore has a significant impact on the ability of ground ambulance entities to stay operational. The COVID-19 PHE placed an enormous burden on ground ambulance services, as public health authorities and hospitals directed them not to transport low- or mid-acuity patients. Recognizing the need to support ground ambulance organizations during this crisis, CMS introduced the treatment in place waiver program.

The waiver allowed EMS practitioners to be reimbursed for treatment in place services at rates equivalent to emergency BLS-E or ALS1-E, depending on the level of service rendered, without requiring patient transportation. The services provided had to be consistent with EMS protocols established by state and/or local laws where the services were furnished.

The waiver program played a crucial role in supporting EMS organizations during the COVID-19 PHE by:

- Allowing reimbursement for treatment in place services, which helped alleviate the financial burden on EMS organizations and allowed them to continue providing essential services.
- Reducing hospital surge by allowing EMS practitioners to treat patients in their homes when it was no longer safe or appropriate to transport them to hospitals.
- Facilitating telehealth services by recognizing ground ambulance entities as legitimate originating sites and reimbursing them for telehealth services they provided.

The Need for Permanent Change

The conclusion of the COVID-19 public health emergency in 2023 signaled the expiration of the associated federal waivers. One of the most significant of these, the COVID-19 treatment-in-place waiver, included in the *American Rescue Plan Act,*[107] had underscored the necessity of reimbursing EMS organizations for medical care provided to patients, without requiring patient transportation to hospitals. Concurrently, the Emergency Triage, Treat, and Transport (ET3) Model, another program allowing for flexibility in EMS services, was terminated prematurely by the Centers for Medicare & Medicaid Services (CMS).

The disappearance of these temporary but transformative programs laid bare a clear demand for permanent change in EMS billing and reimbursement policies. As EMS care continues to innovate, with an increasing shift toward treatment-in-place programs and other advanced care models, a fundamental reassessment of these policies is critical.

The future of EMS reimbursement and funding should encompass several key principles:

- **Financial Sustainability:** Permanent policies should ensure the financial stability of EMS organizations by allowing for reimbursement of treatment-in-place services—an increasingly crucial facet of EMS care.
- **Encouragement for Program Development:** Reimbursement for services provided outside the traditional transport-to-hospital model will encourage the development and expansion of innovative programs. Such programs can not only reduce hospital surge but also improve patient outcomes.
- **Integration of Telehealth Services:** Modern policies should facilitate the incorporation of telehealth services into EMS care. By doing so, they provide more diverse care options and minimize unnecessary contact between patients and healthcare professionals.

The discontinuation of the COVID-19 waiver and ET3 programs has imparted an important lesson—the need for comprehensive and sustainable EMS funding models that recognize the evolving role of EMS practitioners. By championing permanent implementation of treatment-in-place reimbursement, EMS leaders and managers can help shape EMS billing and reimbursement policies to align with the changing dynamics of EMS care. This advocacy will be instrumental in securing the financial sustainability of EMS organizations and continuing to meet patient needs effectively and efficiently.

16

Essential Service Status

"The purpose of government is to enable the people of a nation to live in safety and happiness. Government exists for the interests of the governed, not for the governors."

EMERGENCY MEDICAL SERVICES PLAY A CRUCIAL ROLE IN THE NATION'S healthcare system, providing life-saving care and transport to patients in need. Despite its importance, EMS is not universally designated, recognized, and funded as an essential service by governments, which has significant implications for its funding, organization, and public perception.

Essential services refer to those services deemed critical to the functioning and well-being of society by governments. These services are often considered indispensable for preserving public safety, maintaining order, and ensuring the continuation of vital infrastructure. Examples of essential services typically include police, fire protection, emergency medical services, water, sanitation, and public utilities.

The designation of a service as essential carries an implication that governments have an obligation to guarantee its provision and availability to the public. This responsibility can significantly impact the organization, funding, and regulation of such services, with governments playing a more active role in their oversight. However, the designation of any function of government as "essential" without a corresponding obligation of funding and resources is simply a title.

Recognizing that local governments were not treating EMS as an essential service, an early leader of the profession wrote,

> "Nationwide, emergency medical service remains one of the weakest links in the delivery of health care…local governments must accept responsibility for providing emergency medical services as they do fire and police services. The greatest threat to the average citizen in his own community today is not a fire in the home or a criminal in the street. The greatest threat is the inability to obtain adequate emergency medical care at the time of need-when knowledge, skill, and minutes can save lives." [108]

IMPLICATIONS OF ESSENTIAL SERVICE DESIGNATION

Officially designating any governmental service as essential generally has several implications:

- **Continuity of Service**: Essential services must be provided continuously, regardless of external circumstances such as emergencies, natural disasters, or other crises. This continuity is crucial for maintaining public safety, order, and well-being during challenging times.
- **Funding and Allocation of Resources**: Governments are more likely to allocate dedicated resources, including financial support and personnel, to essential services. This funding can provide a stable and predictable revenue stream for these services, allowing for more effective planning and budgeting.
- **Regulation and Oversight**: Governments often establish standards, requirements, and regulations for essential services to ensure that they are provided effectively and consistently across all jurisdictions. This oversight can include performance benchmarks, quality assurance mechanisms, and reporting requirements to maintain a high level of service.
- **Workforce Implications**: In some cases, designating a service as essential can affect the workforce responsible for providing that service. For example, in some circumstances, the workforce may be subject to specific regulations, education and training requirements, or expectations related to their roles in delivering essential services that did not exist when the service was not designated as "essential".

Criteria for Designating a Service as Essential

Governments use various criteria to determine whether a service should be designated as essential. Some common factors include:

- **Public Safety and Health**: Services that directly impact public safety and health are often considered essential, as they play a vital role in protecting citizens and maintaining order.
- **Basic Needs:** Services that ensure the provision of basic needs, such as clean water, sanitation, and shelter, are typically deemed essential due to their importance in daily life.
- **Infrastructure and Communication**: Services that support the continuation of critical infrastructure, including transportation, energy, and communication systems, are often designated as essential due to their importance in maintaining societal function.
- **Economic Stability**: In some cases, services that contribute to the stability and continuity of the economy may be considered essential, particularly if their disruption could have significant consequences for the broader society.

The process of designating a service as essential varies by jurisdiction and may be subject to political, social, and economic factors that influence policymakers' decisions.

EMS as a Designated Essential Service: Barriers and Misconceptions

Asserting the significance of designating Emergency Medical Services (EMS) as "Essential" may seem like stating the obvious. Amid the COVID-19 pandemic, when only 'essential' workers were authorized to work, the vital role of EMS was universally recognized without dispute. Yet, while the importance of EMS is generally agreed upon, the intricacies involved in officially classifying it as "Essential" may not be fully understood.

To truly recognize EMS as essential, it must be repositioned within governmental structures. This implies ensuring State EMS Offices occupy an equivalent position to other essential services, such as State Police, Fire Marshal Offices, National Guard, and other vital infrastructure. Similarly, financial support must reflect this classification; mere designation without funding fails to alter the current situation.

However, the significance of designating EMS as an essential service is not without contention and varies across jurisdictions. It undoubtedly plays a pivotal role in public health and safety, but this designation carries profound implications, encompassing funding, regulation, and workforce considerations.

Benefits of Designating EMS as an Essential Service

- **Service Continuity**: Generally, essential services must be provided continuously, regardless of external circumstances such as emergencies, natural disasters, or other crises. Ensuring this continuity requires funding, planning, and infrastructure to be committed in advance to ensure all communities will have reliable access to emergency medical care.

- **Funding Stability**: All designated essential services should include reliable and predictable funding. This would allow EMS organizations to maintain their readiness to respond to emergencies.

- **Regulation Standardization**: Governments often establish standards, requirements, and regulations for essential services to ensure that they are provided effectively and consistently across all jurisdictions. This oversight can include performance benchmarks, quality assurance mechanisms, and reporting requirements to maintain a high level of service. For EMS, this would further codify consistent standards and regulations governing emergency medical care, enhancing the quality of service provided.

- **Workforce Support**: Essential service designation, in theory, should lead to improved support for EMS personnel, including training, benefits, and protections, enhancing their job satisfaction and overall performance.

Challenges of Designating EMS as an Essential Service

The key challenge to universally designating EMS as an essential service is the financial burden it would place on state and local governments. A commitment of this magnitude would entail substantial monetary resources, necessitating taxpayers to shoulder the added costs. Roddy Brandes, during his 1973 testimony to Congress, pointed out this dilemma. He noted that local government officials often depend on underfunded EMS agencies operating on goodwill, thereby releasing them from the duty of providing adequate service. [109] Brandes, who was the President of the Ambulance Association of America and the Chair of the National Registry of EMTs in 1970, provided crucial insight into the financial aspects of EMS service provision that remains true today.

Misconceptions and Public Perception

Numerous misconceptions blur the understanding of the Emergency Medical Services system, particularly in relation to its funding, responsibilities, and sustainability.

A widespread misconception is that EMS is already officially deemed an essential service like police and fire departments. This belief suggests that communities are bound to provide and finance these services. However, contrary to popular belief, most U.S. communities lack both a mandate for ambulance services and a requirement to dispatch an ambulance in response to a 911 call. The origins of this misconception might be traced back to the initial development of

EMS, which started as community-based efforts supported by grants, voluntary labor, and other resources.

The constant visibility of ambulances further perpetuates this misconception. Since the 1972 television show "Emergency!" aired, communities have come to expect an advanced life support ambulance to be dispatched as needed. While almost all communities in the United States currently have access to ambulance services, many are unaware that a significant number of these services are facing significant sustainability challenges, and some are constantly on the brink of collapse.

A further misconception is that EMS is universally funded by tax dollars, much like most police and fire departments. Although some EMS agencies are fully tax-funded, many others are only partially funded, and a substantial portion receives no tax funding at all. This misunderstanding regrettably simplifies the intricate funding dynamics of EMS agencies, overlooking the financial difficulties they often encounter.

The public's misconceptions about the nature, obligations, and funding of EMS as an essential service have significant implications for the future efficiency and viability of these crucial services. Therefore, addressing these misconceptions and fostering a more accurate understanding of the EMS system is critical to ensure its sustainability.

THE DISTINCTIVE NATURE OF EMS AMONG ESSENTIAL SERVICES

Emergency Medical Services in all regions of America - urban, suburban, rural, or frontier - are grappling with significant challenges. The critical nature of these challenges, particularly the chronic underfunding and undervaluing of the service, must be communicated to both the public and policy makers.

However, illuminating the challenges is not sufficient. Advocacy needs to transition from merely identifying problems to actively seeking enduring, sustainable solutions. This ensures the long-term effectiveness and reliability of these essential services. EMS occupies a unique position among essential governmental services, primarily due to the lack of universal recognition and funding as such, combined with its inherent public service nature.

Many rural and frontier communities heavily rely on unconventional methods such as volunteer labor, philanthropic grants, donations, and community fundraisers to deliver EMS. This atypical reliance sets EMS apart from other essential services. Communities, for instance, don't usually hold bake sales to fund their snowplows, garbage trucks, or police cars, nor do they depend on volunteer labor to operate critical facilities like water treatment plants, schools, or hospitals.

EMS, having developed organically at the community level, has encountered difficulties transitioning to a modern, sustainable model. The commitment of EMS practitioners to their communities often goes beyond professional boundaries, reflecting deeply ingrained community involvement. However, this profound connection can occasionally prove counterproductive. EMS practitioners frequently address challenges within their profession with the same emergency, life-preserving approach they use for their patients - they manage the metaphorical bleeding and attempt to stabilize the situation.

These heroic efforts, while necessary, often mask the deeper, systemic issues within the service. To the public and elected officials, EMS may appear to be operating adequately, despite the industry's pleas for assistance. As a result, the underlying systemic issues risk being overlooked until they escalate, leading to a potential failure in local EMS systems. It's therefore vital to acknowledge EMS's unique circumstances, address its underlying challenges, and reaffirm its status as an essential service within governmental structures. Action towards sustainability and reliability is required now to prevent the challenges faced by isolated communities from becoming widespread issues.

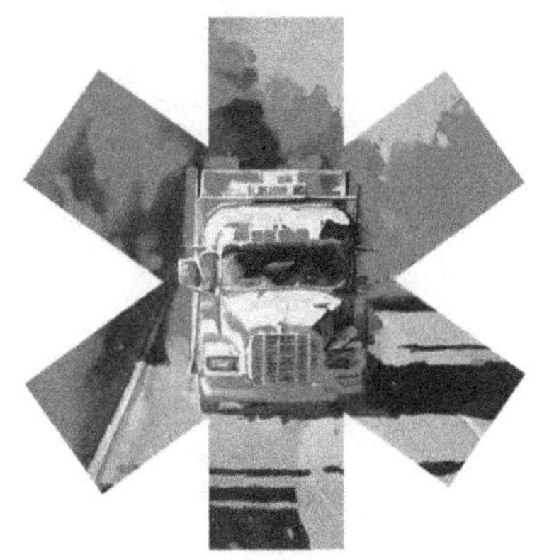

Section 3

EMS PERSONNEL

Emergency Medical Services personnel form the unacknowledged foundation, bearing the weight of our nation's healthcare system delicately. In challenging and unimaginable situations, these medical professionals straddle the line between life and death, delivering specialized emergency medical care. Serving as the first line of defense, their steadfast dedication to emergency care fortifies our healthcare structure. Additionally, EMS clinicians play a crucial role in supporting and shoring up fragile healthcare systems, offering pivotal assistance to public health, underserved high-dependency patients, and those without access to primary or preventive healthcare. As a society, we owe EMS clinicians our utmost respect and boundless gratitude.

- Donnie Woodyard, Jr

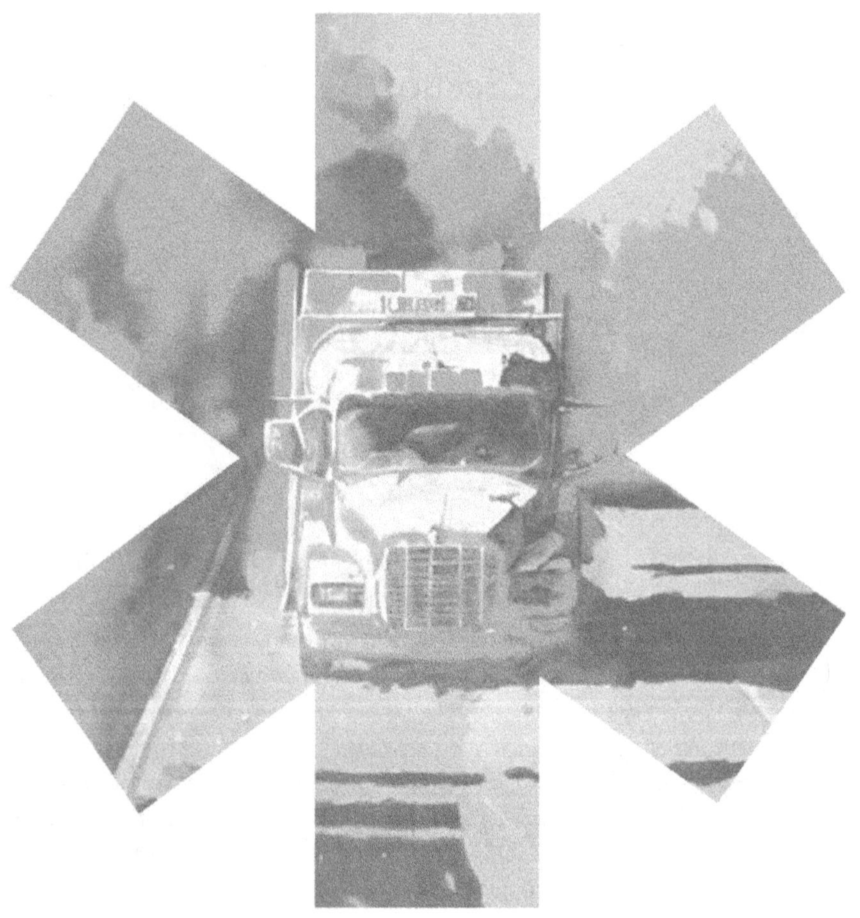

17

Certification, Licensure & Credentialing

"An individual may only perform a skill or role for which that person is:
***EDUCATED**, and*
***CERTIFIED**, and*
***LICENSED**, and*
***CREDENTIALED**."*

- National EMS Scope of Practice Model (2019)[110]

THE COMPETENCE OF PERSONNEL IS A CRUCIAL FACTOR IN ENSURING the delivery of safe and effective patient care. To maintain and enhance the proficiency of EMS practitioners, a systematic and structured approach has been developed. In addition to education, the approach encompasses three key pillars: National Certification, State Licensure, and Credentialing. These pillars serve as the foundation for the professional practice of EMS personnel, providing a framework that supports their ability to deliver high-quality patient care.

A comprehensive understanding of the distinctions between these three pillars, as well as their respective roles and purposes, is vital for EMS personnel, employers, regulatory bodies, and the public. This chapter aims to highlight these differences, clarify the individual and collective roles of Certification, Licensure, and Credentialing, and address common misconceptions related to each. By gaining a comprehensive understanding of these fundamental aspects of EMS practice, the profession can maintain high standards of care, benefiting both the EMS community and the patients they serve.

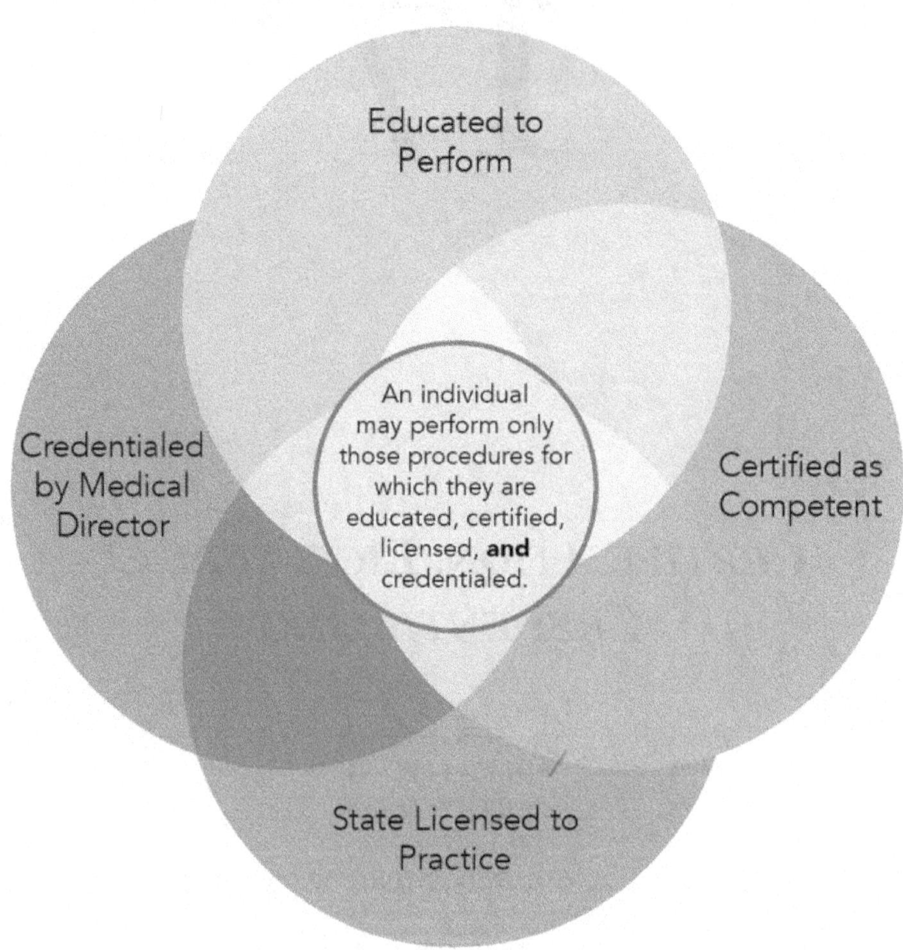

CERTIFICATION

Certification is an evaluation process that assesses an individual's knowledge and skills in a specific domain, ensuring they meet a predetermined set of standards. In the context of EMS, certification is typically granted upon successful completion of standardized, nationally recognized examinations. In 1970, it was determined that a single national body would be responsible for the certification of EMS personnel in the United States and the National Registry of Emergency Medical Technicians (NREMT) was formed. Since its creation, the primary responsibility of the NREMT has been to scientifically evaluate an EMS practitioner's cognitive and psychomotor abilities and determine their level of competence in emergency medical care.

The primary purpose of certification is to demonstrate that an EMS professional has achieved minimum entry-level competency, as defined by the relevant national standards. Certification serves as an assurance to employers, peers, and the public that an individual possesses the requisite knowledge and skills to perform effectively in their designated role. By achieving certification, an individual demonstrates that they have the necessary knowledge and skills to practice safely and effectively within their specific EMS domain. This foundational competency is crucial to ensuring that EMS personnel can fulfill their professional responsibilities, ultimately contributing to the delivery of high-quality patient care.

Common Misconceptions: Certification

- **Certification is not a license**: It is important to recognize that national EMS certification does not grant legal authority to practice. While certification attests to an individual's knowledge and skills, it does not confer the necessary legal privileges to provide patient care. This distinction is important to avoid confusion and ensure that EMS personnel understand the additional steps required to obtain licensure.

- **Certification does not guarantee employmen**t: While certification may be a prerequisite for licensure and employment, it does not guarantee a job in the EMS field. Employment opportunities depend on various factors, such as the availability of positions, the applicant's qualifications, and the hiring policies of employing organizations. Certification is a vital component of professional development but should not be viewed as a guarantee of employment.

- **Certification is not mastery**: Achieving national EMS certification does not imply that an individual is an expert or has mastered the information. Individuals with a national EMS certification, especially a new one, have demonstrated minimum entry-level knowledge. It is crucial to recognize that certification serves as a foundation for further professional development, rather than a definitive indication of expertise or mastery.

- **Certification does not mean qualified to practice**: While certification does signify that an individual possesses entry-level knowledge and skills, it does not automatically mean that they are safe or qualified to practice. Several other factors must be considered before an individual is deemed qualified to practice, highlighting the importance of licensing and credentialing in the process of assessing and verifying an individual's competence.

Exploring The Nuances: EMS Certifications Vs. Licenses

The terms "certification" and "licensure" in the context of Emergency Medical Services often create confusion due to their interchangeable use across different states. This conundrum primarily stems from historical context and terminology evolution as EMS was being developed.

In the 1960s and early 1970s, federal legislation pushed for the development of a national EMS system. During this period, the federal agencies, such as the Department of Transportation and the Department of Health, Education and Welfare (now the Department of Health and Human Services), urged states to create EMS systems and required states to report their progress. One common datapoint was the number of trained personnel operating ambulances. States then started tracking 'certifications' issued by organizations like the American Red Cross, as ambulance attendants at the time generally only had formal first aid training.

As the EMS profession matured and became a recognized Allied Health Profession in the mid-1970s, the practice of states tracking certifications persisted. When states began regulating EMS as a legitimate medical profession, requiring state authorization to practice (a license), they often continued to use the term "certification" due to historical precedents.

However, it's essential to clarify that regardless of what a state agency calls the process, if the occupation has a regulatory or statutory defined scope of practice and only those authorized by the state can perform these functions, such individuals are effectively licensed. Even if the state uses a term other than 'license', the authority granted has the legal effect of a license.

Currently, every state has established a specific, restricted area of medical practice known as Emergency Medical Services. Before practicing patient care as an EMT or Paramedic, state authorization is required. While many states have updated their statutes to use the term 'license', some continue to use 'certification' to refer to the state-issued authority.

For the purposes of this discussion and in line with industry standards, 'certification' refers to the recognition granted to an individual by a non-governmental organization upon meeting predetermined qualifications specified by that organization. On the other hand, 'licensure' refers to the authority to practice issued by a state or jurisdiction. Despite the variances in terminology across states, the essential factor is the state-granted authority to practice, ensuring the service provider meets the required qualifications and standards.

LICENSURE

As the second component of the triad, state licensure involves granting individuals the legal authority to practice a specific profession within a particular jurisdiction. In the EMS field, state or territory regulatory bodies are responsible for issuing licenses and enforcing the relevant practice standards and requirements.

The primary function of licensure is to ensure professional accountability and public protection by regulating the practice of EMS personnel within a specific jurisdiction. During the licensure process, regulatory bodies confirm that individuals have fulfilled the necessary educational and certification requirements, thus guaranteeing their possession of the appropriate knowledge and skills to practice safely within their designated scope. Additionally, jurisdictions hold the authority and responsibility to evaluate an individual's criminal history and weigh the public safety implications associated with issuing a license.

Licensure plays a crucial role in safeguarding the public by granting licensing jurisdictions the ultimate responsibility for deciding who receives a license. Licensing jurisdictions also possess the authority to conduct investigations and, if necessary, impose license discipline. This oversight helps ensure that EMS personnel maintain accountability and adhere to professional standards.

Upon obtaining a license, individuals demonstrate compliance with the requirements set forth by the relevant regulatory body, ensuring accountability and adherence to professional standards. Licensure also delineates the scope of practice for EMS personnel, specifying the authorized interventions and procedures. As individually licensed healthcare providers, EMS personnel accept the responsibility and accountability for their actions and decisions. This professional accountability includes practicing within the established scope, adhering to professional standards, and maintaining responsibility for patient care.

All EMS practitioners must hold a valid license issued by the appropriate jurisdiction. In recent years, many jurisdictions have implemented interstate compacts to reduce the necessity for individuals to secure and maintain multiple licenses across jurisdictions. The Recognition of EMS Personnel Licensure Interstate Compact (REPLICA) streamlines EMS personnel's practice in multiple jurisdictions by granting a legally recognized "privilege to practice." In Compact states, a valid license from one Member State grants EMS personnel the Privilege to Practice in other Member States, provided the Compact conditions are met.

Participating states recognize and accept the privilege to practice, granted by the EMS Compact, as a valid alternative to a separate state license, provided the EMS professional fulfills the Compact's requirements. This recognition simplifies the process for EMS personnel working across multiple jurisdictions while maintaining a high level of professional accountability, public protection, and patient care quality.

Common Misconceptions: Licensure

- **Licensure is not the same as certification**: Although certification is often a prerequisite for licensure, they are not the same thing. Certification demonstrates that an individual has achieved a certain level of knowledge and skills, while licensure grants the legal authority to practice in a specific jurisdiction. For instance, obtaining National EMS Certification (NREMT) does not automatically authorize someone to practice as an EMS clinician. Understanding this crucial distinction is essential for EMS personnel to be aware of the necessary steps required to obtain and maintain their legal right to practice. (As previously discussed, certain states still label the authorization given by the State EMS Office as a "State Certification," which, although confusing and incongruent with other professions, originates from EMS's historical roots.)

- **Licensure requirements may vary by jurisdiction**: While national certification standards exist, licensure requirements are established by individual states and may vary between jurisdictions. EMS personnel should know these variations when pursuing licensure and ensure that they meet the specific requirements of their intended practice location.

CREDENTIALING

The final element of an EMS practitioner's ability to practice is local credentialing. Credentialing is a local process by which an individual is permitted by a specific entity (medical director) to practice in a specific setting (EMS agency)[111]. For EMS practitioners, credentialing is typically conducted by medical directors in collaboration with employing agencies, hospitals, or other healthcare facilities and involves assessing an individual's education, training, certification, licensure, and professional experience.

The primary purpose of credentialing is to ensure that EMS personnel possess the necessary skills and qualifications to perform their assigned duties within their scope of practice. This process helps to maintain the quality of patient care by ensuring that EMS practitioners are competent, well-trained, and able to work effectively in their respective roles.

In 2017, the National Association of EMS Physicians summarized this as "the attestation by an organization's EMS physician medical director that the EMS practitioner possesses required competencies in the domains of cognitive, affective, and psychomotor abilities. These aptitudes must be shown in the application of clinically oriented critical thinking, particularly in situations germane to that organization's local practice of EMS medicine."[112]

For example, a paramedic may be certified and properly licensed in a state that permits paramedics to perform surgical cricothyrotomies. However, just because the skill may be included in the scope of practice, that is not enough. The employer should have established written medical protocols, and if surgical cricothyrotomies are permitted, there should be a protocol for that procedure. Moreover, even with all the necessary protocols in place, the employer (and Medical Director) should keep a record of the individual paramedics that are credentialed to perform the skill and records of training and evaluation of that skill.

The process of credentialing is very common in the medical field. Another example is that of physicians. A licensed medical doctor cannot simply go to any hospital and practice; they must be credentialed. Furthermore, once a physician is credentialed at a specific hospital, they are additionally credentialed for certain types of practice or procedures. While the state-issued medical license may not restrict a certain practice, performing at a specific level requires both licensure and credentialing.

Credentialing allows EMS personnel to perform specific duties within their scope of practice. Employing organizations use credentialing to evaluate an individual's competence in performing certain tasks and procedures, ensuring that they can deliver safe and effective patient care. Credentialing also helps to maintain the ongoing competence of EMS personnel by requiring them to participate in continuing education and professional development activities.

Common Misconceptions: Credentialing

- **Credentialing is not a one-time process**: Credentialing is often mistakenly thought of as a one-time event. However, it is an ongoing process that requires EMS personnel to maintain their skills and knowledge, engage in continuous professional development, and adhere to the evolving standards of practice. Credentialing may involve periodic assessments, as well as the need to complete additional training or certifications, to ensure that EMS practitioners remain competent and up to date in their field. Also, credentialing at one agency does not satisfy the requirements to be credentialed by other employers. It is a professional responsibility of the EMS practitioner to know and understand the role of credentialing.

- **Credentialing is not synonymous with licensure or certification**: Although credentialing may involve verifying an individual's licensure and certification status, it is a distinct process that focuses on assessing an individual's overall qualifications and competencies within a specific organizational context. Credentialing goes beyond the scope of licensure and certification by considering factors such as clinical experience, professional references, and an individual's ability to perform specific tasks and procedures within their employing organization.

INTERPLAY OF CERTIFICATION, LICENSURE, AND CREDENTIALING

The processes of certification, licensure, and credentialing are interconnected, with each step building upon the previous one. Certification serves as the initial step, demonstrating an individual's foundational knowledge and skills. Licensure follows, granting the legal authority to practice within a specific jurisdiction. Finally, credentialing verifies an individual's competence to perform specific duties within their employing organization.

Each pillar of the EMS personnel's ability to practice serves a distinct but complementary role in maintaining professional standards and safeguarding patient care. By ensuring that EMS personnel possess the necessary knowledge, skills, and legal authority to practice, these processes help to create a robust and reliable framework for the delivery of high-quality emergency medical care.

In addition to the foundational processes of certification, licensure, and credentialing, EMS personnel must engage in ongoing education and professional development to maintain and enhance their competence. Continuing education and professional development opportunities, such as workshops, seminars, and online courses, help EMS practitioners stay current with evolving best practices, new technologies, and advancements in the field.

LICENSE RECIPROCITY: CHALLENGES AND OPPORTUNITIES

License reciprocity—the practice whereby states recognize licenses obtained in other states without mandating the full process for acquiring a new license—has been a key element in EMS personnel mobility. Historically, this practice was necessary due to unique education requirements and standards across states. In 1984, NHTSA worked with NASEMSD[a] to develop license reciprocity guidelines[113] as a mechanism to crosswalk these varying standards, thereby facilitating easier movement of licensed EMS personnel between states. However, with recent standardization efforts and the establishment of the EMS Compact, the traditional model of license reciprocity is obsolete.

The EMS Compact, which, as of this writing, has been adopted by 24 states, presents a significant opportunity to further streamline the licensing process. Under the Compact, initial state licensing requirements have been standardized to include National EMS Certification and the completion of a fingerprint background check. This new commitment to standardization provides an opportunity to eliminate the convoluted and often confusing alternate pathways associated with historic license reciprocity.

Given the current state of standardization, whereby all states recognize National EMS Certification, there exists an opportunity to simplify the licensing process. States could adopt uniform initial licensing requirements for EMS personnel, thereby ensuring that any EMS individual possessing a valid license, issued by any State EMS Office, would be universally recognized as meeting the initial entry level education and certification requirements.

However, this streamlined approach is contingent upon all states adopting and maintaining these universal standards for initial licensure. Should a state deviate from national standards, licenses issued by such a state should not be recognized by others. Therefore, commitment to maintaining these universal standards is crucial for the continued effectiveness and efficiency of the EMS system.

CEILING AND FLOOR SCOPE OF PRACTICE MODELS IN EMS

In the landscape of Emergency Medical Services, different states have adopted distinct regulatory frameworks for defining the scope of practice for EMS professionals, such as Emergency Medical Technicians (EMTs) and Paramedics. These frameworks largely fall into two categories: the Ceiling Scope of Practice model and the Floor Scope of Practice model.

Ceiling Scope of Practice Model

In the Ceiling Scope of Practice model, states specify the maximum permitted scope of practice for each EMS level licensed by the state in their statute or administrative code. This essentially puts a 'ceiling' on what EMTs, and/or Paramedics can do in their roles.

[a] The NHTSA contract was with the National Association of State EMS Directors.

For example, a state like Colorado, which follows this model, lays down a clear set of permissible practices and procedures that EMS personnel can perform. Anything beyond this stated scope of practice is considered outside the legal bounds and would necessitate a waiver to the administrative rules. It's crucial to note that under this model, physician medical directors are not allowed to write protocols or provide standing orders for any medication, skill, or procedure that exceeds the specified scope.

Floor Scope of Practice Model

On the other hand, the Floor Scope of Practice model takes a more flexible approach. States like Texas, which follow this model, specify that all licensed Paramedics should at minimum possess the knowledge, skills, and abilities to perform at an approved scope of practice. This provides a 'floor' or minimum standard.

However, unlike the Ceiling model, the Floor model allows for individual medical directors to provide additional training to EMS personnel to operate above the state-specified minimum. This gives EMS practitioners the opportunity to acquire and utilize additional skills, as approved and overseen by their medical director.

Pros and Cons

Each model has its own advantages and disadvantages. The Ceiling Scope of Practice model offers clear boundaries and uniform standards, fostering consistent practice across the state and reducing ambiguity. However, it also limits adaptability to local needs and restricts EMS professionals' ability to expand their skills under the guidance of their medical director.

Conversely, the Floor Scope of Practice model allows for more adaptability to local circumstances and needs. It offers the potential for EMS professionals to grow their skillset and provides a more personalized approach to patient care. However, this model may result in more varied practice standards across different regions and could potentially lead to confusion over what constitutes permitted practice.

The choice between these two models often reflects the balance between standardization and adaptability, both critical aspects of EMS management and leadership. It's essential for aspiring EMS managers and leaders to understand these distinctions and their implications to navigate and operate effectively within their state's EMS regulatory framework.

"THREE LEGS OF THE STOOL"

The interplay between certification, licensing, and credentialing has been described as the three legs of a stool. Understanding the distinctions between certification, licensure, and credentialing, as well as their respective roles in EMS personnel's ability to practice, is essential for ensuring the continued delivery of safe and effective patient care. Each pillar serves a distinct but complementary role in maintaining professional standards and safeguarding patient care. Certification demonstrates foundational knowledge and skills, licensure grants legal authority to practice within a specific jurisdiction, and credentialing verifies an individual's competence to perform specific duties within their employing organization.

The interconnected nature of these processes highlights the importance of a comprehensive approach to assessing and verifying EMS personnel's competence. By clarifying the distinctions and roles of each pillar - National Certification, State Licensure, and Credentialing - the EMS profession can uphold its high standards of care. This comprehensive approach ultimately benefits both the EMS community and the patients they serve, ensuring that EMS personnel possess the necessary skills and qualifications to provide optimal care in emergency situations.

It is also crucial to recognize that the journey to professional competence and expertise in the EMS field does not end with obtaining certification, licensure, or even credentialing. EMS personnel must engage in ongoing education and professional development to maintain and enhance their competence, stay current with evolving best practices, and adapt to new technologies and advancements in the field. In this way, the EMS profession can continue to grow, adapt, and provide the highest level of care to patients in need.

18

NATIONAL EMS CERTIFICATION

"The growing importance of emergency medical services justifies a professional status comparable to that of other existing technical medical services. Individuals who qualify for this vocation through standard certification should be known as Emergency Medical Technicians. This term should be reserved for those who have received adequate education, passed an examination based on the educational program, and achieved certification."[114]

THE 1960s SAW THE IMPLEMENTATION OF EMERGENCY MEDICAL SERVICES pilot projects across the United States, and with this came the demand for a national authority to ensure EMS certification. This need became more pressing with the 1966 publication of "*Accidental Death and Disability: The Neglected Disease of Modern Society*". As a response, the National Academy of Sciences (NAS) and the National Research Council (NRC) initiated a "Task Force on Guidelines for Training of Ambulance Personnel". The duty of this task force was to develop nationwide guidelines for advanced training for ambulance attendants providing emergency care, and to suggest a course of action to establish a nationally recognized training course.[115]

In March 1968, the NAS-NRC Committee on Emergency Medical Services released its inaugural Guidelines and Recommendations report[116]. The committee and task force included prominent future contributors to the National Registry, such as Peter Safar, MD, Joseph D. Farrington, MD, Walter A. Hoyt, Jr., MD, and Rocco Morando. The report emphasized that training programs should produce professional ambulance attendants and emergency department assistants of a caliber comparable to other certified medical technicians, such as x-ray and physical therapy technicians.

Following the report's release, the American College of Surgeons and the American Academy of Orthopedic Surgeons, in partnership with the U.S. Department of Health, hosted a conference titled "Emergency Medical Services: Recommendations for an Approach to an Urgent National Problem". Dr. Safar, together with his colleague Jerry Esposito,[a] proposed an approach towards a national EMS certification system, which eventually led to the formation of the National Registry of Emergency Medical Technicians. They proposed the following:

> The formation of a registry for ambulance attendants... was initiated by the Committee on Acute Medicine of the American Society of Anesthesiologists at its May 22, 1968, meeting in Pittsburgh. This idea was recommended to and approved by the National Academy of Sciences-National Research Council, Committee on Emergency Medical Services, and the American Medical Association's Commission on Emergency Medical Services. The American College of Surgeons and the American Academy of Orthopaedic Surgeons also endorsed this plan. These national organizations felt that the AMA Commission is the appropriate agency to implement a board of schools and a registry for EMTs.
>
> An American Registry of Emergency Medical Technicians (AREMT?) and a Board of Schools to advise the Council on Medical Education should be formed.
>
> Definition of the Registry: A national board for examination and certification of allied health personnel in emergency medical services—personnel involved in lifesaving and life-supporting measures at the scene, during transportation, and in hospitals.
>
> Goals: To provide education, recognition, professional status, and quality control to allied health personnel involved in emergency medical services at the scene, during transportation, and in hospitals.[117]

[a] Gerald ("Jerry") Esposito (1924-2003), after his service as a World War II B-17 navigator purchased a funeral home in Punxsutawney, PA, and founded the first community-based subscription model ambulance service. He later worked with Dr. Peter Safar on the Freedom House Ambulance service and co-authored the first visionary outline for a national registry for EMTs.

At the conclusion of the conference, the Conference Chairman, Dr. Floyd H. Jergesen,[b] "was instructed to take the steps necessary to implement the recommendation for a Presidential Commission and to...bring the recommendation to the attention of an appropriate advisor to the President of the United States."[118]

On January 21, 1970, in partnership with President Lyndon Johnson's Committee on Highway Traffic Safety, the NAS, NRC, and the American Medical Association formed a Task Force to examine the creation of a national EMS certification body. The inaugural meeting of this task force comprised representatives from a range of professional associations, such as the American Medical Association, Ambulance Association of America, International Association of Fire Chiefs, and others.

After three task force meetings, the Registry of EMTs was formed on June 4, 1970. Soon after, the organization rebranded itself as the National Registry of Emergency Medical Technicians (NREMT) to reflect its nationwide reach. Roddy Brandes, the founder of Mecklenburg Emergency Services and the President of the Ambulance Association of America, was elected as the inaugural Chair, and for a brief period, the organization's mailing address was Roddy Brandes' office in Charlotte, North Carolina.

In 1971, Rocco Morando –a member of the 1968 NAS/NRC task force, an invited subject matter expert attendee at the 1969 Airlie House Conference, and the Emergency Rescue Squad Coordinator for The Ohio State University – was hired as the NREMT's first Executive Director. Rocco Morando established the organization's presence in Columbus, Ohio, and quickly started developing the first EMT-Ambulance National EMS Certification examination. A few months later, the first EMT-Ambulance examination was administered simultaneously to 1,520 ambulance personnel at 51 test sites throughout the United States. The role and value of National EMS Certification was quickly adopted and by 1973 the first recertification cycle for the EMT-Ambulances was conducted and by March 1975, over 31,000 EMTs had obtained National EMS Certification[119].

In 1974, recognizing the need for a standardized advanced EMS practitioner level, the NREMT organized a national meeting to develop guidelines for a national EMT-Paramedic curriculum. The following year, Dr. J.D. "Deke" Farrington, a prominent orthopedic surgeon and Chair of the NREMT board, sent a memo to the American Medical Association (AMA) urging them to officially recognize EMT-Paramedic as a distinct medical profession. The American Medical Association's Committee on Health Manpower agreed and designated EMT-Paramedic as an approved allied health profession and initiated the process for the Council of Allied Health Education and Accreditation (CAHEA) to establish accreditation standards.

It was also in 1975 that Rocco Morando recognized the need for an additional national organization to unite and represent the interests of the individual EMTs[120]. Although individual state associations were developing, the emerging profession lacked a unified national voice from individual EMTs. The NREMT organized and funded a meeting on January 8, 1975, to bring

[b] Dr. Jergesen (1910-1990) was an orthopedic surgeon whose published work addressed the management of bone and soft tissue infections.

representatives from the individual state EMT organizations together to address this need. The state representatives participating in the meeting included: Stanley "Butch" Bridges (Oklahoma), Donald Cross (Maine), A. Roger Fox (Oregon), Jeffrey Harris (Massachusetts), Walter Young (Colorado), and Robert and James Van Steenburg (Florida). Following this meeting, the National Registry of EMTs funded five additional meetings that resulted in the establishment of the National Association of EMTs (NAEMT) on November 15, 1975.

In 1977, the Department of Transportation published the *National Training Course: Emergency Medical Technician Paramedic*, the first national standard curriculum for training Paramedics. Nancy Caroline, MD, was the primary author, with assistance from several of the NREMT visionaries, board members, and founders, including:

- J.D. 'Deke' Farrington, MD – American Academy of Orthopedic Surgeons (and chair of the NREMT's board)
- Norman McSwain, Jr., MD – University of Kansas Medical Center (and a later chair of the NREMT's board)
- Rocco V. Morando – Executive Director, NREMT
- Peter Safar, MD – University of Pittsburgh
- Roger White, MD – Mayo Clinic (and a later chair of the NREMT's board)

The first EMT-Paramedic examination, for candidates completing the EMT-Paramedic national standard curriculum training program, was administered in Minneapolis, MN, on February 21, 1978.

Despite the challenges faced in the 1980s due to changing federal priorities and loss of dedicated funding, the NREMT persisted in its mission. By 1984, 24 states required National EMS Certification, and an additional 15 states accepted National EMS Certification as an alternative to state-administered examinations. While the progress was slow with significant challenges along the way, by 2023, 48 states required National EMS Certification as a prerequisite for state licensure, and the two remaining states will accept National EMS Certification as an alternative to the state-only license examination.

Reflecting on the journey that has brought us to the present state of the National Registry of Emergency Medical Technicians (NREMT), it is clear that the pioneering spirit of the 1960s and 1970s played a vital role in shaping emergency medical services in the United States. At the heart of this evolution were numerous influential stakeholders who wisely recognized the need for a national EMS certification body.

Key among these stakeholders were President Lyndon Johnson and the Committee on Highway Traffic Safety, the National Academy of Sciences and the National Research Council, the American Medical Association, the American College of Surgeons, the American College of Orthopedic Surgeons, the Ambulance Association of America, and individual visionaries like Rocco Morando. Their collective endeavor laid the groundwork for what would become a robust system for emergency medical services certification.

Prominent medical professionals like Dr. J.D. Farrington, a leading figure in orthopedic and trauma medicine, and Dr. Peter Safar, known as the 'Father of CPR', used their knowledge and influence to advocate for and develop the national EMS certification body. Their unwavering commitment to enhancing emergency medical care and their direct experience with trauma patients were instrumental in shaping the vision and objectives of the NREMT.

In 1976, Dr. Farrington, serving as the first physician Chairman of the National Registry, co-authored "*The History of EMS in the United States*".[121] This seminal work underscored the foundational vision and purpose of the National Registry of EMTs, positioning it as a unifying body for the education, examination, and certification of EMTs on a national level.

Regrettably, half a century later, much of this rich history has been forgotten, and many in the profession today remain unaware of the origins and purpose of National EMS Certification. The architects of our modern EMS system identified the need for a specialized medical profession that melded rescue and extrication techniques with cardiac medicine, critical care medicine, and emergency medicine. Moreover, they recognized the necessity of establishing this new profession as a recognized medical profession with nationwide standards and consistency.

As the EMS community honors the past and looks towards the future, it is essential to reflect on the collective efforts, dedication, and vision that have shaped the National Registry of Emergency Medical Technicians into what it is today. This serves as a powerful reminder and a call to action to uphold and advance the standards and principles upon which the NREMT was founded. Preserving and building upon this legacy is a shared responsibility, carried not only for the benefit of EMS professionals but also for the countless lives that have been positively impacted by their care. By honoring this responsibility, the EMS community can continue to make a significant difference in the well-being and safety of individuals and communities.

The Task Force charged with developing a single national EMS certification body was led by Oscar P. Hampton, Jr., MD, from the American College of Surgeons Committee on Trauma. The first meeting was on January 21, 1970, with representatives from the following organizations:

- American Medical Association
- Ambulance Association of America
- International Association of Fire Chiefs
- International Rescue and First Aid Association
- National Ambulance and Medical Services Association
- National Forest Service
- National Funeral Directors Association
- National Park Service
- National Safety Council
- National Ski Patrol
- American Heart Association
- International Association of Chiefs of Police

1968 NRC/NAS Committee & Task Force

TRAINING

of ambulance personnel and others responsible for emergency care of the sick and injured at the scene and during transport

Guidelines and Recommendations of the
Committee on Emergency Medical Services
Division of Medical Sciences
National Academy of Sciences
National Research Council

Prepared under SA-896-68 and Contract PH 110-68-1 with the
U.S. DEPARTMENT OF HEALTH, EDUCATION, AND WELFARE
Public Health Service
Health Services and Mental Health Administration
Division of Emergency Health Services
5600 Fishers Lane, Rockville, Md. 20852

COMMITTEE ON EMERGENCY MEDICAL SERVICES

JOHN M. HOWARD, M.D., Hahnemann Medical College and Hospital, Philadelphia, Pa., *Chairman*

OSCAR P. HAMPTON, JR., M.D., American College of Surgeons, Chicago, Ill.

JAMES B. HARTGERING, M.D., Department of Health, Hospitals, and Welfare, City of Cambridge, Cambridge, Mass.

FRANCIS C. JACKSON, M.D., University of Pittsburgh School of Medicine, Pittsburgh, Pa.

JOHN M. KINNEY, M.D., Columbia University College of Physicians and Surgeons, New York, N. Y.

ROSS A. MCFARLAND, M.D., Harvard School of Public Health, Boston, Mass.

ROBERT M. OSWALD, The American National Red Cross, National Headquarters, Washington, D. C.

J. CUTHBERT OWENS, M.D., University of Colorado Medical Center, Denver

PETER SAFAR, M.D., University of Pittsburgh School of Medicine, Pittsburgh, Pa.

SPENCER T. SNEDECOR, M.D., Hackensack, N. J.

JOHN P. STAPP, COL., USAF, M.C., U. S. Department of Transportation, Washington, D. C.

ALAN P. THAL, M.D., University of Kansas Medical Center, Kansas City

TASK FORCE ON GUIDELINES FOR TRAINING OF AMBULANCE PERSONNEL

JOSEPH D. FARRINGTON, M.D., Minocqua, Wisc., *Chairman*

WALTER A. HOYT, JR., M.D., American Academy of Orthopaedic Surgeons, Akron, O.

WALTER S. HUNT, JR., M.D., The Raleigh Orthopaedic Clinic, Raleigh, N. C.

ROCCO MORANDO, Division of Vocational Education, Ohio State University, Columbus

ROBERT M. OSWALD, The American National Red Cross, National Headquarters, Washington, D. C.

PETER SAFAR, M.D., University of Pittsburgh School of Medicine, Pittsburgh, Pa.

JOSEPH R. TERRITO, LT. COL. M.S.C., U. S. Army Medical Training Center, Ft. Sam Houston, Texas

Liaison Members

ROSWELL K. BROWN, M.D., Committee on Trauma Field Program, New York, N.Y.

OSCAR P. HAMPTON, JR., M.D., American College of Surgeons, Chicago, Ill.

JOHN M. HOWARD, M.D., Hahnemann Medical College and Hospital, Philadelphia, Pa.

LOUIS C. KOSSUTH, COL. M.C., USAF, HQ Air Defense Command, Ent Air Force Base, Colorado

JOSEPH K. OWEN, PH.D., Emergency Health Services Branch, Division of Direct Health Services, U. S. Public Health Service, Silver Spring, Md.

JOHN M. WATERS, JR., CAPT., U. S. Coast Guard, National Highway Safety Bureau, Department of Transportation, Washington, D. C.

THEODORE H. WILSON, JR., CAPT., M.C., USN, U. S. Naval Hospital, Bethesda, Md.

Staff

ROBERT J. FITZSIMMONS, Emergency Health Services Branch, Division of Direct Health Services, U. S. Public Health Service, Silver Spring, Md.

SAM F. SEELEY, M.D., National Academy of Sciences-National Research Council Washington, D. C.

NATIONAL REGISTRY PATCHES OVER THE YEARS

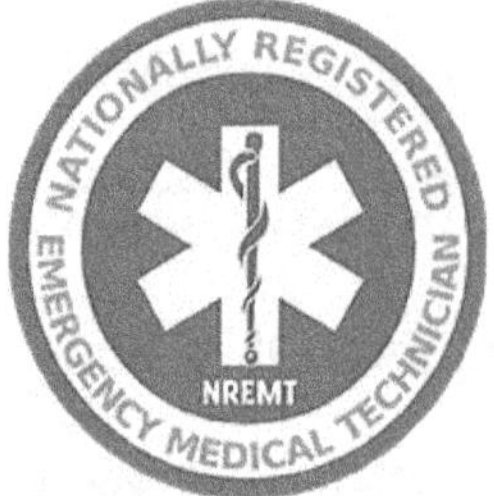

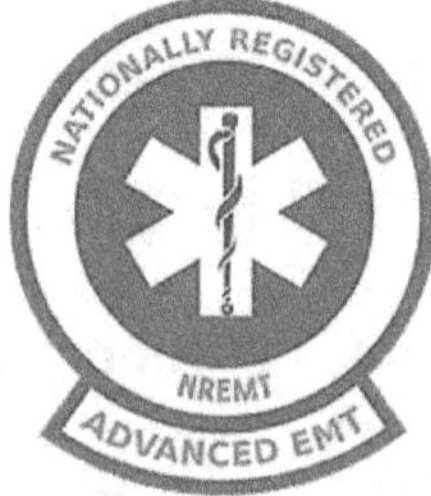

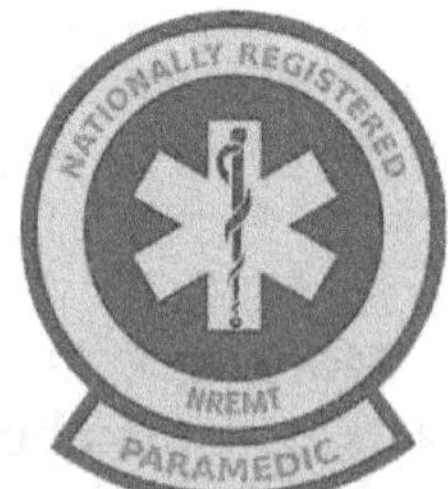

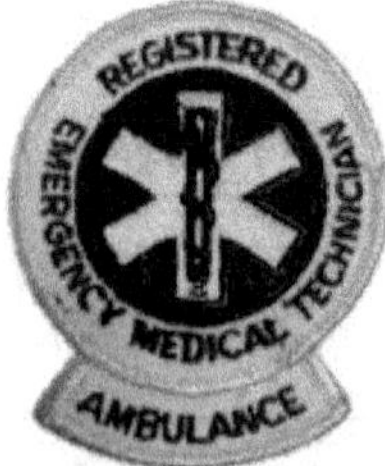

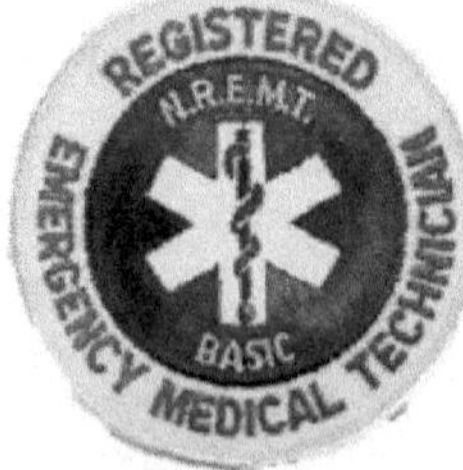

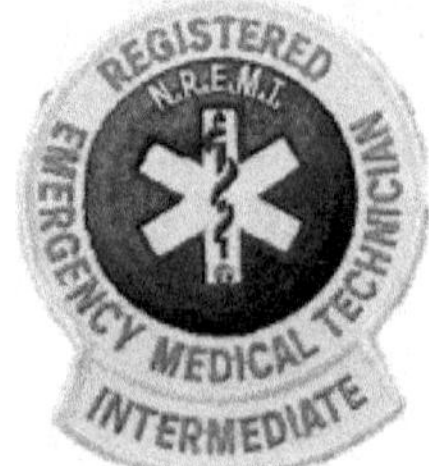

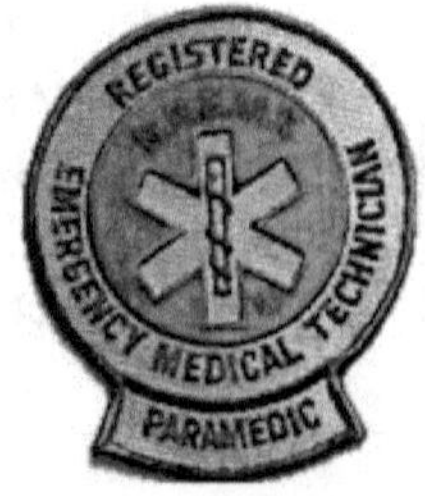

A SINGLE NATIONAL CERTIFICATION BODY: A POLICY CHOICE ROOTED IN HISTORY

The intricate historical background and policy shifts that led to the formation of the National Registry of EMTs have unfortunately been somewhat overlooked as time has progressed. Nonetheless, grasping the origins and reasoning behind this initiative is key to appreciating its importance. The birth of the EMS profession is a testament to the exceptional collaborative work among leading physicians with a shared vision. Distinguished figures including Peter Safar, MD, an innovator in Critical Care Medicine and CPR; R. Adams Cowley, MD, a leader in cardiothoracic and open-heart surgery, and the "Father of Trauma Medicine"; and JD Farrington, MD, a leading orthopedic surgeon of the era, were integral to this process. They wielded significant influence from the White House and Congress to major medical institutions. They had the resolute backing of the American Medical Association, the American College of Surgeons, and the American College of Orthopedic Surgeons, and were united in their aim to transform the disjointed, unregulated, and subpar ambulance services of that era.

Identifying the necessity for a unique medical profession that could extend expertise, skills, and capabilities beyond hospital walls to non-physician professionals, these visionary individuals aimed to ensure this novel profession upheld the highest of standards, while remaining consistent throughout the country.

The inception of the National Registry of EMTs reflected a coordinated national effort:

> The Registry was founded in 1970, following a recommendation by the President's Committee on Highway Safety, to serve as a national certifying body establishing uniform training and personnel standards for ambulance personnel. Its early work was supported by the American Medical Association, Employers Insurance of Wausau, and the American Ambulance Association. Working with the Department of Health, Education, and Welfare, the Department of Transportation, and the broader medical community, the Registry has consistently fulfilled its mission relative to Emergency Medical Technicians.

This historical narration underscores the concerted efforts between various stakeholders, including government agencies and the healthcare community, to form a unified system for EMS professionals. The National Registry of EMTs exemplifies this shared vision, aiming to preserve uniform training, personnel competencies, and overall care quality provided by Emergency Medical Technicians across the nation.

In the face of numerous hurdles that greatly hampered the advocated coordinated national approach to EMS system development in the 1960s and 70s, their vision eventually became a reality. Nevertheless, the 1996 *EMS Agenda for the Future* poignantly highlighted that "over 40 different EMS certification levels exist." Despite these complications, states managed to standardize criteria, including National EMS Certification. As stated in the 2000 *EMS Education Agenda for the Future: A Systems Approach*, a single National EMS Certification is a key component of the national EMS system.

Post-2000, the EMS profession has once more acknowledged and upheld the insight of the profession's founders: national standardization. By 2023, 48 states mandate National EMS Certification as a prerequisite for state licensure. With a highly mobile population, public expectation is straightforward: medical care should adhere to uniform standards irrespective of jurisdictional borders. This notion is further solidified by the quick growth of medical interstate compacts, including robust compacts for nursing, physicians, occupational therapy, psychology, physical therapy, and the EMS Compact.

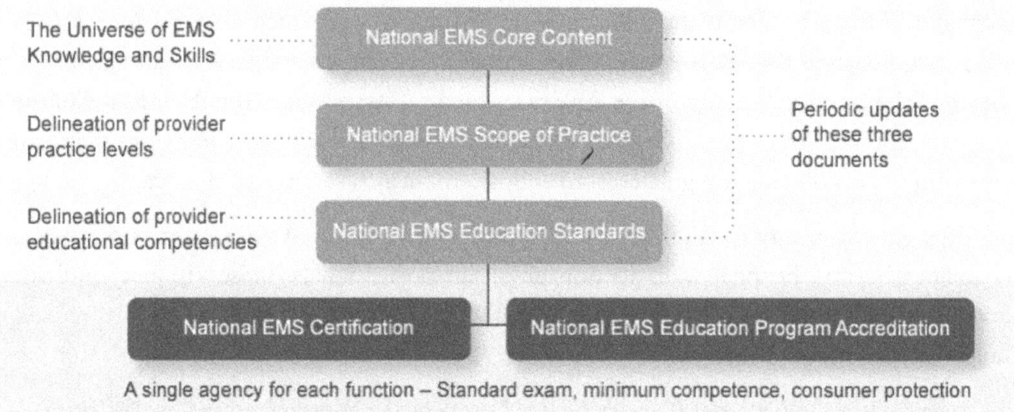

Challenges and Progress in the Adoption of National Standards

While the NREMT continues to make significant strides in unifying the EMS profession under a single national standard, challenges persist in the adoption of these standards, especially in communities with long-standing, unique approaches to EMS training and education. The variability in EMS education has necessitated an ongoing effort from the NREMT to adapt and evolve its certification process, ensuring that all EMS practitioners are sufficiently prepared to provide high-quality care in their communities.

In recent years, the NREMT has taken several steps to address these challenges and further promote the adoption of national standards across the United States. These efforts include:

- **Collaboration with national organizations**: By working closely with organizations such as the National Association of State EMS Officials (NASEMSO) and the National Highway Traffic Safety Administration's (NHTSA) EMS, the NREMT has been able to develop comprehensive national standards for EMS education, certification, and practice. This collaboration ensures that the EMS community is working together to achieve uniformity and consistency in the care provided to patients.
- **Continued refinement of certification programs**: The NREMT regularly reviews and updates its certification standards to align with current best practices in EMS care, while also ensuring compliance with the best practices of the testing and certification industry. By

remaining flexible and adaptable, the NREMT has been able to address the diverse needs of EMS practitioners and better serve communities with unique requirements.

- **Recertification and continuing education**: To maintain the competency of EMS practitioners, the NREMT requires recertification every two years. This process includes meeting continuing education requirements and a validation of continued competency and skills, ensuring that EMS practitioners stay current with advancements in EMS care and continue to meet established standards of practice.

As the NREMT continues to work on overcoming the challenges associated with unifying and maintaining national standards for the EMS profession, its commitment to fostering collaboration, refining certification programs, and supporting EMS research has significantly contributed to the development of a high-quality emergency medical system in the United States.

Standardized Examinations: Essential for State EMS Offices

The National Registry of Emergency Medical Technicians plays a critical role in ensuring legally defensible examinations for the EMS profession. By providing examinations that are secure, unbiased, and adhere to national standards, the NREMT offers states a crucial service that helps maintain public trust and professional credibility. The organization's commitment to developing and administering high-quality examinations supports states in maintaining the highest levels of competence and professionalism among EMS personnel, fostering public confidence in the EMS system.

The creation of these examinations is a meticulous process that involves the collaboration of examination experts, including psychometricians who specialize in the theory and techniques of educational and psychological measurement. These experts ensure that the exams are constructed to accurately measure the knowledge and skills of EMS personnel and meet the highest professional standards. The process begins with a rigorous practice analysis that identifies the essential knowledge and skills required for EMS personnel. This analysis serves as the foundation for the development of examination specifications, which outline the content and structure of the exams.

Once the examination specifications are established, subject matter experts (SMEs) from the EMS community collaborate with examination experts to develop exam questions. SMEs are experienced EMS professionals who represent various geographical regions and diverse backgrounds, ensuring that the exams reflect the knowledge and skills necessary for EMS practitioners across the nation. The collaboration between SMEs and examination experts is crucial to ensure that the exams are both technically sound and relevant to the EMS profession.

After the development of exam questions, a rigorous review process is undertaken to guarantee their clarity, accuracy, and absence of bias. This process entails multiple rounds of revisions, incorporating feedback from independent Subject Matter Experts (SMEs) and psychometricians. Following the finalization of the questions, they undergo pilot testing with numerous EMS candidates in a secure testing environment. Subsequently, psychometricians review the questions to ensure their statistical performance and absence of bias. Questions that do not meet psychometric standards are excluded and never used.

For states, the NREMT's role in providing these examinations is vitally important. Although states have the jurisdictional authority to offer their own license exams, doing so can be both cost-prohibitive and a significant legal liability. The resources and expertise required to develop and maintain legally defensible examinations are burdensome for individual states, and the potential for inconsistencies across jurisdictions can jeopardize the uniformity and credibility of the EMS profession. By relying on the NREMT's examinations, states can ensure a consistent level of competence and professionalism among EMS practitioners.

Moreover, as recognized by the pioneers of the profession, the public expects the EMS profession to be largely standardized across all jurisdictions. The NREMT's commitment to providing high-quality, legally defensible examinations helps to fulfill this expectation and instill public trust in the EMS system. The NREMT's examinations also facilitate mobility of EMS personnel, making it easier for EMS practitioners to transfer state licensure when moving or seeking employment in another state. This, in turn, promotes a more flexible and efficient EMS workforce that can better serve the nation's emergency medical needs.

The NREMT, a non-profit 501(c)3 organization, serves as a vital ally to state EMS offices, providing standardized and legally defensible examinations for the EMS profession. Through collaborations with examination specialists and adherence to national standards, the organization assists states in maintaining high levels of competence and professionalism among EMS personnel. This partnership not only alleviates financial and legal burdens on states but also ensures that the EMS profession meets the public's expectations for consistent and high-quality emergency medical care across all jurisdictions. The NREMT's unwavering dedication to developing and administering reliable and valid examinations contributes significantly to the ongoing enhancement and advancement of emergency medical care nationwide. However, despite its more than fifty years of existence, many professionals in the field remain unaware of the origins and processes involved in creating the examination or the National EMS Certification process.

The National EMS Certification Process

The National EMS Certification process goes far beyond merely writing and administering examinations. The comprehensive process encompasses a range of crucial elements, including a Practice Analysis, creating questions, exam development, and the design and administration of computer adaptive examinations. These components work together to create a robust and dynamic certification process that enables EMS professionals to demonstrate their competence and remain up to date with the ever-evolving field of emergency medical services. Moreover, the certification process must be legally defensible, unbiased, and compliant with the *Standards for Educational and Psychological Testing*[122] to ensure a fair and equitable assessment of EMS practitioners' knowledge and skills. By emphasizing these essential aspects, the National EMS

Certification process maintains its integrity and effectively promotes high-quality care within the EMS community.

Understanding the Practice Analysis

The National Registry of Emergency Medical Technicians (NREMT) places great importance on conducting regular Practice Analyses to ensure that the National EMS Certification examinations accurately assess the knowledge and skills required for EMS practitioners to deliver safe and effective prehospital care. The Practice Analysis serves as a critical mechanism for maintaining the currency and validity of the certification exams by aligning the content with the latest best practices in the field of EMS. Through these analyses, the NREMT ensures that the examinations remain relevant and reflect the evolving demands and advancements in emergency medical services. By consistently updating the examination content based on the findings of the Practice Analysis, the NREMT upholds the integrity and quality of the certification process, ultimately promoting the delivery of high standards of care in the prehospital setting.

Building on its longstanding commitment to legally defensible and fair examinations that adhere to industry standards, the NREMT has consistently conducted rigorous examinations and evaluations for several decades. The 2019 EMS Practice Analysis, which focused on the Advanced Life Support levels (Paramedic and AEMT), was a significant undertaking that involved more than 3,500 EMS professionals, including staff, panel members, and survey respondents. Data from 10,000 EMS agencies was included in the analysis. The study was conducted using multiple sources, including the National Emergency Medical Services Information System (NEMSIS), surveys from active EMS practitioners, and recommendations from EMS subject matter experts. The findings from the 2019 Advanced Life Support EMS Practice Analysis were published in the National Association of EMS Physicians' journal, *Prehospital Emergency Care,*[123] transparently providing the EMS community with a clear vision of current prehospital care, including the tasks performed by EMS practitioners. Similarly, in 2022, the Basic Life Support EMS practice analysis efforts focused on Emergency Medical Responders and Emergency Medical Technicians.

The purpose of the Practice Analysis includes evaluating the EMS profession by examining the tasks, knowledge, and skills required for competent EMS practice, considering the evolving nature of the profession and advancements in emergency medicine. The findings from the Practice Analysis serve as a foundation for developing NREMT certification exams, ensuring that the test content accurately represents the actual responsibilities and capabilities of EMS practitioners at various levels. Additionally, the Practice Analysis includes a comprehensive assessment of the frequency and criticality of clinical skills and interventions observed in actual clinical practice. By analyzing data from surveys, literature reviews, and EMS patient care reports, the NREMT identifies the tasks and procedures that EMS practitioners encounter most frequently and those that have the greatest impact on patient outcomes. This valuable information allows the NREMT to prioritize and emphasize the content of the certification exams, ensuring that they accurately reflect the demands and challenges faced by EMS professionals in their daily practice.

Furthermore, the Practice Analysis provides valuable insights for EMS educators and training programs, enabling them to design curricula that effectively prepare students for the NREMT certification exams and real-world practice. By aligning the education and training programs with the findings of the Practice Analysis, educators can ensure that students acquire the necessary knowledge and skills to succeed in their EMS careers. This integration between the certification process and educational programs promotes a cohesive and comprehensive approach to EMS training, enhancing the overall competence and preparedness of EMS practitioners.

The process of the Practice Analysis involves several key steps. First, the NREMT collaborates with subject matter experts (SMEs), including a diverse group of EMS professionals such as educators, researchers, and practitioners, who provide their expertise and insights. Data collection follows, which encompasses gathering information from various sources like surveys of EMS practitioners, reviews of EMS-related literature and research, and analysis of EMS patient care reports. This collected data is then analyzed to identify the tasks, knowledge, and skills required for competent EMS practice, as well as to recognize trends, emerging practices, and areas where EMS practitioners may need additional training or support. The findings from the Practice Analysis are used to validate and develop the content of the NREMT certification exams, ensuring that the exams remain relevant and accurately assess the knowledge and skills of EMS practitioners.

Lastly, the NREMT regularly conducts practice analyses to stay up-to-date with the changing field of emergency medical services and continuously improve the certification exams. These practice analyses play a vital role in ensuring that EMS practitioners are well-prepared to provide excellent prehospital care. By evaluating the tasks, knowledge, and skills needed for competent EMS practice, the NREMT keeps the certification exams relevant and rigorous. This ongoing process fosters the development of EMS education and practice, making sure that practitioners have the necessary skills to deliver high-quality care.

The Practice Analysis and the CAT Exam: A Crucial Connection

The Practice Analyses and the Computer Adaptive Testing (CAT) exam are closely intertwined in the process of maintaining and updating the certification exams for EMS practitioners. The Practice Analyses are the foundation for developing the test content, while the CAT exam is the innovative method by which the content is delivered and assessed. The connection between the Practice Analysis and the CAT exam becomes evident when considering the following aspects:

- **Informed test development**: The Practice Analyses findings serve as a crucial foundation for developing the content of the CAT exam. By identifying the specific tasks, knowledge, and skills needed for competent EMS practice, these analyses directly inform the creation of test items. The goal is to ensure that the CAT exam accurately reflects the responsibilities and capabilities of EMS practitioners. This commitment to incorporating the Practice

Analyses findings helps to maintain the exam's validity, reliability, psychometric soundness, and legal defensibility.

- **Test item bank**: The data and insights from the Practice Analysis are used to create a large pool of test items, also known as the test item bank. This bank serves as the basis for the CAT exam, enabling the system to select and present test items that are relevant and appropriate for each individual candidate.
- **Adaptive testing**: The CAT exam is designed to adapt to each candidate's demonstrated ability level based on their responses to the test items. The test items are selected from the item bank, which is informed by the Practice Analysis, to ensure that the exam accurately assesses the candidate's knowledge and skills in relation to the established standards of EMS practice.
- **Continuous improvement**: The ongoing updates and refinements to the Practice Analysis help ensure that the CAT exam remains current with the evolving landscape of emergency medical services. As the Practice Analysis identifies new trends, emerging practices, and areas where EMS practitioners may require additional training, the test item bank is updated accordingly, enabling the CAT exam to consistently assess the most relevant knowledge and skills.

By informing the content of the exam and guiding the selection of test items, the Practice Analysis helps ensure that the CAT exam remains an accurate, reliable, and up-to-date assessment tool for EMS practitioners. This connection between the Practice Analysis and the CAT exam ultimately contributes to the overall goal of promoting high-quality EMS education and practice across the United States.

COMPUTER ADAPTIVE EXAMINATIONS

Computer Adaptive Testing (CAT) represents a sophisticated method of examination that modulates the difficulty level of test questions in real time based on the test-taker's responses. In practice, as a candidate navigates through the test, the algorithm intelligently adapts the subsequent questions in accordance with the candidate's performance, making the test customized to their individual ability. If a test-taker correctly answers a question, they are then presented with a slightly more challenging question. Conversely, an incorrect response prompts a slightly less difficult question next.

In the early 2000s, the National Registry of Emergency Medical Technicians (NREMT) and the NCLEX (Registered Nurse examination) were at the forefront of introducing an innovative technology in medical examinations. The NREMT made a significant transition from traditional linear paper examinations for EMT and Paramedic certifications to the Computer Adaptive Testing (CAT) format in 2007. This transition was the result of extensive research and development efforts, aimed at ensuring that CAT examinations offered valid, reliable, and fair evaluations of test-takers' knowledge and competencies.

CAT examinations confer several noteworthy advantages. First and foremost, they offer high levels of reliability and sensitivity. CAT examinations provide an accurate and efficient measure of an examinee's knowledge and skills by selecting the questions most suitable for their level of ability. This method focuses on the candidate's genuine proficiency, thereby enhancing the examination's reliability and sensitivity.

Moreover, CAT examinations promote improved efficiency. By adjusting to the examinee's level of ability, CAT examinations can evaluate competency using fewer questions compared to traditional examinations. This results in a reduced test duration, less resources required for test administration and scoring, and a decrease in the associated costs of test administration.

Finally, CAT examinations provide enhanced test security by minimizing the risk of cheating and exposure of test questions. The selection of items from a broad pool lessens the chance of examinees encountering the same questions, thereby maintaining the integrity of the examination and the validity of the certification. This advanced approach to testing underscores the progress in educational technology and is emblematic of the commitment to fair, efficient, and accurate assessments in the field of emergency medical services.

STANDARD SETTING: WHAT IS PASSING?

Standard setting in computer adaptive examinations signifies the rigorous process of determining a benchmark performance level. Divergent from traditional linear exams which employ a passing percentage, Computer Adaptive Testing (CAT) harnesses the power of logit scores, a fusion of "log" and "odds", to forecast a candidate's success or failure based on their responses.[124]

This process of standard setting includes an independent panel, comprising EMS regulators, practitioners, employers, educators, and community representatives. Their pivotal task is to outline the traits of a minimally competent (entry-level) candidate, and that candidate's knowledge, skills, and abilities (KSA) for each domain of content.

Upon setting these competence benchmarks, the panel is educated on the methodology of standard setting. This includes determining the proportion of minimally competent candidates who would correctly answer each question. This approximation is anchored on the established competencies and the nature of the questions. A group discussion follows the initial round of ratings, during which the panel is presented with an overview of each question's ratings. Panel members are then encouraged to explain their individual ratings, particularly the extreme ones.

Any question demonstrating a large disparity in ratings or a significant deviation between mean ratings and the mean statistics of the item is analyzed thoroughly. The core focus remains on understanding how a minimally competent candidate would fare on these questions. This stage permits panel members to reevaluate their preliminary ratings, based on newly acquired information and feedback, thereby leading to the final ratings for each question.

These final ratings are utilized to establish the passing cutoff score, which is aligned with minimum entry-level competency. Consequently, this ensures that candidates deemed competent indeed possess the necessary knowledge and skills. Upon completion of the standard setting process, psychometricians, who are specialized examination scientists, statistically scrutinize the examination. This is to ensure that the exam is functioning as anticipated, thus adding an additional layer of reliability and validity to the standard setting process.

How CAT Examinations Work and Common Misconceptions

Despite the myriad advantages offered by Computer Adaptive Test exams, there are instances where they are misunderstood by test-takers, EMS managers, and educators, and over the years this has led to confusion, misconceptions, and frustration.

It is imperative to comprehend that the primary objective of CAT exams is to challenge the test-taker's level of competency. As such, even highly proficient and well-informed candidates might be presented with difficult questions. The fundamental goal of the adaptive algorithm is to discern the true level of competency of the test-taker, which can lead to the presentation of challenging questions regardless of their overall performance.

The inherent adaptability of the CAT exams, along with the uncertainty associated with question difficulty and quantity, can sometimes provoke anxiety or confusion among test-takers. This could lead to a scenario where successful candidates might think that they have failed the CAT exam despite having passed it. Therefore, it is vital for candidates to understand the unique characteristics of CAT exams, be prepared for their adaptive nature, and trust in their preparation and knowledge while interpreting their results.

Consider, for example, an EMT or Paramedic student who consistently performs at a high level in the classroom and easily passes traditional linear examinations. Upon encountering challenging topics during the CAT examination and experiencing an abrupt end to the test, this student might incorrectly surmise that they have failed. They may even experience frustration, presuming that their instructor did not sufficiently cover all required material, questioning the inclusion of certain questions. Nevertheless, shortly thereafter, the candidate receives a notification that they have indeed passed the exam, underscoring the potential for misunderstandings surrounding the CAT examination process.

Candidate Feedback: Scaled Score Reports

In 2023, the National Registry of Emergency Medical Technicians implemented Scaled Score Reports to provide unsuccessful candidates additional feedback on their overall examination performance. This innovation aims to enhance the feedback provided on examination attempts, thus better equipping candidates for future testing experiences.

The Scaled Score Report adopts a holistic approach, encapsulating all domains tested and thereby offering a comprehensive portrayal of a candidate's overall performance. This methodology synthesizes performances across the entire spectrum of the exam into one overall score, presenting a complete picture of a candidate's proficiency.

An essential facet of scaled scores is the standardization of performance. Scaled Score Reports introduce a uniform measure that facilitates a straightforward comparison of individual performances. These reports present a standardized scale, thereby enabling candidates to assess their scores in comparison to the passing standard. Such a method ensures a transparent feedback mechanism that supports candidates in identifying their strengths and areas needing improvement.

The adoption of scaled scoring aligns with best practices in the standardized examination industry, providing unsuccessful candidates with accurate, interpretable feedback on their performance. This method enables candidates, including aspiring EMS managers and leaders, to approach future tests with an enhanced understanding of their abilities. It also assures governmental officials of a fair, transparent, and comprehensive evaluation method for the EMS profession.

We regret to inform you that you have failed the cognitive examination. A score of 950 or above is required to pass the examination. Your result was 840, which is below the passing standard of 950.

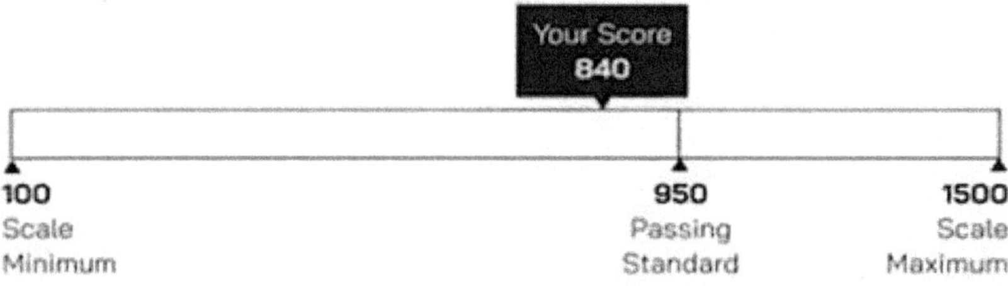

Scale Minimum: 100

Passing Standard: 950

Your Score: 840

THE CAT EXAMINATION PROCESS

1. **Initial question**: The test begins with a question of moderate difficulty, which serves as a baseline to gauge the examinee's proficiency.
2. **Adaptive algorithm**: Based on the examinee's response, the algorithm selects the next question, increasing the difficulty if the initial question was answered correctly or decreasing it if the response was incorrect.
3. **Continuous adjustment**: The CAT examination maintains an adaptive approach by continuously adjusting the difficulty level of questions according to the test-taker's performance. This adaptive process allows the exam to accurately gauge the individual's true ability by presenting questions that challenge their knowledge and skills appropriately.
4. **Termination criteria**: The examination ends when either a pre-determined number of questions have been answered, the allotted time has expired, or the candidate has demonstrated (or not demonstrated) competency with at least a 95% statistical confidence interval.

Chart Demonstrating a Successful and Unsuccessful Candidate.

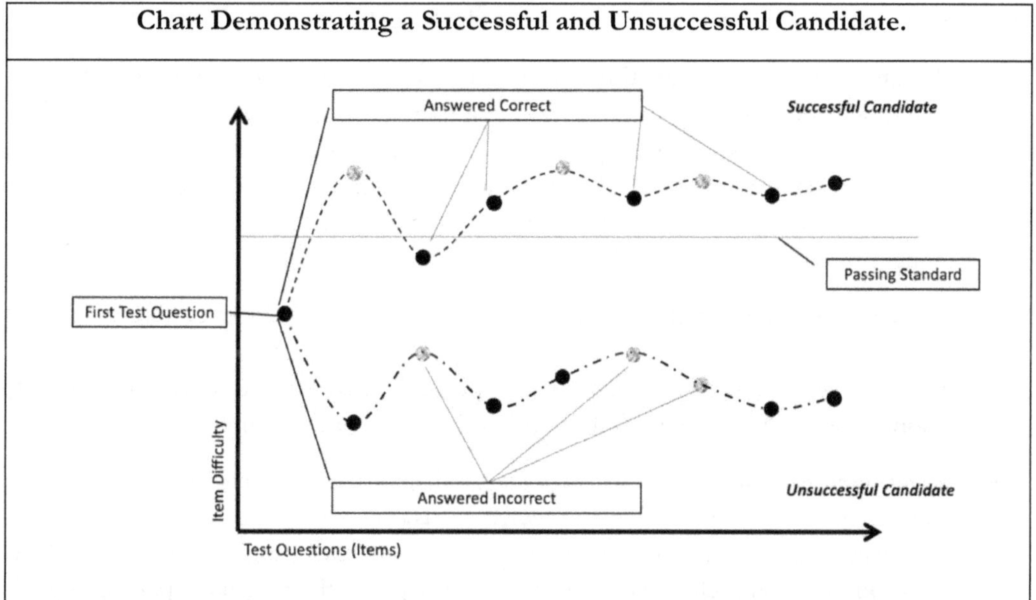

- The examination starts with a calibrated item (question), if the candidate answers the question correctly, the next question will be more difficult.
- When candidates answer questions incorrectly, they will be presented easier questions.
- As the examination progresses, the computer identifies the candidate's ability.

Once the minimum number of questions have been administered, the NREMT examination continues until one of the following:

- There is a 95% confidence that the candidate is ABOVE the established passing standard.
- There is a 95% confidence that the candidate is BELOW the established passing standard.
- The candidate has reached the maximum allowed time, known as ROOT (Run Out Of Time).

Common Misconceptions

- **Misinterpretation of Question Difficulty**: Candidates may erroneously believe that encountering complex questions indicates poor performance, or alternatively, that straightforward questions suggest superior performance. The CAT examination evaluates the test-taker's proficiency level by providing calibrated questions of diverse difficulty until the maximum proficiency level is statistically ascertained. In some instances, if a candidate's proficiency level far exceeds the passing standard, the questions presented may seem extraordinarily difficult.
- **Unequal Number of Questions**: There may be concerns among test-takers that the CAT examination concludes after a variable number of questions for each candidate, which could be perceived as inequitable. Nevertheless, once the candidate has answered a predetermined minimum number of questions, the adaptive nature of the test guarantees accurate and efficient evaluation of all examinees, irrespective of the total number of questions addressed.
- **Perceived Randomness**: The CAT examination may appear arbitrary to test-takers, as questions are selected from a vast pool and the sequence and difficulty of questions may not follow a foreseeable pattern. This perception can induce confusion or anxiety among candidates unfamiliar with the adaptive nature of the examination.
- **Misconception about Passing Scores**: Candidates may inaccurately presume that a specific number or percentage of correct answers is required to pass the CAT examination. The CAT algorithm, however, evaluates the examinee's proficiency level based on their comprehensive performance throughout the test, and a passing score is ascertained by the overall demonstration of competency rather than a fixed quantity of correct responses.

Addressing these common misconceptions and educating test-takers about the CAT process can help mitigate confusion and anxiety, ultimately fostering an enhanced understanding and appreciation of the benefits that CAT examinations offer in accurately and efficiently evaluating knowledge and skills. This comprehensive guidance and communication can assist candidates in adjusting their expectations, minimizing anxiety, and cultivating a more positive mindset when approaching the exam.

Candidate Preparation

When discussing CAT examinations with students, educators and EMS leaders should emphasize the following points:

- **Different Examination Design**: Instructors traditionally use examinations to gauge a student's progress and identify areas for improvement. These tests are typically structured for learning, measuring how much students know about specific topic areas as they progress through different phases of learning. Students are used to receiving item-level feedback and using this feedback for further study. However, licensing and certification examinations differ as they aim to determine whether a candidate's knowledge is at, above, or below the established standard. Once this scientifically valid, reliable, psychometrically sound, and legally defensible determination is made, the assessment ceases.

- **Focus on Competency**: Remind test-takers that the CAT examination aims to assess their competency, rather than their ability to memorize facts or recall information. Candidates should be encouraged to develop a robust foundation of knowledge and skills, enabling them to demonstrate their proficiency during the exam.

- **Understanding the Adaptive Nature**: Explain that the CAT examination modifies the complexity of questions based on the candidate's performance, which allows the computer to rapidly identify the candidate's true ability level. Encountering challenging questions is part of this process and should not be interpreted as indicative of poor performance.

- **Embrace the Variability**: Clarify that the CAT examination is not a traditional linear test and the number of questions, or their sequence may differ for each candidate. Encourage test-takers to concentrate on their individual performance and refrain from comparing their experience with their peers.

- **Trust the Process**: Reiterate that the CAT examination is engineered to provide an accurate and efficient evaluation of their knowledge and skills. Encourage candidates to trust the examination process and to focus on demonstrating their competency, rather than attempting to predict their results or decipher the algorithm.

By promoting a thorough understanding of the CAT examination process, EMS educators and managers can help candidates dispel misconceptions and reduce apprehensions, ultimately leading to a more positive testing experience. As test-takers become more accustomed to the adaptive nature of the CAT examination, they will be better equipped to showcase their knowledge and skills during the assessment. This improved familiarity will contribute to ensuring that EMS professionals across the United States are well-prepared to provide high-quality care to their patients. Furthermore, it supports the ongoing development and refinement of EMS education and practice.

By addressing these misconceptions and increasing transparency about the CAT examination process, the level of confidence among candidates can be elevated. It is vital for EMS educators and managers to understand the concerns and misconceptions that may arise from the unique nature of CAT examinations, to adequately prepare candidates for this distinctive testing experience. Proper guidance and comprehensive communication strategies can ensure that candidates are fully aware of what to expect during a CAT exam, helping them to manage anxiety, adjust their expectations, and approach the exam with a more positive mindset. Education about CAT examinations improves the overall testing experience and ensures a fair and accurate assessment of candidates' knowledge and skills.

ENSURING FAIRNESS AND MINIMIZING BIAS IN CAT EXAMS

Due to the design and mechanism, Computer Adaptive Testing exams are extremely fair and accurately assess the knowledge and skills of EMS practitioners. One of the key strategies employed by the NREMT to achieve this goal is the extensive pilot testing of exam items. Pilot testing plays a crucial role in evaluating and refining the test items to minimize bias and ensure fairness for all candidates. Here's how pilot testing contributes to these objectives:

- **Pretesting of items**: Before a test item is included in the CAT exam, it undergoes a rigorous pretesting process as part of a pilot test. These pilot test items are embedded within the actual CAT exam; however, responses do not contribute to a candidate's final score. Most pretest items are taken by hundreds of candidates. This process allows the NREMT to gather valuable data on the performance of each item, such as difficulty level, discrimination index, and potential sources of bias.

- **Diverse candidate pool**: Pilot testing also involves administering test items to a diverse and representative sample of candidates, ensuring that the items are evaluated by individuals with varying backgrounds, experiences, and perspectives.

- **Item analysis and review**: After the pilot test, the data collected on each test item is analyzed and reviewed by a panel of subject matter experts. This analysis includes examining the item's difficulty, discrimination, and potential sources of bias. If any issues are identified, such as a cultural or regional bias, the item may be revised or removed from the item pool.

- **Ongoing monitoring and refinement**: Pilot testing is an ongoing process, and the test item pool is continuously refreshed based on the feedback and data collected through pilot testing. This ensures that the CAT exam remains fair and unbiased over time, as new items are introduced, and existing items are revised or retired.

By incorporating pilot testing into the development and maintenance of the CAT exam, all high-stakes organizations – including the NREMT - ensure that the assessment is fair and without bias for all EMS practitioners. This process allows the NREMT to identify and address potential issues with test items, resulting in an exam that accurately and reliably measures the knowledge and skills required for competent EMS practice, regardless of a candidate's background or experience.

THE NREMT'S ROLE IN RESEARCH

In addition to its role in administering examinations and national EMS certification, the NREMT has also emerged as the pioneer in EMS research. Acknowledging the importance of rigorous research in the field of Emergency Medical Services, the NREMT has taken significant steps to promote and support research endeavors aimed at studying and enhancing the EMS workforce, improving the quality of care, and evaluating the effectiveness of EMS systems. Among its notable contributions to research is the establishment of the EMS Research Doctorate Fellowship Program. This program serves as a valuable platform for fostering advanced research in EMS and nurturing the development of future leaders and scholars in the field. Through initiatives like these, the NREMT continues to demonstrate its commitment to advancing the knowledge and evidence base in Emergency Medical Services.

The EMS Research Doctorate Fellowship Program was created with the aim of cultivating a new generation of EMS researchers who are dedicated to advancing the field through high-quality, evidence-based research. By providing financial support and mentorship to promising doctoral candidates, the NREMT has played a critical role in fostering the development of research expertise within the EMS community.

The fellowship program offers various benefits to recipients, including:

Financial support: The program provides funding for tuition, fees, and living expenses during the doctoral studies, alleviating the financial burden, and allowing candidates to focus solely on their research endeavors.

Mentorship and guidance: Fellowship recipients receive guidance and mentorship from established EMS researchers and NREMT representatives, which helps them refine their research skills and develop a robust foundation in EMS research methodologies and best practices.

Networking opportunities: Fellows can connect with other researchers and experts in the EMS community, providing valuable networking opportunities that can lead to future collaborations and research projects.

Dissemination of research findings: The NREMT encourages fellows to publish their research findings in peer-reviewed journals and present their work at national and international conferences, helping to disseminate new knowledge and foster discussions about emerging trends and best practices in the EMS profession.

The EMS Research Doctorate Fellowship Program has had a significant impact on the EMS community, contributing to the development of a growing body of research that has influenced best practices, policy decisions, and the overall improvement of EMS systems across the United States. By investing in the education and training of new researchers, the NREMT has played a pivotal role in shaping the future of EMS and ensuring that the profession continues to evolve in response to new evidence and advancements in medical care.

CONTROVERSIES SURROUNDING THE NREMT

As with any organization responsible for setting and maintaining national standards, the National Registry of Emergency Medical Technicians has faced controversies and challenges throughout its half-century history. Some of these controversies include:

Local resistance to national standards: some local communities and states exhibited resistance towards adopting national standards for EMS education and certification. This resistance originated from apprehensions about relinquishing local control over training programs and a perception that national standards might fail to address the unique needs of specific communities. Despite these concerns diminishing over time, resistance persists in some regions. Nevertheless, maintaining a unified minimum professional standard, recognized across the nation, is paramount for the EMS profession to ensure consistent, high-quality emergency care regardless of location.

Variability in pass rates: The adoption of the NREMT standards and examinations led to some communities experiencing unusually low pass rates. Critics argue that this variability highlights potential inconsistencies in EMS education and may point to a need for further standardization and improvement in training programs.

Perceived difficulty of the CAT exam: The NREMT's Computer Adaptive Testing exam has been criticized by some test-takers as being overly difficult or confusing. This perception may be due in part to misunderstandings about how CAT exams work, as well as the unique structure and adaptability of the test.

High-stakes nature of the exam: The NREMT certification exam is a high-stakes test that can significantly impact an individual's career in EMS. As a result, some have raised concerns about the potential for test anxiety, which may affect performance and, consequently, the validity of the exam as a measure of competence.

Recertification requirements: The NREMT's recertification process, which includes continuing education or passing a recertification examination every two years, has been criticized by some as being overly burdensome or unnecessary. However, proponents of the recertification process argue that it is an essential component of maintaining competency and ensuring that EMS practitioners stay current with advancements in the field.

Despite these controversies, the NREMT remains a critical organization in the development and maintenance of national standards for EMS education, certification, and practice. Its commitment to ensuring the quality and competence of EMS practitioners through rigorous examination and ongoing professional development has significantly contributed to the evolution and improvement of the EMS system in the United States.

UPHOLDING NATIONAL STANDARDS

The principle of standardization stands as a cornerstone in the healthcare sector and the domain of professional licensure. Despite the U.S. Constitution empowering states to create their own standards and requirements (as explained in Chapter 25), the broader benefits of national entry-level standards typically surpass state sovereignty rights to establish independent benchmarks. This is particularly evident in the medical field. The EMS profession in the United States serves as an example of this concept. Over the past five decades, following the creation of the National Registry of Emergency Medical Technicians, the EMS profession has witnessed significant standardization and unity. NREMT certification, now obligatory for state licensure in all but two states, further underscores the wide acceptance of national EMS certification.

Despite these strides, challenges continue to endure. There is an unsettling trend among certain legislative bodies, and regrettably, some stakeholders, to abandon national standards as a misdirected shortcut to tackle local inadequacies. Alarmingly, when some jurisdictions grapple with educating EMS clinicians, personnel recruitment, retention, and training, their approach is to dilute the firmly established minimum standards aimed at protecting the public. Such circumventive maneuvers not only impede progress but also destabilize the national profession, undermining the quality and effectiveness of emergency care, and potentially resulting in severe consequences.

States and jurisdictions that deviate from national standards ought to be liable to substantial penalties. Such repercussions should encompass financial implications, including non-reimbursement from federal payors like Medicare and Medicaid for services that fail to meet or surpass the national standard. Regrettably, EMS clinicians licensed to a lesser standard should not be granted licensure in other jurisdictions until they exhibit proficiency in line with the national standard. This underscores the necessity for the EMS profession to unite in preventing states from deviating from the national standard.

Maintaining uniformity in healthcare, with professionals meeting or exceeding a common minimum standard, is essential to bolster public trust and assure consistent, high-quality care. Therefore, it becomes an indispensable professional duty for all EMS industry stakeholders to firmly uphold these foundational standards. Proposals aimed at diluting or abolishing these standards, rather than suitably funding and supporting EMS, must be met with steadfast opposition, comprehensive education, and proactive advocacy.

Furthermore, in instances where jurisdictions propose to lower standards or resort to shortcuts rather than investing in the profession, it becomes crucial for the national EMS profession to respond as a unified body. Professionals from all corners of the nation must work in synergy to enlighten and inform policymakers about the paramount importance of adhering to stringent standards for maintaining the integrity of the EMS profession and safeguarding public welfare.

Low pass rates or issues with recruitment and retention should not be addressed by diminishing standards. Rather, these challenges highlight the urgency for states to intensively invest in EMS education. EMS should be designated as an essential service, and states should allocate appropriate funding reflecting its critical role within the healthcare system. To address workforce shortages, innovative approaches need to be pursued, such as the creation of incentive programs to ensure fair compensation for EMS professionals, as well as motivate them to offer their services in underserved communities. These strategic solutions hold immense potential to not only uphold the high standards of care we aspire to, but also elevate the profession, benefiting the communities they serve.

Adherence to national standards is more than just a mandate—it is the bedrock of quality care, patient safety, and professional integrity, and is the distinguishing line between an occupation and a medical profession, as envisioned by the founders of EMS.

The EMS profession is presented with a formidable challenge: to unyieldingly uphold, safeguard, and advocate for national standards, standing resolute against any attempts to dilute them. The appropriate course of action involves confronting these issues through investment, education, and advocacy. By demonstrating unity, determination, and an unwavering commitment to excellence, the EMS profession can continue to stand as a beacon of trust, competence, and quality care nationwide.

19

Paramedic Accreditation

"Without standardization, there can be no improvement."
- Taiichi Ohno

ACCREDITATION IS A METHOD FOR CONDUCTING NON-GOVERNMENTAL, peer evaluations of educational institutions and programs. It serves as a cornerstone of quality assurance in higher education, including health education. Despite the states having different levels of control over education, higher education institutions generally operate with substantial independence and autonomy, resulting in a wide range of characteristics and quality in their programs.

Accreditation serves to ensure a fundamental level of quality across these diverse institutions. Implemented by private entities, this process revolves around established criteria that embody the qualities of a solid educational program. These entities have also devised procedures for assessing institutions or programs to determine if they meet the required quality benchmarks. In general, the functions of accreditation include:

1. **Standards Verification**: Accreditation verifies that an institution or program meets established standards. This is essential in health education, ensuring programs prepare students adequately for their future careers.
2. **Assisting Prospective Students**: Accreditation helps students identify institutions that are recognized for their quality, thereby safeguarding their educational investment.
3. **Transfer Credits Acceptance**: Accreditation aids institutions in determining the acceptability of transfer credits, allowing for the mobility of students across different schools and programs.

4. **Investment Guide**: Accreditation helps identify suitable institutions and programs for public and private investment, including scholarships and research funding.
5. **Protection Against Harmful Pressures**: Accreditation protects an institution from damaging internal and external pressures that might compromise educational quality.
6. **Improvement and Standard Raising**: Accreditation encourages the self-improvement of weaker programs and stimulates an overall elevation of standards among educational institutions.
7. **Institutional Evaluation and Planning**: Accreditation involves the faculty and staff comprehensively in evaluating and planning, fostering a culture of continuous improvement.
8. **Professional Certification and Licensure Criteria**: Accreditation establishes the criteria for professional certification and licensure in health education. It ensures that courses offering such preparation meet the necessary standards.
9. **Eligibility for Federal Assistance**: Accreditation provides one of several considerations used to determine eligibility for federal assistance, such as student loans.

Accreditation is a non-governmental, peer-evaluation process that ensures a basic level of quality in educational institutions and programs. It plays an instrumental role in health education, maintaining high educational standards, facilitating student mobility, protecting institutions, and helping to identify worthy investments for public and private funds.

Accreditation further branches into two types - institutional and programmatic accreditation.

- **Institutional Accreditation**: This type of accreditation evaluates the institution. It assesses the quality and integrity of all programs and services offered by the institution. It is not specific to any program but evaluates the institution in its entirety, indicating the institution meets certain standards of quality across all its departments and programs.
- **Programmatic Accreditation**: Also known as specialized or professional accreditation, programmatic accreditation focuses on specific programs within an institution. This form of accreditation is often associated with professional education, like health, law, or engineering programs. It indicates that a specific program within the institution meets the standards of the profession.

Both types of accreditations are pivotal but serve different purposes. Institutional accreditation is usually required for participation in federal financial aid programs, while programmatic accreditation is often necessary for licensure and certification in many professions. They collectively contribute to the quality assurance and enhancement of higher education.

PARAMEDIC PROGRAMMATIC ACCREDITATION

The establishment of national benchmarks for paramedic education has been a complex and arduous journey. Although the accreditation process implemented by EMS is markedly different from the nursing profession, which already enjoyed a robust foundation and strong backing from political entities and stakeholders, it followed the accreditation process used by other allied health professions of the 1970s.

In a pivotal moment in 1975, Dr. J.D. Farrington, Chairman of the Board of the National Registry of EMTs, petitioned the American Medical Association (AMA) to recognize "EMT-Paramedic" as a new allied health profession[125]. It is pertinent to note that the AMA was the accrediting authority for all allied health professions at the time. Dr. Farrington's petition underscored that EMT-Paramedics would employ the established process followed by allied health, nursing, and medical education: standardized education, program accreditation, professional certification, and standardized examinations across the United States. In April 1975, the AMA formally acknowledged the National Registry's request, establishing EMT-Paramedic as a legitimate health occupation. [126]

To ensure the new profession developed in compliance with AMA's requirements for allied health professions, the AMA promptly established a "Task Force for Accreditation of Emergency Medical Technicians-Paramedic", chaired by Dr. Norman McSwain[127] and the "Joint Review Committee on Education Programs for the EMT-Paramedic"[128] (JRCEMT-P). The first accreditation standards, known as the "Essentials for EMT-Paramedic Program Accreditation," were approved in late 1978. The University of California, Los Angeles, (UCLA) and Eastern Kentucky University became the first institutions to have their paramedic programs officially reviewed and accredited by 1980. By 1985, twenty paramedic programs in the United States were accredited.

Alongside the AMA's declaration of EMT-Paramedic as an official "health occupation,"– on par with Physician Assistants, Physical Therapy, and Occupational Therapy, at the time – the National Highway Traffic Safety Administration EMS Bureau contracted with Dr. Nancy Caroline from the University of Pittsburgh to develop the first National Standard Curriculum for EMT-Paramedic.[129] In 1978, the first NREMT paramedic examination was administered in Minneapolis, MN.

The early paramedic programs were accredited through the AMA's Council of Allied Health Education and Accreditation (CAHEA). However, in 1992, Congress enacted the Higher Education Amendments of 1992.[130] This Act declared it was a conflict of interest for the AMA to approve and accredit allied health educational programs. To rectify this conflict, the AMA transitioned CAHEA to a new independent organization called the Commission on Accreditation of Allied Health Education Programs (CAAHEP). In 2000, the Joint Review Committee for EMT-P was reorganized as the Committee on Accreditation of Emergency Medical Services Professions (CoAEMSP) and aligned as one of the allied health programs under CAAHEP. As of 2022, over 700 paramedic programs across the United States are accredited or have a letter of review from CoAEMSP.

The Joint Review Committee on Education Programs was not only the standard well-established mechanism for all allied health programs, it was also the required accreditation body. At the time, the U.S. Department of Education guidance for the "Criteria and Procedures for Listing by the U.S. Commissioner of Education and Current List" noted the Committee on Allied Health Education and Accreditation (CAHEA) of the American Medical Association is recognized as a coordinating agency for accreditation of education for the allied health occupations. In carrying out its accreditation activities, CAHEA cooperates with the review committees sponsored by various allied health and medical specialty organizations."[131] When the JRCEMT-P was established, 23 other allied health programs existed, including: [132]

- Joint Review Committee on Education in Occupational Therapy
- Joint Review Committee on Education in Physical Therapy
- Joint Review Committee on Education in Radiologic Technology (JRCERT)
- Joint Review Committee on Educational Programs in Nuclear Medicine Technology (JRCNMT)
- Joint Review Committee on Educational Programs for the Assistant to the Primary Care Physician
- Joint Review Committee on Education for Inhalation Therapy (Respiratory Therapy)
- Joint Review Committee for the Operating Room Technician

A SINGLE ACCREDITATION BODY: A POLICY CHOICE ROOTED IN HISTORY

The issue of why paramedic programs are restricted to a singular accreditation body remains a recurrent and occasionally contentious topic in contemporary dialogues pertaining to the accreditation of paramedic programs. Grasping the historical context and policy decisions driven by stakeholders that sculpted this choice is essential to understanding the reasoning behind this approach.

All medical professions necessitate a high degree of standardization nationally to garner professional recognition. While state-to-state variation is anticipated, the disparity should be minimal. For example, it is expected that a Registered Nurse or a physician in one state should possess comparable qualifications and competencies to their counterparts in other states. In 1974, Ralph C. Kuhli of the American Medical Association's Department of Allied Medical Professions and Services described accreditation as a "professional responsibility" for allied health education programs.

Different medical professions have adopted various approaches and mechanisms to achieve this standardization. For example, the modern nursing profession, which has roots dating back to the 1800s, leveraged the *Nurse Training Act*[133] and later established the National Council of State Boards of Nursing (NCSBN) to provide a unified framework for nursing regulation. Individual state nursing regulators form the governing body of the NCSBN, which produces model Nurse Practice Acts and standards for nursing education. Each state then adopts its own version of the *Nurse Practice Act*, establishing uniform standards for nursing practice and education. Consequently, with the establishment of a uniform standard for nursing education through model legislation, the industry can accommodate multiple accreditation bodies while maintaining uniformity within the profession.

In contrast, the EMS profession adopted the Allied Health single-entity accreditation model that was prevalent at the time for twenty-three other health professions ranging from Physician Assistants to Physical Therapists. Under this model, individual state legislation defining educational standards is unnecessary. Instead, all educational programs seek accreditation from the same body, ensuring uniformity within the profession and reducing legislative and administrative burdens. Moreover, this approach guarantees long-term consistency when standards require updating, as legislative amendments are not needed. Unlike nursing, EMS in the late 1970s emerged as a new, underfunded, and predominantly community-centric field that lacked a unified national voice and the necessary legislative influence to pursue model legislation in all states and territories. The physician founders of the EMS profession, recognizing the need for national standardization, adopted the standard approach for all allied health professions: a single national accreditation organization.

While some Allied Health professions of the 1970s have subsequently modified their accreditation processes and requirements, a single accreditation model remains for most. For example, Physician Assistants seeking to take the Physician Assistant National Certifying Examination (PANCE) must graduate from a program accredited by the Accreditation Review Commission on Education for the Physician Assistant (ARC-PA).

As the EMS profession matured, the decision to maintain a single accreditation standard underwent review and reinforcement on several occasions. Not only was a single accreditation body the de facto standard for allied health professions, the national EMS profession generally lacked the funding, influence and political support required to adopt model legislation in every state. Consequently, national stakeholders and system designers reinforced the single accreditation model, the Commission on Accreditation of Allied Health Education Programs (CAAHEP), paired with a single national certification body, the National Registry of EMTs, to ensure national standardization for paramedics in the United States.

The strategy of relying on a single accreditation body for paramedic education, supplemented by a single national certification examination, theoretically facilitated the swift development of a uniform system for paramedic education without necessitating state-by-state legislation. However, the absence of state-level regulations mandating national EMS certification as a prerequisite for state licensure led to variations in EMS education, license and practice levels, and practices among individual states. The lack of national coordination, compounded by the community's strong desire for access to ambulances staffed with paramedics, led to a fragmented and compartmentalized approach to paramedic education. This situation bred tension and posed challenges for maintaining consistency and quality in paramedic training programs.

The American Medical Association (AMA) formally recognized EMT-Paramedic as an allied health profession in 1975, with the intent that paramedic education would be based at universities, community colleges, or teaching hospitals, like the other approved allied health programs. However, the strong community demand for paramedics, the absence of state regulation, and the readily available National Standard Curriculum led to paramedic programs being developed ad hoc at an accelerated pace around the nation. While many of the programs were accredited and established at colleges and universities, other programs emerged at local ambulance services, fire departments, or community training centers. The result was disparities in the quality of paramedic education and training.

To, yet again, seek to rectify these inconsistencies and the challenges imposed by the fragmented approach, national EMS leaders continually emphasized the importance of standardization in EMS education and practice through ongoing efforts and initiatives. The cornerstone documents establishing the profession, including the *National Standard Curriculum*, the *EMS Agenda for the Future*, the *EMS Education Agenda for the Future*, all reinforce the importance of a single national EMS certification and a single national EMS program accreditation approach.

In response to the growing fragmentation and variation among paramedic programs across the nation, the National Association of State EMS Officials (NASEMSO) passed Resolution 2010-03, in 2010, titled "National EMS Certification and Program Accreditation". This resolution, representing a unified voice of state EMS officials, urged the National Registry of EMTs to modify their requirements and mandate graduation from a CoAEMSP accredited paramedic program as a prerequisite for National EMS Certification at the paramedic level.

The policy change was designed to ensure that current and future paramedic education programs adhered to a single national standard, promoting consistency and quality in paramedic training and education. However, implementing this new requirement generated frustration among some in the industry who felt that it limited their flexibility and imposed additional burden on the development and operation of paramedic education programs. Despite these concerns, the overarching goal of the policy change was to reestablish the original EMS system design and foster a more unified and consistent approach to paramedic education, ultimately benefiting both EMS professionals and the patients they serve.

The history of paramedic accreditation in the United States has been shaped by the unique challenges and constraints faced by the EMS community during its development. The decision to recognize a single accreditation body was a pragmatic solution, grounded in tradition and experience, to ensure a single national standard for paramedic education and accreditation in the absence of unified state-level regulation. While this approach has created a foundation that has served the profession's needs, ongoing efforts are necessary to further promote excellence and standardization in EMS education to ensure the delivery of high-quality care to patients in need.

Over the years, EMS leaders have remained committed to refining and improving paramedic education and accreditation standards. This commitment has helped shape the EMS profession into a respected and vital component of the healthcare system. By continuing to work collaboratively with stakeholders, EMS leaders can address the remaining disparities in education and practice across the United States and enhance the overall quality of emergency medical care for patients.

While other approaches to accreditation and standardization are possible, any transition should be carefully designed with extensive stakeholder input if the unified profession desires a different approach. The first step would include the adoption of model legislation for uniform EMS Practice Acts in every state to ensure a high level of consistency and professionalism within the EMS community. However, this would require a unified and nationally focused effort of the EMS profession to pass model legislation in all states and be prepared to repeat the process when standards require an update.

As the history of paramedic accreditation continues to unfold, the EMS community will persist in evolving and adapting, ensuring that paramedics are well-prepared to provide life-saving care to those in need. By working together, EMS leaders and stakeholders can develop strategies to maintain and enhance the standards of the profession while addressing the challenges and opportunities that lie ahead.

Excerpt from the 2000 EMS Education Agenda for the Future: A Systems Approach

"**A single, nationally recognized accreditation agency** will be created and will establish standards and guidelines for each level of EMS education. **A single agency** will provide a consistent structure, process, and evaluation for all programs. The accreditation process will recognize the special issues involved in evaluating the entire range of EMS programs.

Universal acceptance of National EMS Education Program Accreditation will result in extensive self-assessment of EMS education programs and the implementation of continuous quality improvement initiatives. Having clear standards and guidelines, programs will improve their faculty and the overall quality of instruction. They are structure, process, and outcome oriented. Programs and instructors will use the National EMS Education Standards and commercially available or locally developed instructional support material to develop curriculum materials.

Accreditation standards and guidelines will provide minimum program requirements for sponsorship, resources, students, operational policies, program evaluation, and curriculum. Standards have also been developed for program faculty credentials and qualifications. Program standards will be developed with broad community input, peer review, and professional review. National EMS Education Program Accreditation will be universal and required for each level of EMS provider identified in the National EMS Scope of Practice Model. To be eligible for National EMS Certification and state licensure, a candidate must graduate from an accredited program."[134]

The *EMS Education Agenda for the Future: A Systems Approach* illustrated the relationship between EMS education, program accreditation and national EMS certification in the following graphic:

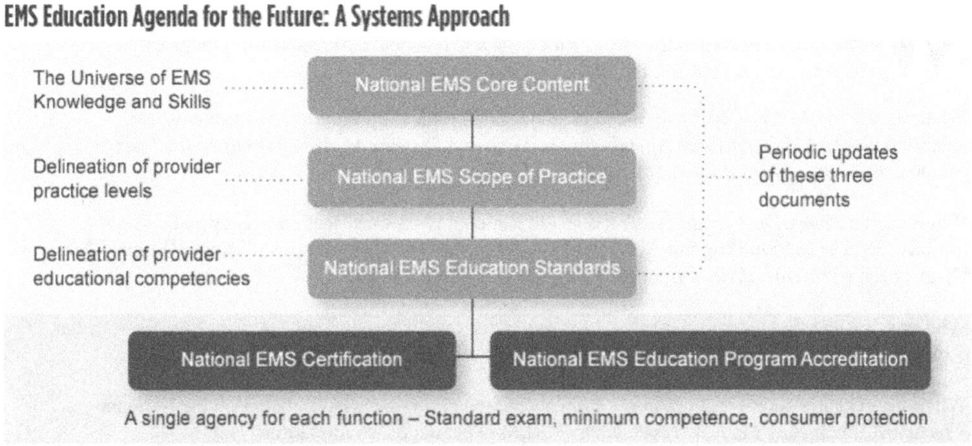

NASEMSO

Resolution 2010-04

National EMS Certification and Program Accreditation

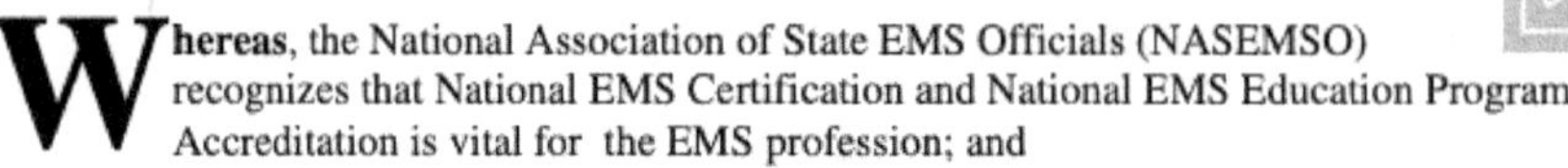

Whereas, the National Association of State EMS Officials (NASEMSO) recognizes that National EMS Certification and National EMS Education Program Accreditation is vital for the EMS profession; and

Whereas, National EMS Certification and National EMS Education Program Accreditation are identified by *The EMS Education Agenda for the Future: A Systems Approach* ("*Education Agenda*") as components of the system for preparing qualified EMS personnel; and

Whereas, the *Education Agenda* calls for a single National EMS Certification agency and a single National EMS Education Program Accreditation agency, and calls for all states to adopt National EMS Certification and National EMS Education Program Accreditation; and

Whereas, NASEMSO recognizes that EMS is one of the few licensed allied health care professions that does not currently require graduation from a nationally accredited educational program; and

Whereas, evidence shows that graduates from accredited programs perform better on the National Registry of Emergency Medical Technicians (NREMT) paramedic examinations; and

Whereas, NASEMSO recently supported a national knowledge, attitudes, and barriers (KAB) survey to evaluate the potential impact of EMS education program accreditation, and most paramedic program directors participating in the 2009 KAB survey support program accreditation; and

Whereas, the Commission on Accreditation of Allied Health Education Programs (CAAHEP) issues the national accreditation to paramedic education programs and CAAHEP's Committee on Accreditation of Educational Programs for the EMS Professions (CoAEMSP), through their many outreach efforts, has made significant progress in assisting paramedic education programs to achieve accreditation; and

Whereas, the NREMT issues National EMS Certification; and

Whereas, the NREMT has established a target date of 2013 by which paramedics applying for National EMS Certification must have graduated from a nationally accredited education program.

Now, therefore be it resolved that NASEMSO supports January 1, 2013 as the beginning date for the NREMT to require graduation from a nationally accredited paramedic education program as a requirement for personnel to gain national EMS certification.

Signed this 15th day of October, 2010.

Steve Blessing
2008-10 President

Jim DeTienne
2009-10 Secretary

National Association of State Emergency Medical Services Officials
201 Park Washington Court ▪ Falls Church, VA 22046 ▪ Phone 703-538-1799 ▪ Fax 702-241-5603 ▪ www.nasemso.org

20

RECRUITMENT & RETENTION

"EMS is a calling, not a job. But it shouldn't be a sacrifice." - Rob Lawrence

THE EMERGENCY MEDICAL SERVICES SYSTEM PLAYS A CRITICAL ROLE in providing emergency care to individuals in need across the United States. However, EMS agencies face significant recruitment and retention challenges that impact the sustainability of their workforce. These challenges include issues related to workforce equity, diversity and inclusion, geographic population distribution, changing employment opportunities, and volunteerism. In addition, while the number of trained EMS personnel is at an all-time high, there is a shortage of available personnel willing to participate in the active workforce. Factors including burnout and compensation remain a significant concern. Addressing these challenges requires innovative solutions, including improving wages and benefits, promoting diversity in the workforce, addressing physical and mental stress, and adapting to changing societal attitudes towards volunteering. By addressing these challenges, the United States can strive towards ensuring a sustainable and skilled EMS workforce that can effectively meet the growing demand for emergency medical services.

Recruitment and retention challenges are significant issues facing the national Emergency Medical Services system. Some of the key challenges impacting EMS recruitment and retention include:

- **Shortage of Qualified Personnel**: A constant demand exists for highly trained and specialized EMS personnel, including paramedics, emergency medical technicians (EMTs), and other distinct roles. Although the total number of nationally certified EMS personnel continues to grow, there is still a deficiency when it comes to fulfilling the traditional, ambulance-based roles. EMS agencies persistently face challenges in recruiting enough qualified personnel to fill vacancies, and many are finding it increasingly difficult to compete in the evolving job market.

- **Increasing Demand for EMS agencies**: The demand for EMS services is on the rise due to various factors, such as post-pandemic changes in access and utilization of healthcare, an aging population, increasing population density in urban areas, and the need for EMS support in rural and remote regions. This increased demand places a strain on EMS agencies to recruit and retain sufficient personnel to meet the growing needs of the community.

- **Competitive Job Market**: The career landscape for EMS professionals is broadening, with opportunities extending far beyond traditional ambulance-based roles. While these expanded possibilities have benefits, they also present challenges. Hospitals, clinics, and private practices are competing with EMS agencies, often offering more enticing opportunities in terms of pay, benefits, and career advancement. This diversified job market intensifies the difficulty for traditional EMS agencies in attracting and retaining qualified personnel.

- **Physical and Mental Stress**: EMS work can be physically and mentally demanding, with long hours, exposure to high-stress situations, and the risk of occupational injuries. This can lead to burnout, fatigue, and mental health issues among EMS personnel, which may impact recruitment and retention efforts.

- **Pay and Benefits**: Despite their high skill level and substantial responsibilities, EMS personnel often earn lower wages than other healthcare professionals. This wage disparity can act as a deterrent in recruitment and retention efforts, as EMS professionals may seek higher-paying opportunities in the increasingly diverse healthcare sector.

- **Lack of Career Development Opportunities**: Traditionally, EMS careers have been viewed as lacking in career advancement opportunities compared to other healthcare professions. With the growing diversification of career paths in EMS, this perception is slowly changing. However, this evolution could also lead to higher turnover rates in more traditional EMS roles, impacting recruitment and retention.

- **Rural and Remote Locations**: Hiring EMS personnel in rural and frontier areas of the United States is challenging due to factors such as limited resources, difficult working conditions, and geographical barriers. This can impact recruitment and retention efforts, as EMS agencies may struggle to attract and retain personnel in these locations.

- **Training and Certification Requirements**: EMS professionals are required to undergo continuous training and maintain certifications to stay current in their field. Meeting these requirements can be time-consuming and costly, which may pose challenges to both recruitment and retention efforts.

Addressing these significant recruitment and retention issues is crucial to the vitality of the national EMS system. Solutions could include improving wages and benefits, providing an array of career development opportunities, managing physical and mental stressors, and addressing the unique challenges presented by rural and remote areas. Innovation and adaptability will be paramount in overcoming these challenges and ensuring a sustainable and proficient EMS workforce capable of meeting the growing demand for emergency medical services.

Changing EMS Workforce Opportunities

In recent years, there have been several new employment opportunities for EMS (Emergency Medical Services) personnel. These opportunities have emerged due to various factors such as changes in healthcare delivery models, increased demand for EMS agencies, advancements in technology, and evolving roles of EMS practitioners. Some of the notable new employment opportunities for EMS personnel in the United States include:

- **Community Paramedicine**: Community paramedicine is an innovative model of care that involves paramedics providing expanded services beyond traditional emergency response, including preventive care, chronic disease management, and community health assessments. Nationally, community paramedicine programs have been implemented in some areas to address healthcare gaps, improve patient outcomes, and reduce healthcare costs. EMS personnel can now find employment opportunities in community paramedicine programs where they can work in collaboration with other healthcare providers to deliver care in non-traditional settings such as patients' homes, schools, and community centers.

- **Telemedicine**: With advancements in technology, telemedicine has become an increasingly popular approach to providing remote medical care. EMS personnel have exciting new employment opportunities in telemedicine programs where they can provide real-time virtual medical consultations, receive medical direction, and assist in triaging patients in the field. Telemedicine has the potential to improve patient care in remote or underserved areas, increase access to specialized care, and enhance communication and collaboration between EMS practitioners and other healthcare providers.

- **Mobile Integrated Healthcare** (MIH): Mobile Integrated Healthcare is another multidisciplinary approach that involves EMS personnel working closely with other healthcare providers to deliver coordinated, patient-centered care. The future role of MIH programs will likely be developed to address the healthcare needs of specific populations, such as frequent utilizers of EMS agencies, individuals with chronic diseases, and vulnerable populations. As MIH is developed, EMS personnel will have new employment opportunities where they can work as part of a team, provide preventive care, health assessments, and follow-up care to patients in the community.
- **Disaster Response and Preparedness**: All states are prone to various natural disasters such as wildfires, floods, and severe weather events. EMS personnel can find employment opportunities in disaster response and preparedness organizations, such as state and local emergency management agencies, where they can play a crucial role in responding to emergencies, providing leadership or medical care in disaster-stricken areas, and coordinating with other first responders and healthcare providers.
- **Tactical EMS**: Not long ago, tactical EMS was primarily reserved for military medics. However, in recent years, there has been a significant expansion of opportunities in tactical EMS both nationally and internationally. These opportunities range from local police department tactical medics to a broad assortment of federal roles. EMS personnel with specialized training and skills in tactical medicine can now find employment opportunities in various tactical teams, law enforcement agencies, federal agencies, and international organizations. These positions involve providing medical support in high-risk and specialized environments, such as active shooter incidents, SWAT operations, and disaster response scenarios. The integration of tactical EMS within these teams enhances the safety of both law enforcement officers and the public, as well as improves the outcomes for individuals involved in these critical incidents.
- **Education and Training**: With the evolving roles and responsibilities of EMS practitioners, there is an increased demand for EMS education and training. EMS personnel can find employment opportunities as instructors, trainers, and educators in EMS educational programs, colleges, universities, and training centers. These roles involve teaching and training future EMS practitioners, providing continuing education programs, and ensuring that EMS personnel maintain their competency and skills.

EXPANDING HOSPITAL AND CLINIC EMPLOYMENT

In addition to the opportunities mentioned above, the opportunities for EMS personnel for employment in hospitals and clinics have expanded dramatically since the COVID-19 pandemic. Many hospitals and clinics employ EMS personnel in various roles to provide direct patient care, support hospital operations, and contribute to the overall functioning of the healthcare system. For EMS personnel, the hospital or clinic environment generally offers competitive pay, less stress, reduced liability exposure, and an overall safer more predictable work environment. These clinical roles include:

- **Emergency Department Technicians**: Many hospitals employ EMS personnel as emergency department technicians. In this role, EMS personnel work alongside other healthcare providers in the emergency department, assisting with patient assessments, procedures, and treatments. They may also provide support in managing equipment, restocking supplies, and transporting patients within the hospital.

- **Urgent Care Centers**: Urgent care centers are becoming increasingly popular as a more convenient and cost-effective alternative to emergency departments for non-life-threatening medical conditions. EMS personnel can find employment opportunities in urgent care centers, providing direct patient care, performing assessments, and assisting with procedures.

- **Clinic-based Roles**: Some clinics, such as primary care clinics, specialty clinics, and outpatient clinics, may employ EMS personnel to provide patient care and support clinic operations. EMS personnel can assist with patient assessments, procedures, and treatments, as well as perform administrative tasks, such as patient intake, triage, and scheduling.

- **Pre-Hospital Liaison Roles**: Many hospitals and healthcare systems employ EMS personnel as pre-hospital liaisons or coordinators. In this role, EMS personnel work as a bridge between the pre-hospital and hospital settings, coordinating patient transfers, providing medical direction, and ensuring smooth communication and collaboration between EMS practitioners and hospital staff.

These roles allow EMS personnel to leverage their skills, education, experience, and knowledge in a different healthcare setting, contribute to patient care, and support the overall functioning of the healthcare system. As healthcare delivery models continue to evolve, EMS personnel may find increasing opportunities to work in hospitals, clinics, and other healthcare settings.

EMS Workforce: Equity, Diversity, and Inclusion Considerations

Equity, diversity, and inclusion (EDI) challenges are important issues impacting the national EMS system. Some of the key EDI challenges that are impacting the national EMS system and workforce include:

- **Lack of Diversity in the Workforce**: The EMS workforce has historically lacked diversity in terms of race, gender, ethnicity, and other identities. This lack of diversity may result in disparities in care and hinder the ability of EMS practitioners to effectively serve diverse communities with varying cultural and linguistic needs.

- **Unconscious Bias and Stereotypes**: Unconscious biases and stereotypes may exist among EMS practitioners, which could impact patient care and interactions with diverse populations. These biases may influence decision-making, treatment choices, and communication, leading to disparities in care and outcomes for underrepresented communities.

- **Language Barriers**: The United States has a diverse population with individuals who may speak different languages. Language barriers can impact effective communication between EMS practitioners and patients, leading to misunderstandings, delays in care, and potential errors in treatment.
- **Limited Access to Care in Underserved Communities**: Underserved communities, such as low-income neighborhoods, rural areas, and communities with limited access to healthcare facilities, may face challenges in accessing timely and quality EMS services. This can result in disparities in care and outcomes, particularly for vulnerable populations.
- **Inequities in EMS Education and Training**: Access to EMS education and training programs, including paramedic and EMT training, may not be equitable across different communities. Rural and frontier communities lack access to the same training opportunities as urban areas. This contributes to disparities in the educational pipeline of EMS practitioners.
- **Lack of Inclusive Policies and Practices**: EMS agencies may lack inclusive policies and practices that promote diversity, equity, and inclusion in the workplace. This could include lack of diversity in leadership roles, absence of inclusive hiring practices, and inadequate representation of underrepresented groups in decision-making processes.
- **Limited Cultural Competence**: Some EMS practitioners may not be trained or experienced in cultural competence to effectively understand and respond to the unique needs and expectations of diverse populations. This could result in miscommunication, misunderstandings, and potential disparities in care.

EDI challenges are significant issues impacting the EMS system and workforce. Addressing these challenges requires efforts such as promoting diversity in the workforce, addressing unconscious biases, improving language access services, ensuring equitable access to education and training, promoting inclusive policies and practices, and enhancing cultural competence among EMS practitioners. By addressing these challenges, the United States EMS system can strive towards providing equitable, inclusive, and culturally competent care to all communities it serves.

GEOGRAPHIC POPULATION DISTRIBUTION & WORKFORCE

According to the U.S. Census Bureau's 2019 American Community Survey (ACS), approximately 82% of the population lives in urban areas.[135] Urban areas are typically defined as densely populated areas with a high concentration of developed land, such as cities and towns. However, according to the U.S. Census Bureau's Urban and Rural Classification, approximately 3% of the United States land area is classified as urban.[136] The remaining 97% of the land area in the United States is classified as rural.

Like the general population, the geographic distribution of the national EMS workforce is uneven, with urban areas having better coverage compared to rural and remote areas. This presents challenges in providing timely and equitable access to EMS agencies throughout the entire United States. Some of the challenges associated with the geographic distribution of the EMS workforce include:

- **Rural and Remote Areas**: The United States has vast rural and remote areas, including mountainous regions and sparsely populated areas, which can present challenges in terms of EMS coverage. These areas often have limited access to healthcare facilities, longer response times, and transportation challenges, which can impact the availability and timeliness of EMS agencies.
- **Population Density**: While the United States has many specific densely populated areas, the general population density in most of the United States is relatively low. This can result in uneven distribution of EMS resources, with areas of high population density having a disproportionate EMS coverage compared to rural and remote areas.
- **Limited Workforce Availability**: The EMS workforce, including paramedics, EMTs, and other EMS practitioners, may be limited in some parts of the United States due to factors such as workforce shortages, high turnover rates, and challenges in recruiting and retaining EMS professionals in certain geographic areas. This can result in gaps in coverage and longer response times, particularly in rural and remote areas.
- **Transportation Challenges**: The geography also poses transportation challenges for EMS practitioners. This can impact response times, access to patients in remote areas, and the ability to transport patients to appropriate healthcare facilities in a timely manner.
- **Emergency Service Infrastructure**: The availability and accessibility of EMS infrastructure, such as ambulance stations, helipads, and medical facilities, can vary across different geographic areas. Rural and remote areas may have limited infrastructure, which can impact the availability and delivery of EMS services.
- **Resource Allocation**: Allocating EMS resources, including personnel, vehicles, and equipment, across different geographic areas in the United States can be challenging. Balancing the needs of densely populated areas with those of rural and remote areas,

and ensuring equitable distribution of EMS resources, can be complex and require careful planning and coordination.

- **Training and Education**: Providing EMS training and education in remote areas has traditionally been challenging due to the limited availability of education programs, distance from education centers, and transportation issues. However, the post-pandemic world has seen a surge in distance education and online courses. While this has undoubtedly improved access to education, disparities persist. For instance, access to practical, clinical education in frontier areas remains problematic. Students may need to drive three or more hours in one direction to reach clinical sites. These educational barriers can impact the recruitment and retention of EMS professionals in these regions and lead to potential gaps in their skills and qualifications.

- **Emergency Preparedness**: Rural and remote areas in the United States may face unique challenges in emergency preparedness, such as limited access to specialized training, resources, and equipment for managing emergencies in remote environments. This can impact the ability of EMS practitioners to effectively respond to emergencies and provide optimal care.

Addressing these challenges, inherent to the geographic distribution of the EMS workforce in the United States, requires careful planning, coordination, and innovative solutions. This effort will ensure equitable access to high-quality EMS services across all geographic regions of the country.

VOLUNTEERISM: DECADES OF UNSUSTAINABLE SUBSIDIES

The historic role of volunteer labor as a subsidy for EMS systems cannot be overstated, as it played a significant role in expanding access to emergency medical services, particularly in rural areas where the cost of providing full-time EMS services can be prohibitive. Volunteer EMS agencies have been responsible for providing life-saving services to their communities, and their contributions have been invaluable.

Unfortunately, the decline in volunteerism in Emergency Medical Services in the United States can be attributed to a variety of factors. In recent decades, there has been a shift in demographics, with more people residing in urban areas and fewer in rural areas. Rural areas often rely heavily on volunteer EMS agencies due to limited availability of paid EMS personnel. However, as rural populations decline or shift, the pool of potential volunteers is also decreasing, posing challenges in recruiting, and retaining volunteers.

Additional contributing factors include:

- **Increased Time Demands**: Volunteering in EMS requires a significant commitment of time and availability, often involving being on-call for extended hours and responding to emergencies during irregular hours. In today's fast-paced and demanding society, individuals may find it increasingly challenging to dedicate the necessary time and availability required for volunteering in EMS, particularly if they have other personal or professional commitments.

- **Increased Expectations**: Over the past few decades, the public's expectations for the quality and level of EMS care have increased dramatically (which is good!), however with the increased expectation there are potentially additional legal liabilities for EMS practitioners and an increased emphasis on certifications, training, and qualifications. The growing complexity of EMS care and the need for advanced medical skills have resulted in more stringent requirements for EMS practitioners, including mandatory certifications and ongoing education. These requirements may deter potential volunteers who may not have the time, resources, or inclination to pursue additional and necessary certifications or education.
- **Economic Factors**: Economic factors, such as increased job opportunities and an increase in paid EMS positions, may impact volunteerism in EMS. In recent years, there has been a trend towards paid EMS positions in many states, offering competitive salaries and benefits. This shift makes it more challenging to recruit and retain volunteers, especially in urban areas, who may have previously been motivated by the opportunity to provide volunteer service and not be compelled to serve full-time or part-time.
- **Increasing Demand on EMS agencies**: EMS agencies are facing increasing demand due to various factors, such as population growth, aging population, and increasing healthcare needs. This increased demand can result in higher call volumes and increased workload for EMS practitioners, potentially leading to volunteer burnout and reduced motivation to continue volunteering.
- **Workplace Safety and Increased Illness Risk**: Especially in the post-pandemic world, the perceived or actual increased risk of illness due to providing patient care has become a significant concern in recruiting and retaining volunteer EMS practitioners. During the pandemic, many of the nation's EMS volunteer workforce were aged, leading to a higher exposure risk. This risk contributed to not just a massive resignation from the traditional workforce but also a significant reduction in the volunteer workforce.
- **Changing Attitudes towards Volunteering**: Attitudes towards volunteering and community involvement have evolved over time. Today's generation may have different priorities and motivations when it comes to volunteering compared to previous generations. Factors such as changing societal values, lifestyle preferences, and competing commitments may influence the willingness of individuals to volunteer in EMS or other community service roles.

- **Changes in Financial Requirements**: Today, many households in the United States require multiple incomes to meet financial obligations, resulting in increased time commitments for work and reduced availability for volunteering in EMS. The need for dual incomes to support a household may limit the ability of individuals to volunteer due to competing financial responsibilities, such as paying bills, supporting dependents, and meeting other financial obligations. This may further impact the availability of volunteers for EMS agencies, as individuals may need to prioritize paid work to meet their financial needs, leaving less time for volunteering. The changing financial landscape and increased financial requirements for families can be a significant factor contributing to the challenges in recruiting and retaining volunteers in EMS agencies across the United States. Addressing these financial challenges may require creative solutions, such as offering flexible volunteer schedules or providing incentives to offset financial burdens, to attract and retain volunteers in the EMS field.

It's important to note that the decline in volunteerism in EMS is not unique to any specific state but is a national trend in the United States. Many EMS agencies across the country are facing similar challenges in recruiting and retaining volunteers. Addressing these challenges requires a multi-faceted approach, including efforts to promote the value of volunteering in EMS, provide support and resources for volunteer EMS practitioners, and adapt to changing demographics and societal attitudes towards volunteering.

Available and Engaged EMS Work Force Differences

While the number of EMS personnel in the United States is at an all-time high, traditional EMS and ambulance services are struggling to fill vacancies, especially since the pandemic. The shortage of employable personnel is a complex, layered issue due to several reasons, including:

- **Career Diversity**: EMS personnel now have access to many non-traditional career pathways, including hospital and clinical work, research, industrial health, and other healthcare fields. As the EMS profession continues to evolve, many EMS personnel are seeking out new opportunities that offer better pay, benefits, and career advancement options. This shift away from traditional EMS and ambulance services can further impact the availability of personnel to fill vacancies in these areas, leading to a relative shortage of available personnel.

- **Workforce Attrition**: EMS personnel, like any other profession, may experience attrition due to retirement, career changes, relocation, or other personal reasons. This attrition can create vacancies that may not be immediately filled, resulting in a shortage of available personnel despite the overall number of trained and certified EMS personnel being high.

- **Burnout and Fatigue**: EMS personnel often work in high-stress and demanding environments, and the pandemic has only exacerbated these challenges, leading to increased burnout and fatigue. This may result in EMS personnel leaving the profession or reducing their work hours, leading to a shortage of available personnel to fill shifts and meet the demand for EMS agencies.

- **Geographic Disparities**: The availability of EMS personnel can also be impacted by geographic disparities, with certain regions or areas facing more challenges in recruiting and retaining EMS personnel compared to others. Rural and frontier areas may have limited access to healthcare resources, lower pay scales, and challenges with work-life balance, which can further impact the availability of EMS personnel.

- **Compensation and Benefits**: Compensation and benefits play a crucial role in attracting and retaining EMS personnel. If ambulance services are not offering competitive compensation packages or benefits, they may struggle to attract and retain qualified personnel, leading to a shortage of available personnel.

- **Increasing Demand**: The demand for EMS agencies has been on the rise due to various factors such as an aging population, increased healthcare utilization, and changing patterns of emergencies and disasters. This increased demand for EMS agencies may outpace the growth in the number of available EMS personnel, resulting in a shortage to meet the demand.

- **Management and Leadership Challenges**: Another significant issue within the EMS workforce is the scarcity of management and leadership skills. Tragically, many EMS managers, promoted for their exceptional clinical skills, lack formal training or experience in management. This deficit often leads to their failure in management roles, contributing further to the workforce challenges.

The 2019 annual EMS Employee Retention survey, conducted by the American Ambulance Association, underscores the need for innovative human resource approaches and strategies to bolster employee engagement.[137] The data suggest that enhanced management training could potentially reduce EMS employee turnover. According to the survey, organizations with 100 employees should budget over $200,000 per year to replace employees leaving voluntarily or involuntarily. Given the high voluntary turnover rates of up to 38%, and the fact that 20% of new hires leave during the on-boarding or probationary period, nearly an entire workforce of 100 employees would need to be replaced within four years!

Addressing these issues necessitates the implementation of strategies to recruit, retain, and support EMS personnel, ensuring an adequate and sustainable workforce for traditional EMS and ambulance services across the United States.

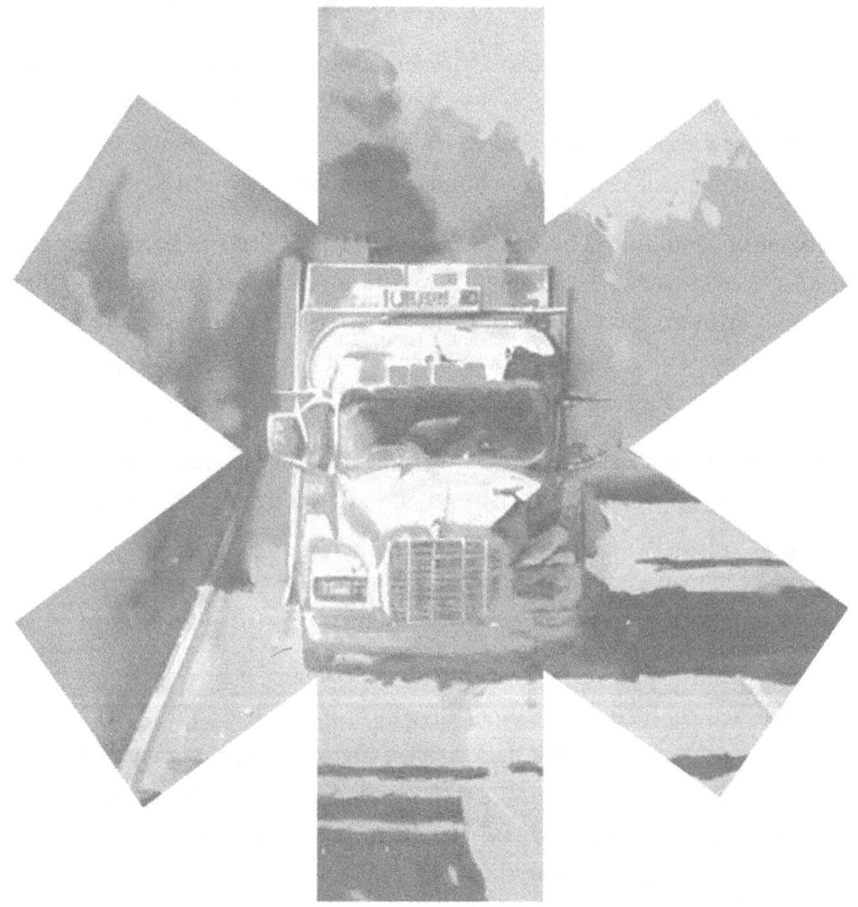

21

EMS PRACTITIONER MENTAL HEALTH: PROTECTING OUR OWN

"First responders are not superhuman. They are human." - Karen Solomon

EMS PROVIDERS IN THE UNITED STATES, LIKE IN MANY OTHER PARTS OF the world, face significant mental health challenges due to the nature of their work. The high-stress, fast-paced, and emotionally demanding environment of EMS can take a toll on the mental health and well-being of EMS practitioners, and these challenges are often underreported, under-recognized, and under-diagnosed. Some of the mental health challenges impacting EMS practitioners nationwide may include:

- **Compassion fatigue**: EMS practitioners are frequently exposed to traumatic events, suffering, and death, which can result in compassion fatigue. This can manifest as emotional exhaustion, a decreased ability to empathize, and a sense of detachment from others.

- **Post-traumatic stress disorder** (PTSD): EMS practitioners may develop PTSD as a result of experiencing or witnessing traumatic events, such as severe accidents, violence, or other critical incidents. However, due to the nature of their work and the culture of the EMS industry, PTSD may be underrecognized, underdiagnosed, and undertreated among EMS practitioners.

- **Burnout**: EMS practitioners often work long hours, have irregular schedules, and face high levels of job demands, which can lead to burnout. Burnout is characterized by emotional exhaustion, depersonalization, and a reduced sense of value and personal accomplishment. However, burnout in EMS practitioners may be underreported and not always recognized as a mental health issue.
- **Depression and anxiety**: The constant off and on exposure to high-stress situations, chronic fatigue, and sleep deprivation can contribute to the development of depression and anxiety among EMS practitioners. However, these mental health issues may be underreported or attributed to other factors, such as work-related stress or fatigue.
- **Substance abuse**: EMS practitioners may be at an increased risk of turning to substances as a coping mechanism to deal with the stress and emotional challenges of their work. However, substance abuse issues among EMS practitioners may be underrecognized and may not be addressed appropriately.
- **Increased risk of suicide**: EMS practitioners face high levels of stress, traumatic experiences, and other risk factors that contribute to an increased risk of suicide. The demanding nature of their work, exposure to critical incidents, and the cumulative effects of chronic stress can take a toll on their mental and emotional health and well-being. However, suicide risk among EMS practitioners may be underreported and not always addressed proactively.

Research has shown that EMS practitioners have higher rates of mental health issues, including depression, anxiety, PTSD, and substance abuse, compared to the general population. However, these issues are often underreported, under-recognized, and under-diagnosed in EMS practitioners. Therefore, it is crucial to raise awareness about the mental health challenges faced by EMS practitioners and promote early intervention, destigmatize the struggles, and provide access to mental health resources and support programs nationwide.

BARRIERS TO MENTAL HEALTH CARE FOR EMS PRACTITIONERS

There are several barriers that have historically prevented EMS personnel from seeking needed support and care. These barriers can include:

- **Stigma**: There is a persistent stigma associated with mental health issues in many societies, including among EMS practitioners. EMS practitioners may fear that seeking mental health support or care could be perceived as a sign of weakness or incompetence, and may worry about the potential negative consequences, such as being ostracized, judged, or even losing their job. This stigma can discourage EMS practitioners from seeking help and can prevent open conversations about mental health in the EMS culture.

- **Lack of Awareness and Education**: Many EMS practitioners may lack awareness and education about mental health issues, including their signs and symptoms, and the importance of seeking timely care. They may not recognize the signs of mental health issues in themselves or others and may not be aware of available resources for mental health support. This lack of awareness and education can be a barrier to seeking help.

- **Work Culture and Norms**: The work culture and norms within the EMS industry can also be a barrier to seeking mental health support. EMS practitioners often work in high-stress and fast-paced environments, where prioritizing self-care and mental health may be seen as secondary to patient care. There may be expectations to "tough it out" or "deal with it" as a part of the job and seeking help for mental health issues may be perceived as a sign of weakness or failure to meet these expectations.

- **Fear of Repercussions**: EMS practitioners may fear that seeking mental health support or care could have negative repercussions on their job, career advancement, or professional reputation. There may be concerns about confidentiality and privacy and worries about how seeking help for mental health issues could impact their ability to continue working in the EMS industry.

- **Limited Access to Mental Health Resources**: EMS practitioners may face challenges in accessing mental health resources, such as cost, availability, and convenience of services. They may work long hours, have irregular schedules, and face financial constraints, which can make it difficult to prioritize and access mental health care. In rural or remote areas, access to mental health resources may be further limited.

- **Lack of Peer Support**: EMS practitioners often have a strong sense of camaraderie and may prefer to seek support from their peers. However, in a work environment where mental health is stigmatized or not openly discussed, EMS practitioners may be reluctant to seek support from their colleagues, fearing potential judgment or repercussions.

- **Personal Beliefs and Attitudes**: EMS practitioners, like anyone else, may hold personal beliefs and attitudes towards mental health, seeking help, and the efficacy of mental health care. These beliefs and attitudes can be influenced by cultural, religious, or familial factors, and can impact their willingness to seek mental health support or care.

It's important to note that these barriers are not insurmountable, and efforts are being made to address them. Initiatives such as the Path4EMS program and other mental health support programs aim to reduce stigma, raise awareness, provide education, and improve access to mental health resources for EMS practitioners. By addressing these barriers, it is possible to encourage EMS practitioners to prioritize their mental health and seek the care and support they need.

OVERCOMING BARRIERS TO CARE

In recent years, there have been efforts to implement mechanisms to overcome the barriers that prevent EMS personnel from seeking mental health support and care. Some of these mechanisms include:

- **Mental Health Education and Awareness Programs**: Many EMS agencies and organizations have implemented mental health education and awareness programs to increase knowledge about mental health issues, reduce stigma, and promote a culture of mental health wellness. These programs can include training sessions, workshops, seminars, and informational materials that provide EMS practitioners with information about mental health, signs and symptoms of mental health issues, and available resources for seeking help.

- **Peer Support Programs**: Peer support programs involve trained peers, such as fellow EMS practitioners, who provide confidential and non-judgmental support to their colleagues. These programs create a safe space for EMS practitioners to discuss mental health concerns and seek advice, guidance, and emotional support from their peers who can relate to their experiences. Peer support programs can be formal or informal, and can be implemented at the organizational, regional, or national levels.

- **Mental Health Screening Programs**: Some EMS agencies and organizations have implemented mental health screening programs to identify EMS practitioners who may be at risk for mental health issues. These programs often use validated screening tools to assess mental health symptoms and provide early intervention and support. Mental health screening programs can help identify EMS practitioners who may need additional support and connect them to appropriate resources for care.

- **Access to Mental Health Resources**: Efforts have been made to improve access to mental health resources for EMS practitioners. This can include providing information about available mental health services, ensuring that mental health services are covered by employee health insurance plans, offering employee assistance programs (EAPs) that provide confidential counseling services, and partnering with mental health professionals or organizations to provide specialized mental health care for EMS practitioners.

- **Changing Organizational Culture**: EMS agencies and organizations have been working to change the organizational culture to promote mental health wellness. This can include leadership initiatives that prioritize mental health, open communication channels that encourage discussions about mental health, and creating a supportive and non-stigmatizing environment where EMS practitioners feel comfortable seeking mental health support without fear of repercussions.

- **Advocacy and Policy Efforts**: There have been advocacy and policy efforts at local, regional, and national levels to raise awareness about mental health issues among EMS practitioners and advocate for changes in policies and regulations that support mental health care for EMS personnel. This can include lobbying for increased funding for mental health resources, pushing for changes in workplace policies to better support mental health, and advocating for mental health awareness campaigns.

- **Collaborations and Partnerships**: EMS agencies and organizations have been partnering with mental health professionals, mental health organizations, and other stakeholders to develop and implement mental health support programs. These collaborations can help increase access to mental health resources, provide specialized care for EMS practitioners, and create a network of support for those in need.
- **Telehealth Services**: An emerging viable option is the leveraging of telehealth online helplines. Telehealth can offer crucial mental health support services to EMS practitioners, making it possible to access care in a flexible and convenient manner. This flexibility can be particularly beneficial for EMS personnel who work non-traditional hours or find it challenging to schedule in-person appointments. Telehealth can also facilitate more frequent touchpoints with healthcare providers, which can be instrumental in managing ongoing mental health conditions.

It's important to note that these mechanisms may vary depending on the region, organization, or agency, and ongoing efforts are being made to identify and implement effective strategies to overcome barriers and promote mental health wellness among EMS practitioners.

CASE STUDY: COLORADO'S PATH4EMS PROGRAM

In 2019, the Colorado EMS Peer Assistance Program was established via Senate Bill 19-065, serving as a proactive health policy model for Emergency Medical Service providers. This initiative underscores the significance of mental health support for EMS personnel, considering the distinctive challenges and stressors inherent in their professional roles.

Before the introduction of this legislation, a structured peer health assistance program was absent for numerous EMS practitioners. Senate Bill 19-065 filled this void by instituting a specialized program, which the Colorado Department of Public Health and Environment (CDPHE) effectively coordinated and administered. In this role, CDPHE identified and collaborated with proficient mental health professionals and peer health assistance programs, ensuring they satisfied criteria. These included offering education on identifying and preventing physical, emotional, and psychological problems; providing assistance for problem identification; ensuring evaluation and appropriate referrals for treatment; monitoring the status of referred providers; offering counseling and support for providers and their families; and maintaining availability for departmental referrals.

This strategy is comprehensive, focusing on both the recognition and treatment of issues as well as their prevention. It provides a dual advantage by safeguarding the personal well-being of EMS practitioners and enhancing their professional performance, subsequently improving overall public health services.

Upon the program's establishment, CDPHE appreciated the necessity of promoting Path4EMS to EMS practitioners. A logo, website, and educational materials were developed to market the program under the 'Path4EMS' moniker. Communication efforts extended to every licensed EMS practitioner in Colorado via emails, and information about the program was incorporated into routine business correspondences, such as license application status emails and letters from the investigation and enforcement team.

Among the most successful marketing strategies was the creation of a generic magnetic business card featuring the Path4EMS logo, website, and phone number. While awareness of Path4EMS services was prevalent among EMS practitioners, the generic business card was unobtrusive, helping to overcome barriers related to the stigma often associated with mental health support services.

While the Path4EMS program presented a novel statewide approach to EMS mental health services, the initial program design was hindered by a lack of adequate funding to ensure sustainability. Acknowledging the program's importance, CDPHE provided financial support from designated grant funds until dedicated funding mechanisms were established.

The Colorado EMS Peer Assistance Program marks a significant progression in recognizing and addressing the mental health challenges confronting EMS professionals. By facilitating education, intervention, and support, the program contributes to a healthier work environment for EMS practitioners and sets a commendable example for other states to prioritize the well-being of their emergency service personnel. The enactment of SB19-065 and the subsequent establishment of the Colorado EMS Peer Assistance Program indicate a positive policy change. This shift underscores the importance of mental health within the emergency services sector and provides a replicable model for other regions.

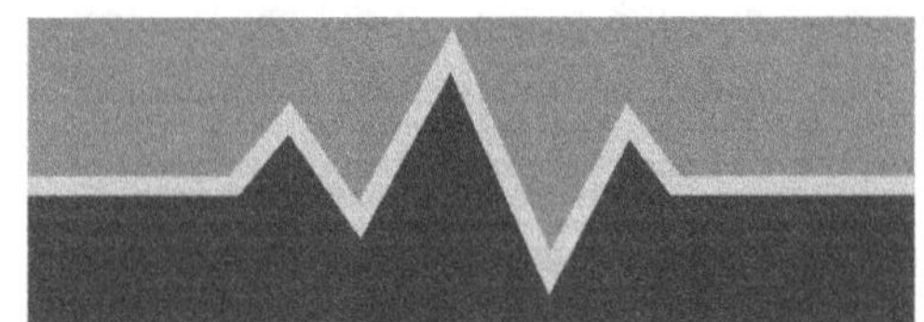

www.Path4EMS.org

22

A PROFESSIONAL CODE OF CONDUCT

"Accountability breeds response-ability."
-Stephen Covey

MEDICAL PROFESSIONS GENERALLY HAVE A CODE OF CONDUCT TO establish and maintain professional standards of behavior and ethical conduct among their members. These codes serve as guidelines that outline the expected conduct, responsibilities, and ethical principles that healthcare professionals should adhere to in their practice. The Hippocratic Oath, which is one of the oldest and most well-known codes of conduct in healthcare, has been a guiding principle for physicians for centuries. Its emphasis on ethical principles such as confidentiality, honesty, and respect for patients has influenced the development of modern codes of conduct for healthcare professionals.

As EMS continues its professional development, there is an urgent need for a unified code of conduct that is adopted and implemented by all states and jurisdictions licensing EMS personnel. Codes of conduct help in ensuring high standards of behavior and ethical conduct in the field and they serve as a critical tool in maintaining public trust in the profession.

The reasons for having a code of conduct in medical professions include:

- **Patient safety**: The primary focus of healthcare is the well-being of patients. A code of conduct helps ensure that healthcare professionals prioritize patient safety, provide competent care, and maintain professional boundaries, which are essential for the welfare of patients.

- **Professionalism**: A code of conduct promotes professionalism among healthcare professionals. It sets expectations for professional behavior, including communication, respect, integrity, and accountability, and helps establish a positive and trusted relationship between healthcare providers and patients.

- **Ethical decision-making**: Medical practice often involves complex ethical dilemmas, and a code of conduct provides a framework for healthcare professionals to make ethical decisions. It helps them navigate challenging situations with integrity, honesty, and in the best interests of the patients.

- **Legal and regulatory compliance**: Healthcare is a regulated field, and a code of conduct helps healthcare professionals comply with laws, regulations, and professional standards. It serves as a guide for adhering to legal and regulatory requirements and helps prevent professional misconduct or violations that may lead to legal or disciplinary action.

- **Professional accountability**: A code of conduct establishes a sense of professional accountability among healthcare professionals. It emphasizes the importance of maintaining competence, continuing education, and upholding professional standards, and encourages self-regulation and accountability within the profession.

- **Reputation and trust**: Healthcare professions are held in high regard by the public, and a code of conduct helps protect the reputation and trustworthiness of the profession. It promotes ethical and responsible behavior, which enhances public trust in healthcare professionals and the healthcare system.

A code of conduct serves as a guiding framework for healthcare professionals, outlining the expected standards of behavior, ethical principles, and professional responsibilities. It helps ensure patient safety, professionalism, ethical decision-making, compliance with laws and regulations, professional accountability, and the reputation of the overall healthcare profession.

The Hippocratic Oath

The Hippocratic Oath is one of the oldest and most well-known codes of conduct in healthcare. It is named after Hippocrates, a Greek physician who lived in the 5th century BCE and is considered the father of modern medicine. The oath is a solemn pledge that physicians take at the beginning of their careers to uphold ethical principles and standards in their practice.

The oath emphasizes the importance of the physician-patient relationship, confidentiality, honesty, and respect for patients. It also includes a commitment to lifelong learning and a promise to use medical knowledge and skills for the benefit of patients and society.

While the original version of the Hippocratic Oath has been modified over time, its core principles have influenced the development of modern codes of conduct for healthcare professionals. The oath continues to be a symbol of the ethical responsibilities of physicians and the importance of maintaining high standards of behavior and ethical conduct in the field of medicine.

EMS Code of Conduct

A professional code of conduct is essential for Emergency Medical Services professionals as it outlines the expectations and standards of behavior that guide their practice. EMS practitioners play a crucial role in providing emergency medical care to individuals in need, often in high-stress situations. A code of conduct serves as a framework for ethical and professional behavior, ensuring that EMS practitioners deliver safe, competent, and compassionate care to patients while upholding the integrity and reputation of the profession.

The EMS profession requires a high level of skill, knowledge, and judgment, as well as adherence to legal and regulatory requirements. A code of conduct provides a set of principles that EMS practitioners should follow in their interactions with patients, colleagues, and the community. It serves as a compass, guiding EMS professionals in making ethical decisions and upholding the highest standards of professionalism.

In addition, a code of conduct helps establish trust and rapport between EMS practitioners and patients, as well as fosters effective collaboration and teamwork among healthcare professionals. It reinforces the importance of maintaining confidentiality, respecting diversity, and advocating for the best interests of patients. Furthermore, a code of conduct serves as a reference for EMS practitioners to understand their rights and responsibilities, as well as the consequences of not adhering to professional standards.

Overall, a well-defined and comprehensive code of conduct is crucial in ensuring that EMS professionals provide the highest quality of care, maintain professionalism, and uphold the ethical and legal standards of the EMS profession.

Although a standardized EMS Code of Conduct has not been adopted, a sample EMS Code of Conduct is provided below.

SAMPLE EMS CODE OF CONDUCT

As a professional EMS Practitioner, I commit to upholding the following code of conduct:

- Promote professionalism and provide competent emergency medical care to all people.
- Use my professional knowledge and skills to promote health, alleviate suffering, and do no harm.
- Treat all patients with respect, compassion, and dignity.
- Assume responsibility to uphold professional standards and education, striving to provide competent medical care to every patient that I encounter.
- Advocate for patients that lack medical decision capacity and ensure equal access to medical services.
- Act responsibly, ethically, and lawfully to enhance the reputation of the profession.
- Work cooperatively with other healthcare professionals in the best interests of our patients.
- Act with honesty by being objective, truthful, and complete. I will include all relevant information in data collection and reporting, statements, applications, and testimony.
- Acknowledge errors and will not distort or alter facts.
- Exercise a level of care and judgment consistent with my level of licensure, certification, and training.
- Abide by all applicable state and federal laws, rules, regulations, and permits.

Furthermore, I understand that as an EMS Practitioner licensed in the state[a] of << State >>:

- It is my professional responsibility and obligation to read, understand, and comply with all << State >> statutes and regulations related to the provision of Emergency Medical Services.
- I can only function as an EMS Practitioner if my license is current, and I have authorization from a physician EMS Medical Director.
- Maintaining my license and tracking my expiration date is my individual responsibility.

As an EMS Practitioner, I acknowledge and understand that:

The State may review and request further information for consideration about any violation of any state or federal law, rules, regulations including but not limited to violations that have been dismissed, deferred, or sealed when determining my fitness to practice as an EMS Practitioner.

Failure to follow this code of conduct provides just cause for disciplinary action by the Department.

Sanctions or discipline imposed on my license will be a public record and final dispositions will be reported to the National Practitioner Data Bank, the Interstate Commission for EMS Personnel Practice, and the National Registry of Emergency Medical Technicians.

---

[a] State or Commonwealth.

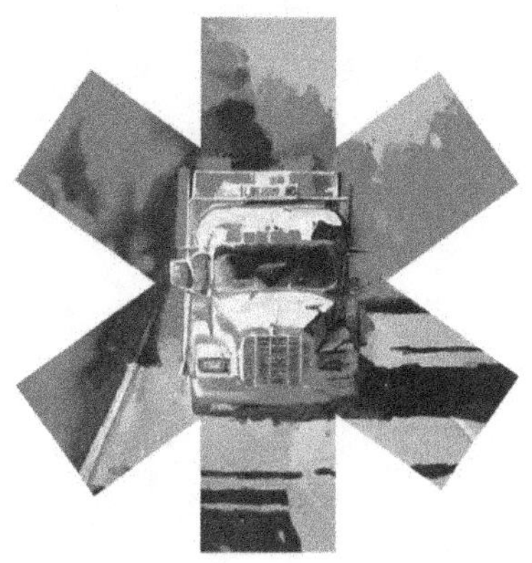

Section 4

STATE REGULATION & ADMINISTRATION OF EMS

"The nine most terrifying words in the English language are: 'I'm from the government, and I'm here to help.'"
– President Ronald Reagan

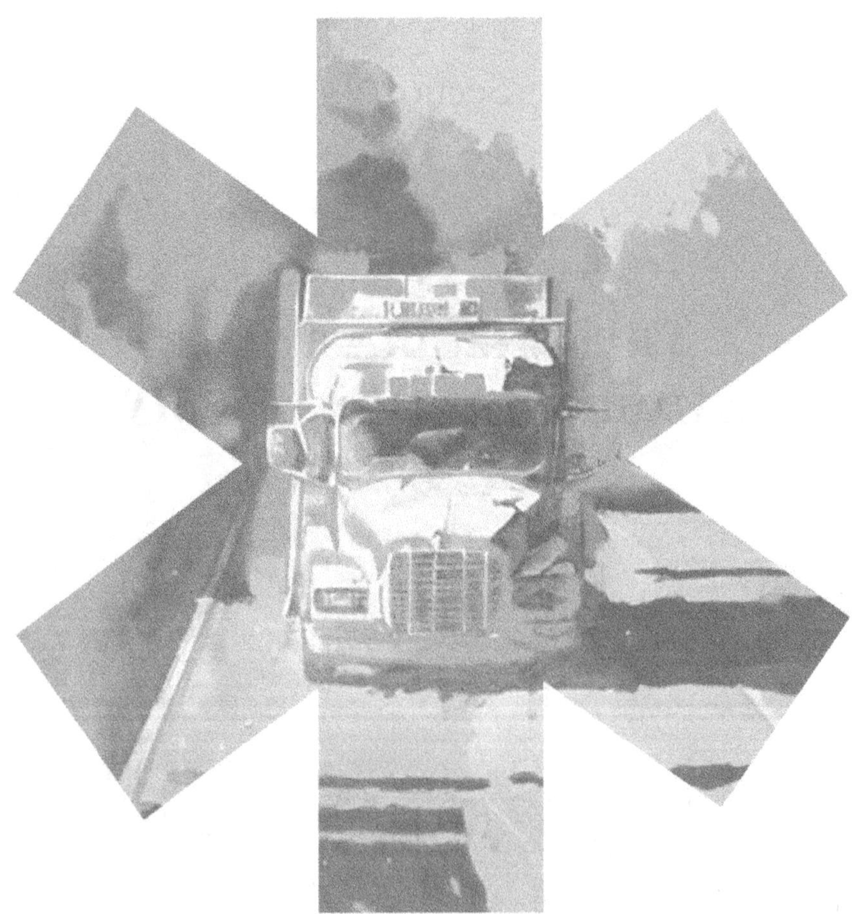

23

An Introduction To Interstate Compacts

"Interstate compacts are the most powerful, durable, and adaptive tools for ensuring cooperative action among the states... [providing] a state-developed structure for collaborative and dynamic action, while building consensus among the states."
- Council of State Governments

INTERSTATE COMPACTS ARE LEGAL AGREEMENTS, GROUNDED IN THE colonial era, that states employ to address issues of common concern. The original thirteen colonies devised agreements, precursors to today's compacts, to manage disputes, particularly those related to boundaries. To resolve such disputes, the colonies and the British Crown developed a process of negotiation and presentation of these disagreements to the Crown through the Privy Council for final judgment.[a] This method set the precedent for resolving state disputes through negotiation and submitting the proposed resolution to a central authority for approval.

[a] The Privy Council served as an advisory body to the British monarchy and played a significant role in governing and overseeing the affairs of the 13 colonies during the colonial period.

The contemporary "Compact Process" was formalized under the *Articles of Confederation.*[138] Specifically, Article VI prevented any two or more states from establishing any alliance or treaty without the explicit approval of the United States Congress. This provision arose out of concerns about managing interstate relations and preventing the formation of influential political and regional alliances.

The Founding Fathers explicitly prevented states from entering "any treaty, confederation or alliance whatever" without congressional approval. Additionally, they devised a comprehensive system for addressing interstate disputes. Under Article IX of the *Articles of Confederation* (1777), Congress was designated as the ultimate authority in all disputes and differences between states, addressing a variety of issues including boundaries and jurisdiction.[139]

Nonetheless, as the *U.S. Constitution* was being drafted, the worry about unchecked interstate cooperation persisted. This concern led to the integration of the "Compact Clause," in Article I, Section 10, Clause 3. This clause states that, "No state shall, without the consent of Congress...enter into any agreement or Compact with another state, or with a foreign power." Although the Constitution does not explicitly empower states to enter Compacts, it does prohibit states from doing so without Congressional approval. Unlike the Articles of Confederation, the Constitution appoints the Supreme Court as the final authority in resolving interstate disputes, either under its original jurisdiction or through the appeals process. However, in 1893, the Supreme Court ruled that the only interstate compacts that would necessitate congressional approval are those that could potentially infringe upon federal authority or affect the balance of power between states and the federal government.[140] Presently, hundreds of valid interstate compact agreements are active without congressional approval.

Today, interstate compacts are legally binding agreements between states, sanctioned by the *U.S. Constitution.* These compacts are not merely statutory laws but also contracts between states that establish collaboration and coordination[141]. Their utilization has broadened from handling boundary disputes to managing many cross-border concerns such as transportation, education, water rights, law enforcement, and healthcare, including emergency medical services. The binding nature of interstate compacts arises from their contractual character and the judicial acknowledgment that for compacts to be effective under the Constitution, they must override conflicting state laws.

THE LEGISLATIVE PROCESS

Interstate Compacts necessitate the adoption of model Compact legislation by individual states as state laws. This system fosters the alignment of legal and regulatory standards across the participating states, facilitating cooperation and shared governance. The process for passing these laws, however, can differ by state due to variations in legislative structures and procedures. Despite these variations, there are general steps that are usually followed.

- **Proposal**: A law often starts as an idea or proposal that a legislator believes will be beneficial to the state's residents. This proposal needs to be sponsored by a lawmaker—usually the one who came up with the idea—for it to be considered.

- **Drafting**: Once a lawmaker sponsors the proposal, it becomes a bill. This bill is meticulously drafted to incorporate all the necessary legal language to put the proposal into action. This process frequently involves legislative counsel and can be lengthy and detailed, with precise language used to prevent ambiguity or future legal challenges. Importantly, in the case of Interstate Compacts, these Compacts also function akin to contractual agreements between states. Therefore, it is vital that the model legislation is adopted without alterations to its substantive content. This ensures the uniform application of the Compact across all member states.

- **Committee Review**: After drafting, the bill is submitted to one or more relevant legislative committees for review. The committee(s) typically consists of lawmakers who specialize in or have an interest in the subject matter of the bill. The committee may debate, amend, or even rewrite the bill before voting on it. Only bills approved by the committee(s) can advance in the process.

- **Legislative Debate and Voting**: If the bill clears the committee stage, it proceeds to the entire legislative body for debate and voting. In a bicameral system, the bill begins in one chamber—House, Senate, or Assembly, depending on the state—where all legislators can discuss its merits, propose amendments, and finally, vote. If the bill passes this initial chamber, it is then transmitted to the second chamber to undergo a similar process.

- **Governor's Approval**: Once the bill receives approval from both chambers of the legislature, it is sent to the governor. The governor can sign the bill into law, allow it to become law without signing, or veto it. If the governor vetoes the bill, the legislature can still make it law by overriding the veto, usually requiring a two-thirds majority vote in each chamber.

- **Enactment**: After the governor's signature, or if the veto is overridden, the bill becomes law and is incorporated into the state's statutes. It's the duty of relevant state departments to enforce this new law. It's critical to note that, in the case of Compacts, once the model legislation is adopted as state law, it becomes the law of that state, carrying all the authority and enforceability of any other state law.

This legislative process provides a checks-and-balances system to ensure that the law serves the best interests of the state's citizens and complies with the state's constitution. For Interstate Compacts, this process also promotes coordination and collaboration across state lines, while respecting the rights and responsibilities of individual states.

EXAMPLE INTERSTATE COMPACTS

This section provides an overview of four common interstate compacts relevant to the broader context of emergency medical services, healthcare, and public safety. Each of these compacts exemplifies the diverse ways in which states collaborate to address shared challenges and improve the quality and efficiency of services provided to their residents.

Emergency Management Assistance Compact (EMAC)

In 1992, Hurricane Andrew wreaked havoc in Florida, highlighting the need for states to collaborate and assist each other during emergencies, even with federal resources. Consequently, the Southern Governors' Association collaborated with Virginia's Department of Emergency Services, leading to the development of a state-to-state mutual aid agreement known as the Southern Regional Emergency Management Assistance Compact (SREMAC) in 1993. Recognizing the potential value of this model beyond the southern region, the compact underwent reorganization in 1994 and became the Emergency Management Assistance Compact (EMAC).

In 1996, Congress ratified the Emergency Management Assistance Compact (EMAC) to facilitate mutual aid and resource sharing among states in times of disaster and emergency.[142] As of September 2021, all 50 states, the District of Columbia, Puerto Rico, Guam, and the U.S. Virgin Islands have adopted EMAC. The National Emergency Management Association (NEMA) administers this compact.

EMAC establishes a legally binding framework that allows states to request and receive assistance from other member states in the event of natural or man-made disasters, public health emergencies, or other crises. The compact delineates the procedures for requesting aid, reimbursement protocols, liability protections, and licensure reciprocity for emergency responders, including EMS personnel. By streamlining the sharing of resources, personnel, and expertise, EMAC enhances states' ability to respond effectively to disasters and emergencies, while ensuring that assisting states are duly reimbursed for their support.

Nurse Licensure Compact (NLC)

The history of the Nurse Licensure Compact (NLC) is a transformative journey that not only changed traditional state-based nursing licensure, but also established the foundation for future interstate medical compacts. For decades, nurses were burdened by the need to obtain individual licenses in every state they wished to practice, leading to bureaucratic complexities and barriers to mobility. This fragmented system also lacked the authority to hold nurses accountable if patients in a state were harmed by nurses practicing remotely from another state.

In 1989, the Pew Health Professions Commission was established with a mission to assist healthcare professionals, policymakers, and educational institutions in addressing the evolving healthcare landscape.[143] As part of its efforts, the Commission evaluated healthcare workforce regulation and proposed recommendations to enhance public protection. In 1995, the Commission released a comprehensive report titled "*Reforming Health Care Workforce Regulation: Policy Considerations for the 21st Century.*"[144] This report highlighted the lack of standardization in entry-to-practice requirements among states, which created unreasonable barriers to interstate mobility for healthcare professionals.

Recognizing the need for reform, the Commission recommended states standardize entry-to-practice requirements and limit them to competence assessments, facilitating the mobility of healthcare professionals. The National Council of State Boards of Nursing (NCSBN) Delegate Assembly unanimously endorsed a mutual recognition model of nursing regulation in 1997. This model promoted cooperation, information exchange, and accountability among state nursing boards in licensure, regulation, investigation, and disciplinary actions.

Building upon this foundation, the Nurse Licensure Compact (NLC) was formally established on January 1, 2000, when Maryland, Texas, Utah, and Wisconsin passed it into law. This was a significant milestone in healthcare licensure and introduced a paradigm shift from individual state licenses to a multistate licensure framework. Nurses could now practice across state lines without the need for additional licenses, under the provision that they adhered to the nursing practice laws of the state where the patient was located.

The NLC not only streamlined licensure but also fostered collaboration among member states, enhancing access to nursing care and reducing regulatory barriers. However, as the NLC gained momentum, concerns emerged regarding the assurance of competence among nurses practicing in multiple states. Consequently, membership in the NLC stalled after the twenty-fifth state joined.

In response to these concerns, the National Council of State Boards of Nursing (NCSBN) developed the Enhanced Nursing Licensure Compact (eNLC). The eNLC, implemented in 2015, was designed to repeal and replace the existing NLC while addressing stakeholder feedback and improving confidence in the compact. It introduced new requirements and safeguards to ensure the competence and accountability of nurses practicing across state lines. As of 2023, 40 states have joined the eNLC, (now again known as the NLC) with more states considering adoption.

The history of the NLC underscores a dynamic and evolving process driven by the goal of enhancing nursing practice and patient care. It reflects a collective effort to overcome the limitations of the traditional licensure model, promote mobility, and align with the changing healthcare landscape. The NLC and its subsequent iterations stand as innovative solutions, empowering nurses with a single multistate license while maintaining the highest standards of nursing practice and public protection.

Driver License Compact (DLC)

The Driver License Compact (DLC) is an interstate compact aimed at promoting highway safety and enhancing information sharing among states regarding driver licensing and traffic violations. Established in 1961, the DLC requires member states to report traffic convictions of out-of-state drivers to their home state and to treat these convictions as if they had occurred within the home state's jurisdiction.

The DLC enables states to share information on traffic violations and suspensions, ensuring that drivers who commit serious traffic offenses in one state do not escape the consequences by moving to another state. This compact helps maintain safer roadways and promotes consistent enforcement of traffic laws across state lines. Although the DLC does not directly involve EMS, it is relevant to EMS leaders and managers as safer roadways and improved traffic safety contribute to a reduction in motor vehicle accidents, resulting in fewer emergency responses and potentially saving lives.

Recognition of EMS Personnel Licensure Interstate Compact (REPLICA)

The Recognition of EMS Personnel Licensure Interstate Compact is the first EMS-specific interstate compact in the United States. Officially established in 2017, REPLICA offers a solution to the complex web of varying state licensure requirements that have traditionally made it difficult for EMS personnel to provide services outside their home state.

REPLICA provides a legal framework for participating states to recognize the EMS licenses of personnel from other member states through a Privilege to Practice in remote states, ensuring that the qualifications and standards of care are consistent across state lines. The compact also establishes a coordinated database for tracking EMS personnel licensure, disciplinary actions, and other relevant information. As of July 2023, 24 states have joined REPLICA, with more states considering adoption. (Read more about the EMS Compact in the following chapter.)

These four interstate compacts demonstrate the broad range of applications and benefits that such agreements can offer in fostering collaboration and improving services across states. By addressing the unique challenges and needs of various sectors, including emergency medical services, healthcare, and public safety, these compacts help to create a more efficient, effective, and cohesive system for delivering essential services to the residents of the United States. For EMS leaders and managers, understanding these common interstate compacts provides valuable insight into the potential advantages of interstate collaboration and the ways in which these agreements can contribute to improved emergency medical care on a national level.

Interstate Compact Administration and Governance

The administration and governance of interstate compacts involve several key components, including their formation and ratification, management structures, and oversight mechanisms. This section provides an overview of these aspects, offering insight into how interstate compacts are established, maintained, and managed to ensure effective cooperation among member states.

Formation and Ratification Process

The process of forming an interstate compact typically begins with the identification of a shared problem or issue that requires collaboration and coordination among states. Stakeholders, such as state agencies, professional associations, or subject matter experts, come together to draft the compact language, outlining its purpose, objectives, and the administrative structures required to implement the compact. The drafted compact is then presented to each state legislature for consideration.

For a state to join the compact, its legislature must pass model legislation to adopt the compact's terms and conditions. In some cases, compacts may require a minimum number of states to join before the compact becomes effective. Once the required number of states has ratified the compact, it may need to be approved by the U.S. Congress, depending on the subject matter and potential impact on federal authority. However, many compacts do not require congressional consent, as they do not encroach on federal powers or responsibilities.

Compact Management Structures and Committees

Interstate compacts often establish management structures and committees to oversee their administration and ensure compliance with the compact's provisions. These structures vary depending on the specific compact but may include a governing body or commission composed of representatives from each member state. This governing body is typically responsible for developing and implementing policies, rules, and procedures that align with the compact's objectives.

In addition to the governing body, interstate compacts may establish various committees or working groups to address specific aspects of the compact, such as finance, legal matters, or technical issues. These committees typically consist of subject matter experts and representatives from member states who work together to develop recommendations, guidelines, and best practices for the compact's implementation.

Some compacts may also establish a compact administrator or executive director, responsible for overseeing the day-to-day operations and management of the compact. This individual usually serves as a liaison between the compact's governing body, member states, and other stakeholders, ensuring that the compact's objectives are met and that communication and collaboration among member states are maintained.

Federal Support and Involvement

Although interstate compacts are primarily agreements among states, the federal government can play a supportive role in the administration and governance of these agreements. For example, federal agencies may provide technical assistance, guidance, or funding to support the compact's objectives and initiatives. Additionally, the federal government may participate in compact meetings or serve as a liaison between the compact and other federal entities to ensure alignment with national priorities and policies.

In some cases, interstate compacts may require congressional consent or approval, particularly if the compact impacts federal authority or involves matters that fall under federal jurisdiction. In these instances, the federal government plays a more direct role in the compact's governance and oversight, ensuring that the compact's provisions are consistent with federal laws and regulations.

Ensuring Transparency and Accountability

To maintain public trust and ensure the effectiveness of interstate compacts, transparency and accountability are essential components of their administration and governance. Compacts should establish processes and mechanisms that promote openness, such as holding public meetings, providing access to compact documents and records, and regularly reporting on the compact's activities, progress, and outcomes.

Accountability is achieved through a combination of internal and external oversight, as well as the establishment of clear performance metrics and evaluation processes. By monitoring and assessing the compact's performance against its stated objectives, stakeholders can identify areas for improvement, address challenges, and demonstrate the compact's value to the public and member states.

Dispute Resolution and Compliance Mechanisms

Interstate compacts must also establish mechanisms for resolving disputes and ensuring compliance among member states. Dispute resolution procedures may include negotiation, mediation, or arbitration, depending on the nature of the disagreement and the compact's provisions. These procedures provide a structured and impartial process for addressing conflicts that may arise among member states during the compact's implementation.

Compliance mechanisms are critical to ensuring that member states adhere to the compact's provisions and uphold their commitments. These mechanisms may involve monitoring and enforcement actions, such as inspections, audits, or sanctions for non-compliance. By establishing clear consequences for non-compliance, compacts promote accountability and encourage member states to fulfill their obligations under the agreement.

The administration and governance of interstate compacts involve a complex interplay of processes, structures, and stakeholders working together to achieve the compact's objectives. Through effective governance, compacts can promote collaboration, standardization, and resource-sharing among states, ultimately leading to improved services and outcomes for the residents they serve. For EMS leaders and managers, understanding the intricacies of compact administration and governance is essential for shaping the development and success of interstate compacts in the ever-evolving landscape of emergency medical services.

LEGAL AND REGULATORY CONSIDERATIONS

Interstate compacts present unique legal and regulatory considerations that are not well understood – even amongst policy makers and many lawyers. This section provides a high-level overview of key issues, including state sovereignty and the Compact Clause, interstate compact litigation and disputes, balancing state and regional interests, and ensuring compliance and enforcement.

State Sovereignty and the Compact Clause

As mentioned earlier, the U.S. Constitution, under Article I, Section 10, Clause 3 (known as the Compact Clause), provides the legal basis for interstate compacts. This clause stipulates that no state shall enter into an agreement or compact with another state without the consent of Congress. However, the U.S. Supreme Court[145] determined that not all interstate compacts require congressional approval, particularly those that do not infringe upon federal authority or impact the balance of power between states and the federal government.

The Compact Clause serves to protect state sovereignty by ensuring that states retain the authority to enter into legally binding agreements with other states while preserving the federal government's role in overseeing matters of national importance. Interstate compacts, therefore, must strike a delicate balance between state autonomy and federal oversight, navigating the complex interplay of legal and regulatory considerations.

Interstate Compact Litigation and Disputes

Interstate compacts, like any contractual agreement, may give rise to disputes and litigation among member states. Disputes may arise from various issues, such as differing interpretations of compact provisions, non-compliance with compact obligations, or conflicts between compact requirements and state laws or regulations. In such cases, the compact's dispute resolution mechanisms help ensure the compact's continued effectiveness.

However, if disputes cannot be resolved through the compact's established procedures, parties may resort to litigation, seeking resolution through the courts. Interstate compact litigation can involve complex legal questions, such as the interpretation of the compact's provisions, the applicability of state or federal laws, or the enforcement of the compact's terms.

Balancing State and Regional Interests

One of the challenges inherent in interstate compacts is the delicate balance between the interests of individual states and the broader regional or national interests that the compact seeks to address. Each state possesses distinct laws, regulations, and priorities that warrant consideration during the development and implementation of compact provisions. Concurrently, interstate compacts strive to foster uniformity, cooperation, and resource-sharing among states, which may necessitate a degree of harmonization and compromise.

However, when a state enacts Compact legislation, such as the EMS Compact, that legislation becomes integrated into the state's laws. For example, upon Colorado's adoption of the REPLICA legislation, the EMS Compact legislation became part of the Colorado Revised Statutes. Consequently, the Compact legislation **is** a Colorado law that instructs the Colorado Department of Public Health and Environment to recognize EMS licenses issued by other EMS Compact states, and due to Colorado's own law, Colorado *shall* also extend a Privilege to Practice, provided that any other requirements specified by the Compact are met. [146]

The crucial distinction lies in the fact that external authorities are not directing a state to take an action; rather, it is the state's own law, enacted according to the state's standard legislative process, which directs the state action. This underscores the autonomy of individual states in the implementation and administration of interstate compacts. Although compacts seek to establish uniformity and cooperation among member states, the ultimate authority for enacting and enforcing compact provisions resides within the state's own legal framework.

EMS leaders and managers hold a pivotal role in maintaining this balance through meaningful dialogue, negotiation, and collaboration with their counterparts in other states. By comprehending the diverse interests and concerns of member states and working to devise mutually beneficial solutions, EMS leaders can contribute to the compact's success and the delivery of effective, high-quality emergency medical services across state borders.

Navigating the Intersection of State and Federal Laws

Interstate compacts must operate within the context of existing state and federal laws, which can create challenges and complexities for EMS leaders and managers. In some cases, the compact's provisions may conflict with or require changes to existing state laws or regulations. To address these issues, states may need to amend or harmonize their legislation to ensure consistency with the compact's requirements.

Furthermore, interstate compacts must navigate the complex interplay between state and federal laws in areas where federal regulations apply. EMS leaders and managers must be aware of the relevant federal laws and regulations that may impact the implementation of any compact, such as the *Health Insurance Portability and Accountability Act*[147] (HIPAA), the *Emergency Medical Treatment and Labor Act*[148] (EMTALA), and the Centers for Medicare and Medicaid Services (CMS) reimbursement rules. By understanding the legal and regulatory landscape within which interstate compacts operate, EMS leaders and managers can work proactively to address potential conflicts and ensure seamless integration of the compact's provisions with existing state and federal laws.

Evolving Legal and Regulatory Landscape

The legal and regulatory landscape surrounding interstate compacts and emergency medical services is constantly evolving. Changes in state or federal laws, court decisions, and regulatory developments can all impact the implementation and effectiveness of any compact. EMS leaders and managers should stay informed of these changes and adapt their practices and policies as needed to maintain compliance with the compact's provisions and the broader legal and regulatory environment.

Legal and regulatory considerations play a critical role in the development, implementation, and success of interstate compacts. EMS leaders and managers must navigate the complexities of state sovereignty, interstate compact litigation, balancing state and regional interests, and ensuring compliance and enforcement while operating within the context of existing state and federal laws. By understanding and addressing these legal and regulatory challenges, EMS leaders can contribute to the effective administration and governance of interstate compacts, ultimately leading to improved emergency medical services and outcomes for the residents they serve.

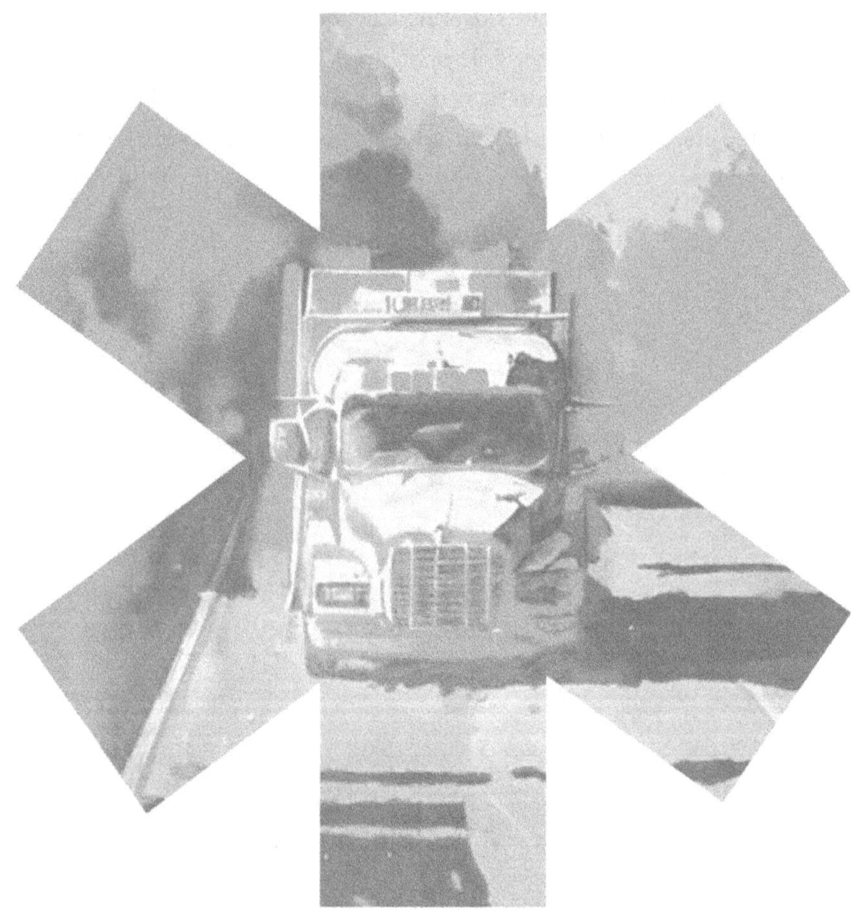

24

THE EMS COMPACT

"Interstate compacts are the most powerful, durable, and adaptive tools for ensuring cooperative action among the states... [providing] a state-developed structure for collaborative and dynamic action, while building consensus among the states."
- Council of State Governments

THE EMS COMPACT, OFFICIALLY TITLED THE *RECOGNITION OF Emergency Medical Services Personnel Licensure Interstate Compact* (REPLICA), is a groundbreaking initiative in the annals of emergency medical services in the United States. First launched as a conceptual project of the National Association of State EMS Officials and funded by the Department of Homeland Security in 2012, the initiative was designed to tackle the issues stemming from an increasingly mobile EMS workforce and the escalating demand for EMS personnel who can operate across state boundaries.

By 2023, 24 states had enacted legislation to adopt this mechanism, indicating a strong shift towards increased flexibility for EMS personnel. The EMS Compact functions as an interstate agreement, a tried-and-true approach for resolving cross-border challenges. Through this agreement, the process of licensing for EMS personnel is streamlined, enabling them to practice in any participating state without having to obtain individual licenses for each one. This significant development paves the way for improved mobility, efficiency, and responsiveness in the delivery of emergency medical services nationwide.

The Components of the EMS Compact

The Emergency Medical Services Compact is composed of several distinct components, each possessing a unique designation or acronym and serving a specific function.

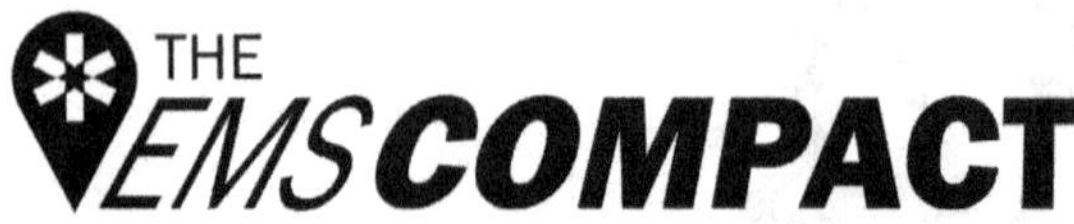

EMS Compact – The phrase "EMS Compact" is the commonly used designation for the "Recognition of EMS Personnel Licensure Interstate Compact".

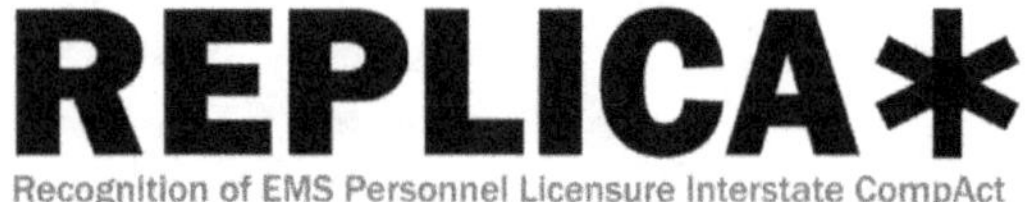

Recognition of EMS Personnel Licensure Interstate CompAct (REPLICA) - REPLICA is the official model legislation ratified by the states. It signifies the mutual acceptance of EMS licensure across state lines.

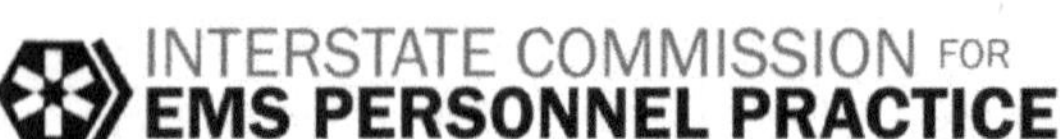

Interstate Commission for EMS Personnel Practice (ICEMSPP) - The ICEMSPP is a governing body formed pursuant to the REPLICA legislation. It oversees the administration and governance of the Compact. Like most interstate compacts, the ICEMSPP is constituted by one Commissioner from each of the member states.

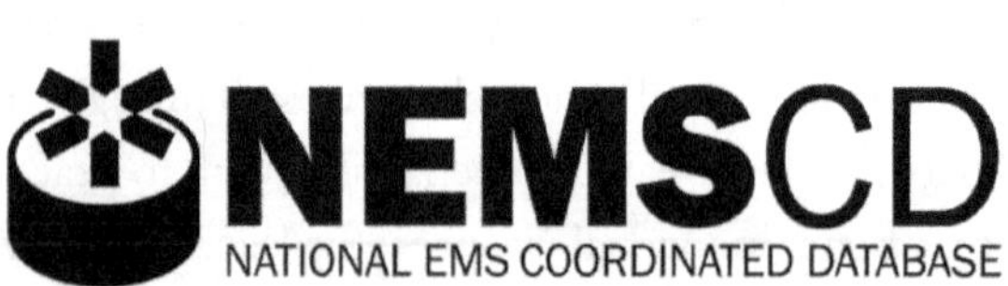

National EMS Coordinated Database (NEMSCD) - The Compact mandates member states to share licensure information. The NEMSCD was consequently established to enable this requirement, serving as a centralized repository of such data.

HISTORY OF THE EMS COMPACT

The establishment of the Emergency Medical Services Compact traces back to 2012. The Compact was necessitated by the mounting need for improved collaboration and coordination between states in the regulation and licensing of EMS personnel. Further challenges were presented by EMS personnel working across multiple states, contributing to the formation of the Compact. The National Association of State EMS Officials (NASEMSO) spearheaded the REPLICA project, receiving significant support from the Department of Homeland Security, state EMS offices, professional associations, and other federal partners. REPLICA formally began operations in 2017 when Georgia, the 10th state, ratified the Compact.

In the preliminary phases of Compact development, the National Advisory Panel convened twice: once in January and again in March of 2013. The Panel was tasked with guiding the developmental process, conducting policy analysis, and proposing recommendations. Their goal was to aid in the creation of a Compact that upheld state sovereignty and collective control, effectively establishing a self-regulating system for states. The structure of the EMS Compact was established in tight coordination with the Council of State Governments' National Center for Interstate Compacts.

The Panel comprised 23 members representing a wide range of stakeholder organizations, including the EMS industry, EMS agencies, and federal partners. Some of these organizations included the American Ambulance Association, American College of Emergency Physicians, Association of Air Medical Services, Bureau of Land Management, International Association of Fire Chiefs, International Association of Fire Fighters, Federation of State Medical Boards, and the Federal Bureau of Investigation, among others.

Once the need for the EMS Compact and its structural framework was established, a Drafting Team of Compact and subject matter experts from various backgrounds was assembled. This team started working in June, 2013, and the final version of the model legislation was unveiled a year later, in June, 2014. (The final version of the Model Legislation is included in this book's Appendix.) The team incorporated representatives from the International Association of Fire Fighters, National Association of State EMS Officials, Council of State Governments, Association of Air Medical Services, and other organizations.

The EMS Compact's model legislation (available in the Appendix of this book) was officially published in June, 2014. Colorado led the way in adopting the EMS Compact legislation, signing Colorado HB 15-1015 into law on May 8, 2015. This was followed by Texas, which enacted its legislation on September 1, 2015.

As per the model legislation, at least ten state legislatures needed to enact the EMS Compact for its formal inception. To meet this requirement, an advocate was appointed by the NASEMSO to educate stakeholders and assist in devising strategies for introducing, passing, and securing gubernatorial approval of the REPLICA legislation in each state.

The EMS Compact's governing body, the Interstate Commission for EMS Personnel Practice, held its first meeting on October 7-8, 2017, in Oklahoma City, OK. The meeting was attended by representatives from several states, including Alabama, Colorado, Delaware, Georgia, Idaho, and others.

Apart from the Commissioners, Douglas Wolfberg, JD, acted as the Commission's Interim Chair, Rick Masters served as Special Counsel, and Sue Prentiss was the Commission's Advocate and Educator. The Commission also had three honorary Chairpersons: Debra Cason,[a] Rick Patrick,[b] and Dia Gainor.[c]

Following the recognition and seating of each state-appointed Commissioner, Commissioner Joseph Schmider of Texas was unanimously elected as the Commission's first Chairman. Douglas Wolfberg, JD, of Page, Wolfberg & Wirth, LLC was designated as counsel for the Commission.

From October 2017 to March 2020, the Commission worked to establish the governance framework, rules, and technology necessary to fully implement and operationalize the EMS Compact. Then, on March 10, 2020, in acknowledgment of the public benefit provided by the Compact as EMS personnel responded to the COVID-19 pandemic, the EMS Compact was formally activated.

The EMS Compact's formation, development, and subsequent operation signify a monumental shift in the way emergency medical services personnel are licensed and regulated across state lines. This change has provided a unique solution to the long-standing challenge of personnel mobility, fostering a system of cooperation and mutual aid that serves the public interest. The Compact also exemplifies the capacity for states to maintain their sovereignty while collaboratively addressing shared concerns.

The history of the EMS Compact is a testament to the strength of collaborative efforts in addressing national issues. It also stands as a significant achievement in interstate cooperation and self-regulation, embodying a successful model that could inform similar initiatives in the future.

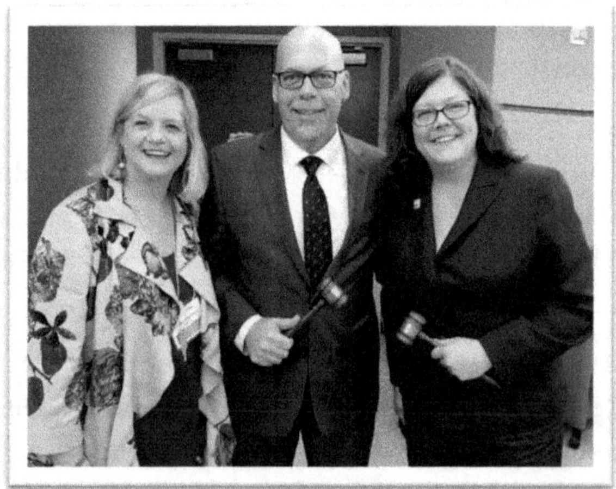

[a] Debra Cason was the Chair of the Board of the National Registry of EMTs
[b] Rick Patrick, Senior Advisor, Department of Homeland Security, Office of Health Affairs
[c] Dia Gainor was the Executive Director of the National Association of EMS Officials

The three honorary Chairpersons: Debra Cason, Rick Patrick, and Dia Gainor.

NATIONAL ADVISORY PANEL (2013)

- American Ambulance Association
- American College of Emergency Physicians
- Association of Air Medical Services
- Association of Critical Care Transport
- Bureau of Land Management
- EMS Labor Alliance
- Federal Bureau of Investigation
- Federation of State Medical Boards
- International Association of EMS Chiefs
- International Association of Fire Chiefs
- International Association of Fire Fighters
- International Association of Flight & Critical Care Paramedics
- International Paramedic
- National Association of EMS Educators
- National Association of EMS Physicians
- National Association of EMTs
- National Association of State EMS Officials
- National EMS Management Association
- National Governors Association
- National Registry of EMTs
- National Volunteer Fire Council

Model Legislation Drafting Team- Guided by technical and legal advice from the Vedder Price Law Firm, the drafting team included:

- National Association of State EMS Officials
- Council of State Governments
- Association of Air Medical Services
- International Association of Flight and Critical Care Paramedics
- International Association of Fire Fighters
- National EMS Management Association
- National Association of EMTs

INAUGURAL COMMISSIONERS FOR THE EMS COMPACT (2017)

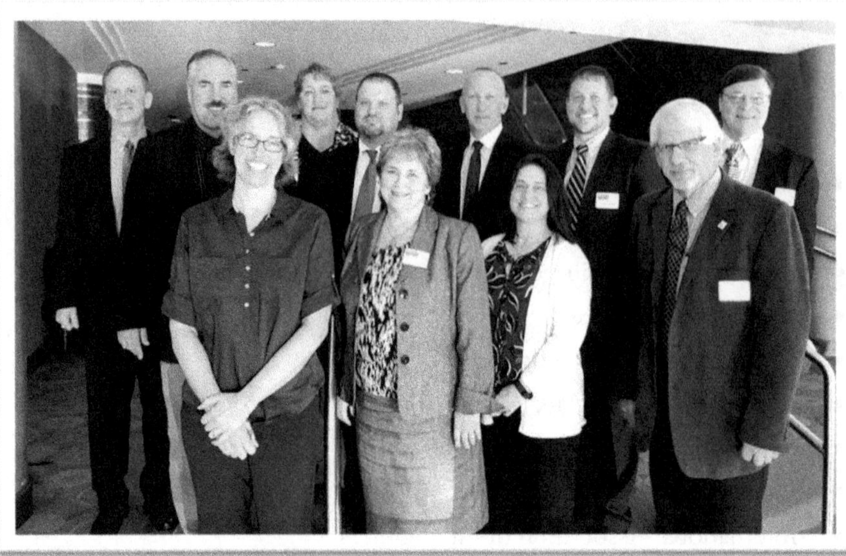

Back: Wayne Denny (Idaho), Guy Dansie (Utah), Diane McGinnis Hainsworth (Delaware), Stephen Wilson (Alabama), Andy Gienapp (Wyoming), Joseph House (Kansas), Gary Brown (Virginia). Front: Jeanne-Marie Bakehouse (Colorado), Donna G. Tidwell (Tennessee), Alisa Williams (Mississippi), Joseph Schmider (Texas). Not pictured: Keith Wages (Georgia).

PURPOSE OF THE EMS COMPACT

The primary purpose of the EMS Compact is to enhance the mobility of EMS personnel across state borders, providing a more efficient and effective system for the delivery of emergency medical services. The compact achieves this goal by unifying common licensure requirements across multiple states and streamlining the licensure process for EMS personnel. EMS personnel licensed in one member state can practice in other member states without needing to obtain separate licenses for each jurisdiction.

The EMS Compact also serves several secondary objectives, including:

- Facilitating the exchange of licensure, investigative, and disciplinary information among participating states.
- Fostering cooperation and coordination among state EMS regulatory bodies.
- Promoting the development of uniform and consistent standards for licensure and practice of EMS personnel.
- Improving access to EMS services for rural, underserved, and border communities.
- Supporting emergency response efforts during interstate disasters by enabling swift deployment of EMS personnel across state boundaries.
- Assisting in the expedited licensing of military personnel.

UNDERSTANDING HOW THE EMS COMPACT WORKS

The Interstate Commission for EMS Personnel Practice (the "Commission") is a governmental body that operates and manages the Emergency Medical Services Compact. The Commission, composed of one delegate from each Compact member state, is tasked with ensuring the successful execution of the Compact, formulating and enforcing its regulations and policies, and fostering communication and cooperation among member states.

To participate in the EMS Compact, EMS personnel are required to hold a valid, unencumbered license from a member state—referred to as a home state. Upon obtaining licensure in their home state, qualified EMS personnel are granted a "privilege to practice" in other member states. This permits them to deliver emergency medical services across state lines without necessitating additional licenses. Nonetheless, the "Privilege to Practice" is subject to certain constraints and restrictions as stipulated by the EMS Compact and its rules. For example, EMS personnel must abide by the laws and regulations of the state in which they are practicing, and they can be subjected to disciplinary actions by their home state for any misconduct occurring in another member state.

A parallel can be drawn between the EMS Compact and the Driver License Compact in terms of the "Privilege to Practice" and the privilege to drive in another state, respectively. Both compacts allow individuals to operate in a remote state under the premise that they bear the responsibility for understanding and complying with the laws and regulations of that state. Moreover, both compacts enable the remote state to investigate and hold the individual accountable for any violations that may occur while operating under these privileges.

The establishment and efficacy of the Driver License Compact served as a template for the formation and structure of the EMS Compact, showcasing the advantages of interstate collaboration in addressing shared challenges. Both compacts underscore the significance of state sovereignty, collective control, and self-regulation, while offering a platform for enhanced cooperation and coordination among states.

Besides facilitating the practice of EMS personnel across state lines, the EMS Compact also institutes mechanisms for sharing licensure, investigative, and disciplinary information among member states. This data sharing fosters transparency and accountability, ensuring that EMS personnel meet the necessary standards for licensure and practice across all participating jurisdictions.

While the EMS Compact provides a framework for the interstate practice of EMS personnel, it is vital to delineate its boundaries and comprehend what the Compact does not encompass. Specifically, the EMS Compact does not extend to EMS agencies or ambulances; it focuses solely on individual EMS personnel, such as EMTs, Advanced-EMTs, and Paramedics.

Currently, ambulances and EMS agencies are not part of any compact and remain subject to existing state laws and regulations. Consequently, they are required to adhere to the distinct rules and requirements of each state in which they operate. The EMS Compact does not confer exemptions, privileges, or expanded legal protections to EMS agencies or ambulances, as it does for individual EMS personnel.

MULTI-STATE PRIVILEGE TO PRACTICE

The EMS Compact grants qualified EMS personnel licensed by a Compact Member State ("home state") a Privilege to Practice in other Compact states ("remote state"). This privilege has specific requirements defined by Section 4 of the REPLICA legislation. To exercise this privilege, EMS practitioners must meet the following conditions:

1. Be at least 18 years of age;
2. Hold a current unrestricted license as an EMT, AEMT, Paramedic, or a state-recognized and licensed level with a scope of practice and authority between EMT and Paramedic, issued by an EMS Compact Member State; and
3. Practice under the supervision of a physician medical director.

Importantly, while the Compact utilizes the term license, an "EMS certification" issued by a member state is treated as equivalent to an EMS license for the purposes of the EMS Compact.

SCOPE OF PRACTICE IN A REMOTE STATE

EMS practitioners working in a remote state under the privilege to practice are generally expected to function within the Scope of Practice authorized by their Home State. Nevertheless, the scope of practice may be modified by an appropriate authority in the remote state under certain circumstances, such as extended deployments, special events, local physician medical direction, and surge staffing situations. This flexibility recognizes the variety of scenarios that may necessitate adjustments to the standard practice parameters. It is important to note that all EMS providers operating in a remote state are required to maintain valid medical direction and be affiliated with a recognized EMS agency, as defined by the remote state's regulations.

To illustrate, consider a flight medic based in Texas who responds to Colorado to pick up a patient. In this scenario, it is logical and more efficient for the medic to adhere to one set of protocols and a single source of medical direction for the entire duration of patient transport. Switching protocols or medical directors mid-transport could introduce unnecessary complexity and potential for error.

On the other hand, consider a Colorado EMT who travels to Utah to assist with a large event. In this instance, they would affiliate with a properly recognized Utah EMS agency and comply with that agency's established credentialing process, including local medical direction and protocols. This ensures that their practices align with the local standards of care and expectations, contributing to a coordinated and effective response to the event.

These examples underscore the necessity for both consistency and adaptability in the Scope of Practice for EMS personnel operating under the EMS Compact, always ensuring optimal patient care and safety are maintained.

Restricted License or Restricted Privilege to Practice

The EMS Compact stipulates that the Privilege to Practice can be restricted by any Compact State, as defined in Section 8 of the REPLICA legislation. In such cases, only the state that suspended or revoked the Privilege to Practice can modify or remove the restriction. Any suspension of a Privilege to Practice in one state results in the removal of the Privilege to Practice in all Compact states. However, individuals with a suspended EMS Compact Privilege to Practice may still seek licensure in any state.

De-duplication of Data: National EMS Identification Number

During the development of the EMS Compact, one challenge that surfaced was the absence of a unified and consistent identification system for EMS personnel across various state licensing systems. Despite states issuing unique license numbers and the widespread utilization of the National Registry of Emergency Medical Technicians, these systems lacked uniform "keys" that could be linked across multiple databases. For example, the NREMT number, although unique, is not permanent. The number changes with each certification alteration, such as progressing from EMT to Paramedic, or when certification lapses. Similarly, state licensing numbers are non-standardized and frequently subject to change.

This inconsistency posed numerous issues, including an inability to accurately determine the total number of unique EMS personnel in the United States. While it was possible to inquire about the number of licensed personnel in each state, many EMS practitioners hold multiple state licenses—with flight medics and federal agents often needing to hold licenses in several states at once. The EMS Compact, therefore, necessitated a mechanism for sharing licensure information, privilege to practice details, and disciplinary and investigative information between states. To address this issue, the National Registry collaborated with EMS Compact leadership, state representatives, and stakeholders to develop a solution. The result was the creation of the National EMS ID number.

The National EMS ID is a unique 12-digit identification number that is automatically generated for all EMS professionals and students aspiring to join the profession. When an individual first creates an account with the National Registry, an EMS ID number is produced. For EMS clinicians who were licensed before a NREMT requirement came into effect, states have established a mechanism for generating a National EMS ID number. For nearly two million EMS professionals with pre-existing NREMT accounts, EMS ID numbers were retroactively generated, requiring no action on their part. The EMS ID number, randomly generated, does not contain any encoded data about the EMS professional. It was modeled after the National Provider Identifier (NPI) issued by the Centers for Medicare and Medicaid Services for physicians. In contrast to state license numbers or the National Registry number, which change as an individual's certification evolves, the EMS ID number is assigned once and remains constant, never expiring. This number acts as a master account number, under which individual certification numbers are linked. The design of the EMS ID number thus ensures a consistent identifier that stays with the EMS professional throughout their career, regardless of changes in their certification status.

The National EMS ID number functions as the primary database key nationwide that connects state licensure information, National Registry information, and EMS Compact information. Looking ahead, the EMS ID is set to streamline the tracking of EMS personnel education and minimize duplication of efforts among states, employers, and systems. Furthermore, during disaster scenarios, the EMS ID number will expedite personnel credentialing, contributing to the swift deployment of qualified personnel where they are needed most. The implementation of the National EMS ID number fulfilled the need for a unified and consistent identification system, thereby bolstering the EMS Compact's capability to foster cross-state cooperation and information sharing.

COMPACT GOVERNANCE

Like other interstate compacts, the governance of the EMS Compact is established by the model legislation. The model legislation created the *Interstate Commission for EMS Personnel Practice* (ICEMSPP), also known as the Commission, which is a body-politic composed of one delegate (Commissioner) from each Compact member state. The Commission is responsible for administering the Compact, which includes maintaining the database, hiring staff, and working with member states.

Limitations of the EMS Compact

While the EMS Compact offers several benefits, it is important to understand its limitations. The Compact specifically focuses on individual EMS personnel, including EMTs, Advanced-EMTs (and EMT-Intermediates), and Paramedics. The EMS Compact does not apply to EMS agencies.

EMS agencies and ambulances must comply with the unique rules and requirements of each state in which they operate. The EMS Compact does not grant exemptions, privileges, or expanded legal protections to EMS agencies or ambulances as it does for individual EMS personnel.

25

STATE SOVEREIGNTY

"The powers delegated by the proposed Constitution to the federal government, are few and defined. Those which are to remain in the State governments are numerous and indefinite."
- President James Madison

THE REGULATION OF EMERGENCY MEDICAL SERVICES IN THE UNITED States is primarily the responsibility of individual states under the U.S. Constitution. This is due to the principle of state sovereignty, which is enshrined in the Tenth Amendment to the Constitution. This amendment explicitly states that "the powers not delegated to the United States by the Constitution, nor prohibited by it to the States, are reserved to the States respectively, or to the people." This means that the federal government has only those powers that are specifically granted to it by the Constitution, while the states retain all other powers.

The concept of state sovereignty is a core element of federalism, which is the division of power between a central authority (in this case, the federal government) and constituent political units (in this case, the states). In a federal system, the states have a degree of autonomy to regulate their internal affairs, while the federal government has authority over matters that affect the country. This balance of power is important to protect individual states from federal overreach and to allow them to tailor their policies to local needs and resources.

While there are federal agencies such as the National Highway Traffic Safety Administration (NHTSA), the Federal Emergency Management Agency (FEMA), the Department of Homeland Security (DHS) and other federal offices that provide guidance, funding, and support for EMS, they do not have the authority to regulate EMS at the state or local level. Instead, each state has its own system of EMS regulation and oversight, which is typically administered by the executive branch of government: the department of health, department of public safety, or another similar state agency.

One advantage of this decentralized approach to EMS regulation is that states can tailor their local EMS systems to meet the unique needs of their communities and populations. States establish their own standards for EMS personnel, education and training, and response protocols, based on local needs and resources. Additionally, the decentralized approach allows for innovation and experimentation with new models of EMS care and service delivery, which can be shared and adapted across states as appropriate.

However, one major disadvantage of having states regulate their own EMS systems in a silo is the potential for significant variation in EMS standards, terminology, and education across different states. Historically this has resulted in confusion and inconsistencies in EMS education, license levels, and public expectations, particularly in situations where EMS practitioners from different states are working together.

Furthermore, the historic lack of uniformity in EMS standards and practices has made it difficult for EMS practitioners to move between states, or work across state lines. For example, an EMT or paramedic who is licensed in one state generally is not authorized to practice in other states due to differences in licensing requirements or scope of practice (the EMS Compact provides a solution for this and is discussed in other chapters). These jurisdictional variations not only create challenges for EMS agencies and providers that work or train in different states, but they also create unnecessary barriers in addressing regional disasters or emergencies that require assistance from other states.

The lack of standardization also creates interoperability issues between EMS agencies and systems, particularly in situations where EMS practitioners need to communicate or share patient information across different jurisdictions. This can result in delays in care and potentially negative outcomes for patients.

Ultimately, the lack of standardization can contribute to disparities in EMS care and response across different communities, particularly in rural or underserved areas where resources may be limited. This can lead to unequal access to quality EMS care and potentially negative health outcomes for patients.

In recent years, the push for greater standardization and interoperability in EMS has grown stronger. This is due in part to the fact that the public is not only highly mobile but with the real-time sharing of information made possible with the internet, the public expectation for uniformity in standards and medical care has increased. Patients expect that they will receive the same quality of care regardless of where they are located and that their medical records will be easily accessible to any healthcare provider who needs them. This has led to calls for greater standardization and interoperability in EMS, particularly in the areas of training, certification, and licensure.

Another area where greater standardization is needed is in the licensure of EMS personnel. Despite over fifty years having elapsed since the inception of the National Registry of EMTs—a body formed explicitly to institute a uniform framework for the certification of EMS personnel—some states[a] have persisted in utilizing state-specific examinations. For the advancement of the profession, it is imperative that every state recognizes the importance of adopting a unified national model for the education and examination of EMTs, Advanced-EMTs, and Paramedics.

While the decentralized approach to EMS regulation allows states to tailor their EMS systems to local needs and resources, it can also create challenges with standardization, interoperability, and efficiency in EMS operations. The push for greater standardization and interoperability in EMS has grown stronger in recent years, driven in part by the increasing mobility of the public and the expectation for uniformity in standards and medical care. While there are no easy solutions to these challenges, the industry needs to embrace national EMS education and training standards, national EMS certification, and standardized licensure processes.

Balancing State Sovereignty and National Standards

A significant challenge within the United States healthcare system involves navigating the equilibrium between state sovereignty and national standards. Other medical professions, including physicians and nurses, have adopted successful strategies for unifying standards across states. Centralized platforms such as the Federation of State Medical Boards (FSMB) and the National Council of State Boards of Nursing (NCSBN) exemplify such efforts. These organizations streamline licensing, disciplinary information, and established nursing practice standards across states.

These professional bodies not only develop and uphold uniform licensure, education, and practice standards across states but also foster continuing education and professional development, contributing to the elevation of healthcare quality. Nonetheless, this balance is a complex, ever-present issue, given the historical role and extensive authority states hold in regulating healthcare within their borders. This authority enables vast diversity in healthcare policies and practices, reflecting regional values, priorities, and fostering experimentation with novel approaches.

However, uniform national healthcare standards offer undeniable advantages. The absence of a uniform standard can generate confusion, inefficiency, and disparities in care, stemming from variations in state resources and standards. This concern is particularly poignant regarding the licensing and certification of healthcare professionals. While states have traditionally maintained jurisdiction over medical practice regulation within their borders, mounting pressure for

[a] At the time of publication, North Carolina and New York still maintained state-specific examinations for EMS personnel.

uniform standards has surfaced, spurred by workforce shortages and the necessity for healthcare professionals to practice across state lines.

In response, national licensure and certification standards have received increasing support, as evidenced by the Nurse Licensure Compact developed by the NCSBN and the Interstate Medical Licensure Compact. These initiatives allow healthcare professionals to practice in multiple states under a single license through a streamlined process.

Notwithstanding, concerns persist regarding potential infringements on state sovereignty and states' capacity to tailor healthcare regulations to local values and priorities. Critics suggest that national standards could catalyze a homogenization of healthcare practices, neglecting the unique requirements and conditions of individual states and communities.

National Standards in Nursing Education and Licensure

The NCSBN, a nonprofit organization, unites nursing regulators from each state and territory to formulate and implement national standards for nursing education, training, licensure, and regulation. This council not only champions best practices for nursing education and regulation but also provides continuous education opportunities for nurses and regulators. Collaboration with healthcare industry stakeholders also ensures quality and safety in nursing practice.

When the NCSBN establishes national standards, each state typically adopts regulations congruent with these standards. As such, state boards of nursing leverage the NCSBN's standards to shape regulations and policies pertaining to nursing education, licensure, and practice. This uniformity ensures that nurses, regardless of their practicing location, are adequately prepared to offer safe and effective patient care.

To further standardize the profession, all states administer the National Council Licensure Examination (NCLEX). This mandatory standardized exam, based on the NCSBN's test plans, assesses the knowledge and skills necessary for safe and effective nursing practice. Consequently, the NCSBN fosters uniformity in nursing education and regulation across states, promoting safe and high-quality patient care.

Tenth Amendment and the Regulation of EMS

In the context of EMS, state sovereignty refers to the ability and responsibility of individual states to regulate and oversee EMS within their borders. The power to regulate EMS is not explicitly delegated to the federal government in the Constitution, so according to the Tenth Amendment, it is reserved for the states. Thus, each state has its own standards and systems for EMS, and there is a great deal of variability in these systems across the country.

This variability can lead to confusion and inconsistencies, particularly when EMS practitioners from different states need to work together, or when EMS personnel want to work across state lines. These differences can also lead to inefficiencies and redundancies, and they can result in disparities in EMS care and response.

However, there is a growing push for greater standardization and interoperability in EMS. This is driven in part by the increasing mobility of the public and the expectation for uniformity in standards and medical care, regardless of location. The development of national EMS education and training standards, a national EMS certification or licensure process, and regional or national EMS systems could help address these challenges.

This chapter also discusses how other medical professions, such as physicians and nurses, have implemented strategies to unify standards across states while respecting state sovereignty. For example, the Federation of State Medical Boards (FSMB) provides a centralized platform for licensing and disciplinary information for physicians, and the National Council of State Boards of Nursing (NCSBN) has established standards for nursing practice and education.

Both organizations, while maintaining the balance of state sovereignty, have created effective ways to ensure consistent, high-quality care across states. They have done this through the creation of standardized practices and procedures, ongoing professional development, and collaboration with other stakeholders in healthcare.

Learning from these examples, the EMS community might explore similar methods for balancing state sovereignty with national standards. This might involve implementing a national licensure or certification system that still respects the individual needs and resources of each state or developing regional or national EMS systems that use uniform standards while allowing for local customization.

These efforts can help to ensure that all patients, regardless of where they are, have access to high-quality EMS care and can contribute to a more efficient and effective EMS system on a national level. However, the potential impact on state sovereignty and the need to respect local values and priorities must always be considered in these discussions.

While the principle of state sovereignty allows each state to tailor its EMS system to local needs and resources, it also creates challenges with standardization and efficiency. Addressing these challenges will require thoughtful consideration and collaboration among all stakeholders in EMS, with the goal of ensuring the best possible care for patients.

STATE SOVEREIGNTY AND MEDICAL LICENSING

Dent v. West Virginia[149] was a significant United States Supreme Court case in the late 19th century that explored the intersection of state laws and the practice of physicians. The case presented a direct challenge to West Virginia's physician licensing law, enacted in the early 1880s.

Case Background: Frank Dent, a self-declared physician who worked alongside his father and grandfather in Newburg, West Virginia, faced legal consequences when the state passed the Board of Health Act in 1881. This act required medical practitioners to hold either a diploma from a reputable medical college, a certificate proving ten years of practice, or successful completion of a state-administered examination. Dent, having apprenticed with his father and practiced for six years, submitted a diploma from the American Eclectic Medical College in Cincinnati in 1882. However, the Board of Health considered this diploma to be from a fraudulent institution. Dent continued practicing, leading to his arrest. Dent sought the assistance of his cousin, Marmaduke H. Dent, a West Virginia attorney and the first graduate of the University of West Virginia, to defend his case. In 1883, Frank Dent was found guilty of practicing without a medical license, prompting an appeal of the decision to the West Virginia Supreme Court.

In 1884, the West Virginia Supreme Court of Appeals upheld the conviction. Dent filed an appeal to the U.S. Supreme Court in 1885, asserting that his rights under the due process clause of the 14th Amendment of the U.S. Constitution had been violated.

Justice Stephen J. Field delivered the unanimous opinion of the Court on January 14, 1889, affirming the validity of the West Virginia statute. Justice Field emphasized that while citizens possessed the right to engage in any lawful profession, certain natural and reasonable restrictions, imposed by the state, applied. The Court recognized the unique nature of medical practice, requiring extensive training, comprehensive knowledge of the human body, and the ability to handle life-and-death situations. Consequently, the Court endorsed the importance of a licensing system, which assured the competence of medical professionals. States were justified in excluding individuals without licenses from practicing medicine under specific circumstances.

The Court's decision in *Dent v. West Virginia* had lasting implications. In the subsequent case of *Hawker v. New York*[150] (1898), the Court extended its ruling by considering character as a crucial qualification for obtaining a medical license. *Dent v. West Virginia* has been frequently cited in legal discourse, particularly in discussions pertaining to the appropriate balance between state regulation and Constitutional restrictions on Bills of Attainder.

State Authority to License Medical Personnel

The Supreme Court decisions in *Dent v. West Virginia* (1889) and *Hawker v. New York* (1898) have significant implications for state sovereignty regarding the licensing of Emergency Medical Services personnel. These cases clarified the scope of state authority in regulating the qualifications and character requirements for individuals seeking medical licenses, which extended to the licensing of EMS professionals.

Dent v. West Virginia established the principle that states have the right to impose reasonable restrictions on the practice of medicine to ensure public safety and the competency of healthcare providers. The Court recognized the unique nature of medical practice, which involves complex knowledge of the human body and high-stakes situations. As a result, the Court upheld West Virginia's physician licensing law, emphasizing the importance of a licensing system as an assurance of competence.

Hawker v. New York further extended the Court's ruling in *Dent v. West Virginia* by emphasizing the significance of character as a qualification for obtaining a medical license. This decision highlighted that not only medical knowledge but also the moral character and integrity of healthcare professionals were essential considerations in granting licenses. The Court recognized that the public's trust in medical practitioners relied on both their competence and ethical conduct.

These principles set forth by the Supreme Court in Dent and Hawker cases can be applied to the licensing of EMS personnel. States have the authority to regulate and establish licensing requirements for EMS professionals, ensuring they possess the necessary skills, knowledge, and character traits to provide emergency medical care effectively and safely. By incorporating character evaluations into the licensing process, states can promote professionalism, integrity, and ethical behavior within the EMS workforce.

State sovereignty in licensing EMS personnel allows individual states to tailor their requirements to address specific local needs and circumstances. This flexibility enables states to establish standards that align with their healthcare systems, population demographics, and unique challenges in delivering emergency medical services. It also ensures that EMS personnel are well-prepared to handle the critical situations they may encounter, contributing to the overall quality of emergency medical care within each state.

However, it is important to strike a balance between state regulation and ensuring that licensing requirements do not unduly burden qualified individuals from entering the EMS profession. States must carefully consider the necessity and reasonableness of their licensing regulations to prevent arbitrary barriers to entry while upholding public safety and the quality of healthcare services.

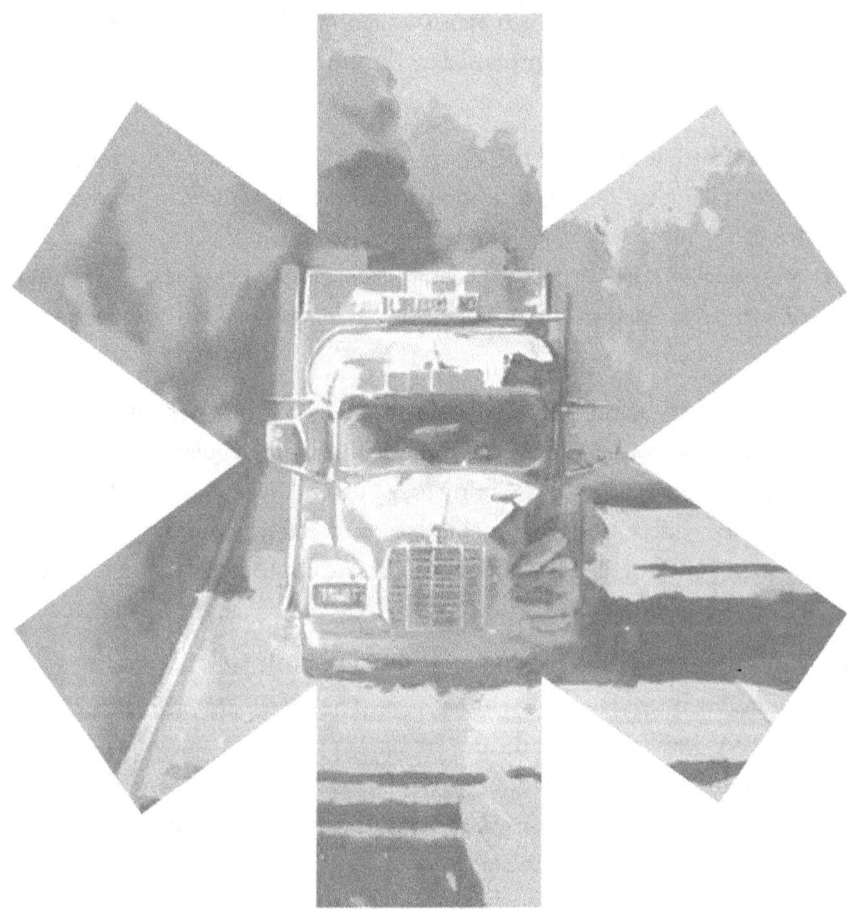

26

STATE EMS OFFICES

"EMS is not a job; it is a calling."
-Unknown

STATE EMS OFFICES ARE ESSENTIAL IN LEADING AND COORDINATING Emergency Medical Services within their jurisdictions. Every state and territory within the United States possesses a designated lead EMS agency, operating as part of the executive branch of government. In numerous instances, this office is situated within the state health department, public safety department, or functions as an independent state agency. These state EMS offices carry the responsibility for planning, coordinating, regulating the state EMS system, and licensing EMS personnel and agencies, which encompass air and ground ambulances.

In 2010, the National Association of State EMS Officials, along with the NHTSA Office of EMS, published a guide outlining the structure of State EMS Offices.[151] According to this model, all State EMS Offices should perform two core functions: Technical Assistance and Regulatory. Successful State EMS Offices strike a balance between these often-competing functions.

- **Technical Assistance**: This role involves providing comprehensive support and guidance to EMS agencies and personnel. This may include offering advice on policy and operational matters, facilitating training and education, and assisting with the implementation of new protocols or technologies. Essentially, the aim is to improve the performance and effectiveness of EMS services within the state.
- **Regulatory Functions**: These relate to the enforcement of laws, rules, and standards within the EMS system. Regulatory tasks include granting licenses to EMS personnel and agencies, ensuring compliance with professional standards and protocols, and conducting investigations into alleged breaches of these standards. The overarching goal is to maintain a high standard of EMS practice and service delivery to ensure public safety and trust.

The NASEMSO model further organizes state EMS responsibilities into ten subsystems:

- **System Leadership, Organization, Regulation & Policy Subsystem**: This subsystem oversees the comprehensive functioning of the EMS system, including the enforcement of regulations and policy formulation.
- **Resource Management Subsystems–Financial**: This subsystem ensures the efficient utilization and management of financial resources within the EMS system.
- **Resource Management Subsystems–Human Resources**: This subsystem manages matters pertaining to personnel, including hiring, training, and personnel welfare.
- **Resource Management Subsystems–Transportation:** This subsystem supervises all facets of patient transportation, ranging from ground ambulances to air transport services.
- **Resource Management Subsystems–Facility and Specialty Care Regionalization**: This subsystem coordinates and manages healthcare facilities and specialized care services.
- **Public Access and Communications Subsystem**: This subsystem ensures the effectiveness of communication systems within the EMS operations and the public's accessibility to these services.
- **Public Information, Education, and Prevention**: This subsystem informs the public about EMS services, promoting awareness and preventive practices.
- **Clinical Care, Integration of Care, and Medical Direction**: This subsystem oversees patient care, integrates various care services, and provides medical guidance.
- **Information, Evaluation, and Research Subsystem**: This subsystem collects and analyzes data for system improvement and supports research in EMS-related areas.
- **Large Scale Event Preparedness and Response Subsystem**: This subsystem prepares for and responds to large-scale events or emergencies.

The ten subsystems identified by the NASEMSO model provide a comprehensive framework for understanding the multifaceted functions and responsibilities of State EMS Offices. Through their diverse roles, State EMS Offices ensure the effective functioning and continual improvement of EMS systems while advocating for the interests of the public and the advancement of emergency medical services. Some of the specific roles and responsibilities of State EMS Offices include, but are not limited to, the following:

- **Licensure of Personnel and Agencies**: State EMS offices ensure proper licensing (or certification) of all EMS personnel within the state and authorize and license EMS agencies, including ground and air ambulances and, in many states, non-transporting first response EMS agencies.
- **EMS Education**: The State EMS Offices administer and oversee EMS education programs offered within the state, ensuring adherence to national standards and providing technical assistance.
- **System Design**: The State EMS office has the responsibility for designing and implementing a comprehensive EMS system that caters to the needs of the state's residents. (In states where EMS systems are ad hoc, it is the responsibility of the state EMS office to advocate for change to ensure EMS systems are designed and implemented.)
- **Consumer Protection and Complaint Investigation**: The state EMS office upholds public safety by guarding against unsafe or unethical EMS practices. This entails fielding and scrutinizing complaints, formulating administrative and/or court orders, levying penalties and instituting restrictions when necessary, and advocating for the interests of the public and the state in legal proceedings.
- **Data Collection and Analysis**: They collect and analyze vital metrics data, including syndromic surveillance data, especially critical in events like the COVID-19 pandemic. They play a significant role in public health monitoring, using data to identify improvement areas within the EMS system and measure the effectiveness of implemented changes.
- **Disaster Response Coordination**: The state EMS office takes on a leadership role, marshaling resources and offering support to local and state emergency management partners during emergencies and disasters. Depending on the specific organization of the state, this role might encompass leading or staffing one or more formal Emergency Support Functions (ESFs) within Emergency Operations Centers, or alternatively, it might involve providing essential support services.
- **System Funding:** Many state EMS offices administer statewide grants and other funding programs to support the EMS system.

- **Public Education**: The state EMS office educates the public on EMS agencies and the importance of emergency preparedness. One example of public education is the annual EMS Week designation and proclamation issued by the White House and state governors.

- **Interagency Collaboration**: State EMS offices play a significant role in collaborating and coordinating with other state and local agencies.

- **Legislation**: State EMS offices are critical in reviewing and molding the legislative framework that influences the operation of EMS systems. This includes a broad array of aspects including licensure and certification of EMS professionals and agencies. Working alongside legislative bodies, the EMS offices help create, review, and amend laws to align with evolving medical practices, technological advancements, and societal needs. They often serve as expert consultants, providing valuable insights on the practical implications of proposed laws, helping legislators understand the unique needs and challenges of EMS operations. Furthermore, State EMS offices also play a pivotal role in implementing new legislation by translating legal mandates into practical regulations and guidelines, facilitating compliance among EMS agencies and personnel, and updating the state administrative code accordingly.

- **Administrative Code & Regulations**: State EMS Offices are responsible for developing and updating the administrative code, a comprehensive set of rules and regulations that govern EMS operations within the state. These rules span areas such as personnel licensing, patient care standards, EMS agency protocols, vehicle and equipment requirements, and data reporting. These codes are kept current with evolving national standards, local needs, and advancements in technology and medical science. The process involves collaboration with various stakeholders for feedback and finalization, effective communication of these rules to relevant parties, enforcement of compliance, and integration of legislative changes impacting EMS operations into the administrative code.

- **Quality Improvement**: State EMS offices drive continuous quality improvement initiatives for EMS. These programs often involve systematically collecting and analyzing data on various aspects of EMS performance, identifying areas of potential improvement, and implementing changes aimed at enhancing service delivery. State EMS offices also facilitate training programs for EMS personnel focused on quality improvement methods, encouraging a culture of continuous learning and improvement within the EMS community.

- **Bridging Rural and Urban Differences**: Acknowledging the unique challenges and needs posed by both urban and rural settings, State EMS offices play a critical role in ensuring that EMS services are equitably distributed and effectively delivered across diverse geographic landscapes. In urban areas, they address issues such as high call volumes, traffic congestion, and a diverse patient population, while in rural areas, they tackle challenges such as longer response times, fewer resources, and limited access to advanced healthcare facilities. State EMS offices work collaboratively with local agencies, hospitals, and healthcare providers to design and implement strategies that account for these differences. They may advocate for legislation and funding to support rural EMS agencies, or they could create programs to facilitate resource sharing and mutual aid between urban and rural agencies. By bridging these differences, they aim to ensure that all residents, regardless of their location, receive timely, effective, and high-quality EMS care.

- **Training and Continued Education**: State EMS offices oversee and regulate EMS training programs, ensuring they meet state and national standards. They also coordinate with education providers, including universities, colleges, and professional organizations, to ensure the availability of relevant and high-quality courses. State EMS offices might maintain databases of approved training programs, coordinate statewide training events, and disseminate information about educational opportunities. They also play a role in tracking the ongoing education of licensed EMS professionals, ensuring they complete required continued education to maintain their licenses.
- **Public Health Integration**: State EMS offices facilitate the integration of EMS personnel into the broader public health system. This involves forging collaborative relationships with public health departments, hospitals, and healthcare providers to establish a comprehensive and coordinated approach to emergency healthcare. It also means aligning EMS practices with public health goals and strategies, such as improving population health, reducing health disparities, and responding effectively to public health crises. This integration may involve participation in public health planning and initiatives, sharing of data and resources, and contributing to public health education and prevention efforts. By aligning EMS services with broader public health objectives, State EMS offices help ensure a cohesive, efficient, and patient-centered approach to emergency care.
- **Technological Innovations**: State EMS offices lead the way in the adoption and implementation of technological innovations to enhance the performance of the EMS system. This role involves staying abreast of advancements in medical and communications technology, data analytics, and software solutions that could enhance the efficiency, effectiveness, and responsiveness of EMS services. The state EMS office may pilot or facilitate the testing of these new technologies, create guidelines for their implementation, and provide technical support and training to EMS agencies for their adoption. They may also advocate for funding or regulatory changes to support the adoption of these innovations. By leveraging technology, State EMS offices can help EMS services deliver faster, more accurate, and more effective emergency care. Some examples include Health Information Exchanges (HIEs), Automated External Defibrillator (AED)registries, and patient tracking solutions.

- **Mental Health and Wellness Programs for EMS Personnel:** State EMS offices support EMS personnel's mental health, often by providing resources like Colorado's Path4EMS program. This initiative offers comprehensive mental health services, reduces stigma, and integrates wellness strategies into the broader EMS education framework, underscoring the importance of self-care in the demanding field of EMS.
- **Performance Metrics**: State EMS offices employ performance metrics as a means of evaluating the efficacy of EMS systems. By quantitatively measuring aspects like response times, patient outcomes, and protocol adherence, these offices can identify areas of strength and potential improvement within the system, driving data-informed decision making and continuously enhancing the quality of emergency medical services delivered.
- **Stakeholder Engagement:** State EMS offices actively engage with a multitude of stakeholder boards, often appointed by the governor. Their roles in these interactions can vary, depending on the state, from advisory to fiduciary. Effective stakeholder management is crucial, as it facilitates the alignment of diverse perspectives and interests, fostering collaboration and ensuring that the EMS system caters to the needs of the various constituents it serves. By coordinating these boards, state EMS offices help to ensure balanced decision-making and representation within their jurisdictions.
- **Reporting**: State EMS offices have the responsibility to generate and submit reports to the legislative and executive branches of government. These reports typically encompass financial summaries, operational updates, strategic initiatives, compliance verification, and tracking of EMS system performance, thereby ensuring transparency and accountability.

While the above comprehensive list outlines the ideal functions that state EMS offices should fulfill, and indeed some are managing to meet these high standards, it's crucial to acknowledge that not all state EMS offices are equal in their resource availability. Regrettably, certain state EMS offices are chronically under-resourced, leading to gaps in executing these core functions. The fallout from these shortcomings can be profound, resulting in EMS systems that operate less as coordinated entities and more as disjointed, independent operations. This disunity contributes to problems in sustainability and resiliency; ultimately exacerbating disparities in access to EMS services. Also, these disparities often disproportionately affect rural, frontier and marginalized communities, where emergency services are most needed. Thus, adequately resourced, and effective state EMS offices are critical to ensure safe, effective, and efficient EMS systems. By diligently performing a broad spectrum of responsibilities, these offices can enhance the quality of care provided by EMS practitioners and contribute significantly to improved health outcomes for their state's residents.

NAVIGATING CHALLENGES IN STATE EMS OFFICES

State EMS offices are essential in managing and coordinating emergency medical services, a pivotal component of the healthcare system. Despite their indispensable function, these offices frequently grapple with a series of profound and persistent challenges, including but not limited to:

- **Structural Misplacement within Government Agencies:** In the wake of modifications to federal funding strategies in the early 1980s, many state EMS offices faced dramatic reductions in federal support. This loss of funding led to a demotion of these offices within their respective state government hierarchies. The resulting structural misplacement can undermine the prominence, priority, and recognition of state EMS offices, crucial elements for maximizing their effectiveness and influence.
- **Persistent Underfunding:** With the repeal of the 1970s *EMS Systems Act*, federal funding for EMS offices was integrated into broader Block Grants. This restructuring left a significant number of states without designated funding mechanisms to ensure their EMS offices are adequately funded, thereby hindering their capacity to carry out their vital responsibilities effectively. Persistent underfunding can strain EMS offices, diminishing their operational efficiency, impairing their ability to attract and retain qualified personnel, and potentially threatening their long-term sustainability.
- **Legislative Disparity:** State EMS offices often confront a disconnect between their legislated responsibilities and the actual authority and accountability they wield. This incongruity can create operational difficulties, spawning inefficiencies, and contributing to suboptimal outcomes in the delivery of emergency medical services. Furthermore, it can fuel frustration and dissatisfaction among office personnel, further complicating office management.
- **High Attrition Rates:** The position of State EMS Director, representing the highest executive branch role of EMS leadership in each state, is afflicted with persistently high rates of annual attrition. Such high turnover creates a volatile environment, disrupting continuity of leadership and vision. This instability can undermine long-term strategic planning and execution, and hinder progress in improving service delivery and patient care.
- **Inconsistency and Lack of Standardization:** State EMS offices are frequently appended to diverse government departments, from public health to public safety, fire administration, and even education. This lack of standardization leads to inconsistencies in the management and oversight of EMS services, complicating inter-state collaboration and communication, and making the development and application of national best practices and standards more difficult.

Tackling these challenges necessitates a comprehensive, multi-faceted approach. Both state and federal governments must play an active role in devising and implementing solutions. These solutions might encompass a reevaluation of funding structures and the redirection of resources; legislative reforms to realign responsibility, authority, and accountability; initiatives aimed at workforce stabilization and reducing attrition; and national efforts to foster greater standardization and consistency across states. These strategies will not only help mitigate the challenges but also augment the resilience and effectiveness of state EMS offices in delivering their mission-critical services.

Funding Models for State EMS Offices

State EMS offices' financial health significantly impacts the state's ability to provide robust and quality emergency medical services. The funding model, or lack thereof, greatly influences the effectiveness and stability of a state's EMS system. Unfortunately, many state EMS offices grapple with chronic underfunding, hindering their ability to optimally execute their roles.

According to a 2016 report by the National Association of State EMS Officials, an alarming 64% of state EMS offices do not receive funds dedicated by statute, severely limiting their ability to operate effectively. In just 7% of states, dedicated funds make up the entirety of the EMS office's annual budget.

Different funding models adopted by states include:

- **Motor Vehicle Registrations:** In states like Virginia, Maryland, and Colorado, a notable portion of funding for state (and regional) EMS offices is derived from motor vehicle registration fees. Specifically, Colorado charges $2, Maryland charges $17, and Virginia levies a $4 per vehicle registration. The collected funds in Virginia, under the banner of the Four-for-Life Fund, are allocated for training of EMS personnel, equipment purchases, EMS development, and local funding for EMS services. This model offers a reliable and predictable revenue stream.

  However, a significant drawback of this model is that it places the funding burden disproportionately on state residents who own vehicles, despite EMS services being utilized by all state residents and visitors. For instance, in a state like Colorado, there are fewer than 6 million residents but over 88 million annual tourists. This model does not account for the administrative and system management requirements of the transient population, thereby potentially limiting the system's reach and effectiveness.

- **EMS Personnel Licensure Fees:** Some state EMS offices primarily rely on EMS personnel licensure fees for their revenue. Although this model might seem fair, as it ensures that the costs associated with the licensing of EMS personnel are covered by those being licensed, it often falls short in funding the comprehensive responsibilities of state EMS offices. For instance, most states have fewer than 20,000 EMS practitioners, and some significantly less, with many operating on a 2 or 3-year licensing cycle. To illustrate, if 6,500 EMS personnel renew their licenses annually, each paying a licensure fee of $50 (already a substantial fee), it would generate only $325,000 in annual revenue. This sum likely wouldn't cover core operations like personnel licensure, complaint processing, and investigations. Therefore, relying exclusively on EMS licensure fees may hinder a state EMS office's ability to deliver essential, effective, and efficient services.

- **Traffic Violation Fees:** Some states, like Minnesota and Pennsylvania, allocate a portion of traffic violation fees to fund their EMS systems. For instance, in Minnesota, funds collected from seatbelt fines are deposited into the EMS relief account.[152] This account then funds regional EMS systems, provides for personnel education and training, and supports equipment purchases and operational expenses of emergency life support transportation services. In Pennsylvania, a $20 surcharge on traffic violations forms part of the funds allocated for EMS training, system development, and medical equipment purchases.[153] This approach creates an additional and somewhat steady source of revenue, yet the unpredictable nature of fine collection may lead to financial instability.
- **Federal Grants:** A range of federal grants is available to state EMS offices, including the Highway Safety Improvement Program (HSIP) Funding, the NHTSA Section 402 (State and Community Highway Safety Grant Program), and the NHTSA Section 405 (National Priority Safety Program). While these grants can stimulate progress and innovation, they come with their own challenges. The funds are neither sustainable nor guaranteed, often being time-limited and administratively complex. Furthermore, they may require the state to provide matching funds, which could prove difficult for states with budget constraints. Therefore, while valuable, these grants are not a reliable standalone funding solution.
- **State General Funds and Dedicated Funds**: A general fund serves as the primary fund for government entities, encompassing all resource inflows and outflows unrelated to special-purpose funds. It encompasses the core administrative and operational tasks undertaken by the government entity. These funds, generated from tax revenues, offer flexibility but are susceptible to economic fluctuations and political changes. According to the NASEMSO report, the utilization of dedicated funds varies significantly, with some states heavily reliant on them while others refrain from their usage entirely. In numerous states, the EMS Office lacks adequate positioning within the executive branch hierarchy, thereby lacking the necessary authority and visibility to ensure appropriate funding allocation for the EMS office. Additionally, EMS is not legally designated as an essential service in many states, nor is it funded as one, further complicating the matter.

The funding mechanism of a state EMS office has a direct impact on the overall state EMS system. Despite the widespread perception of EMS as an essential service, influenced by the popular portrayal of emergency medical services in shows like "Emergency!", many states do not prioritize or adequately fund their EMS offices. It is crucial to educate the public and policymakers about the crucial role of state EMS offices and advocate for a diversified funding approach that combines multiple sources. Such an approach would enhance financial stability and ultimately improve the quality of public services provided by these vital entities.

LIST OF STATE EMS OFFICES

The following table demonstrates the variability in how state EMS offices are positioned within the executive branch of state government.

State / Jurisdiction	Organization
Alaska	Alaska Department of Health
American Samoa	American Samoa Department of Health
Arizona	Arizona Department of Health Services
Arkansas	Arkansas Department of Health
California	California Emergency Medical Services Authority
Colorado	Colorado Department of Public Health and Environment
Connecticut	Connecticut Department of Public Health
Delaware[a]	Delaware Department of Public Health
District of Columbia	District of Columbia Department of Health
Florida	Florida Department of Health
Georgia	Georgia Department of Public Health
Guam	Guam EMS, Department of Public Health and Social Services
Hawaii	Hawaii State Department of Health
Idaho	Idaho Department of Health & Welfare
Illinois	Illinois Department of Public Health
Indiana	Indiana Department of Homeland Security
Iowa	Iowa Department of Public Health
Kansas	Kansas Board of Emergency Medical Services
Kentucky	Kentucky Board of EMS
Louisiana	Louisiana Department of Health

[a] The Delaware State Fire Prevention Commission certifies EMTs, while operating under the State Medical Director's medical license. Paramedics are issued their certification by the Division of Public Regulation, Board of Medical Licensure and Discipline.

Maine	Maine Department of Public Safety
Maryland	Maryland Institute for Emergency Medical Services Systems
Massachusetts	Massachusetts Department of Public Health
Michigan	Michigan Department of Health and Human Services
Minnesota	Minnesota EMS Regulatory Board
Mississippi	Mississippi Department of Health
Missouri	Missouri Department of Health and Senior Services
Montana[b]	Montana Department of Public Health and Human Services
Nebraska	Nebraska Department of Health and Human Services
Nevada	Nevada Department of Health and Human Services
New Hampshire	New Hampshire Department of Safety
New Jersey	New Jersey Department of Health
New Mexico	New Mexico Department of Health
New York	New York State Department of Health
North Carolina	North Carolina Office of EMS
North Dakota	North Dakota Department of Health
Ohio	Ohio Department of Public Safety
Oklahoma	Oklahoma State Department of Health
Oregon	Oregon Health Authority
Pennsylvania	Pennsylvania Department of Health
Rhode Island	Rhode Island Department of Health
South Carolina	South Carolina Department of Health and Environmental Control
South Dakota[c]	South Dakota Department of Health

[b] The Board of Medical Examiners licenses Paramedics and EMTs
[c] Paramedics are licensed by the Board of Medical and Osteopathic Examiners

Tennessee	Tennessee Department of Health
Texas	Texas Department of State Health Services
Utah[d]	Utah Department of Public Safety
Vermont	Vermont Department of Health
Virginia	Virginia Office of EMS
Washington	Washington State Department of Health
West Virginia	West Virginia Department of Health and Human Resources
Wisconsin	Wisconsin Department of Health Services
Wyoming	Wyoming Department of Health

[d] 2023 legislation transferred the Utah EMS Office from the Department of Health and Human Services to the Department of Public Safety.

27

INVESTIGATIONS & ENFORCEMENT

"The moral test of government is how it treats those who are in the dawn of life, the children; those who are in the twilight of life, the aged; and those in the shadows of life, the sick, the needy and the handicapped." – Vice President Hubert H. Humphrey

STATE EMERGENCY MEDICAL SERVICES OFFICES ARE ESSENTIAL regulatory entities that govern the operation of EMS agencies and personnel within their respective jurisdictions. Their mandate is to enforce the norms of professionalism, quality of care, and regulatory compliance expected of EMS practitioners. While disciplinary actions are within their purview, the primary focus for all State EMS Officials should be system improvement by offering technical assistance to EMS personnel, agencies, and education providers. This approach fosters a culture of continual growth and improvement. State EMS Offices are part of the executive branch of government, established by state laws or regulations, with the primary aim of ensuring safe, effective delivery of EMS services to the public.

State EMS offices carry a crucial responsibility to maintain the integrity of the EMS system. This responsibility involves evaluating complaints or reports related to EMS practitioners, including both personnel and agencies. Providers may come under scrutiny for alleged violations, such as substandard or unsafe practices, professional overreach, or breaches of established protocols. Complaints generally originate from stakeholders such as patients, their relatives, healthcare practitioners, or through routine audits and inspections. These offices are tasked with evidence collection, conducting witness interviews, and record examination to establish the veracity of complaints and determine appropriate corrective measures.

Investigation outcomes may lead state EMS offices to enact disciplinary actions against EMS practitioners found guilty of violations or misconduct. Such actions could include suspension or revocation of EMS licenses or certifications, imposition of fines, or other disciplinary sanctions. Providers may also be required to undergo additional training or remedial education to maintain their credentials. All disciplinary actions follow due process, allowing providers the chance to present their defense and appeal decisions.

The roles of state EMS offices extend beyond regulatory enforcement. They play a pivotal part in nurturing professionalism within the EMS community. Given the dynamic and complex nature of the EMS field, providers must demonstrate high levels of clinical competency, ethical behavior, and interpersonal skills. State EMS offices can establish and enforce professional standards, ethical codes, and regulations that guide EMS practitioners' practice, ensuring their ongoing professional development and proficiency.

State EMS offices often collaborate with other stakeholders, such as EMS education programs, EMS agencies, and professional associations, to develop and implement professional standards, guidelines, and policies. They also provide guidance and support to EMS practitioners, helping them navigate complex ethical or legal dilemmas, resolve disputes, and tackle other professional challenges.

These offices play a crucial role in consumer protection. EMS practitioners, both personnel and agencies, are responsible for caring for patients in their most vulnerable states. State EMS offices can investigate grievances or reports of patient harm, misconduct, or other infringements by EMS practitioners. Based on these investigations, they can execute appropriate disciplinary measures, holding providers accountable for their actions, thus deterring unethical or unsafe behavior.

State EMS offices also engage in public education about the EMS system, patient rights, and the process for filing complaints or reporting misconduct. They can develop educational resources, help patients and their families, and conduct public awareness campaigns, promoting transparency and accountability.

Complaints

Investigations into consumer complaints carried out by state Emergency Medical Services offices should ideally involve a comprehensive, equitable, and transparent process adhering to established guidelines and protocols. The following are the general steps often included in a typical investigation:

- **Receipt of Complaint**: A complaint is submitted to the state EMS office by a consumer, patient, or other party. The complaint may allege misconduct, harm, or other violations by an EMS practitioner, and can be submitted in various formats, such as in writing, through a formal complaint form, or via phone or email.

- **Initial Assessment**: The state EMS office examines the complaint to ascertain whether it falls within their jurisdiction and if it warrants further investigation. This assessment may involve confirming the identity of the complainant, scrutinizing the details of the complaint, and conducting a preliminary evaluation of the gravity and credibility of the allegations.

- **Collection of Evidence**: If the complaint merits further investigation, the state EMS office may proceed with the collection of additional evidence. This evidence may encompass medical records, witness statements, EMS practitioner records, and other pertinent documents. The collection of evidence must be conducted in a thorough and impartial manner, safeguarding the confidentiality and integrity of the information.

- **Interviews and Statements**: Interviews may be conducted with the complainant, the EMS practitioner, witnesses, and other relevant parties to garner more information and perspectives. These interviews follow established documentation protocols and are conducted professionally and impartially.

- **Review and Analysis**: After collecting all relevant evidence and information, the state EMS office conducts a comprehensive review and analysis of the findings. This process involves comparing the evidence with established standards, regulations, and protocols to determine if there has been a violation and evaluating the severity of the said violation.

- **Conclusion and Report**: Based on the investigation's findings, the state EMS office will draw conclusions and prepare a report summarizing the investigation's outcomes. This report must be objective, thorough, and grounded in the evidence collected as part of the investigation.

- **Technical Assistance**: One underutilized tool available to state EMS offices during the enforcement process is the provision of technical assistance. While disciplinary actions maintain accountability, they are inherently punitive. Offering technical assistance, on the other hand, demonstrates a proactive and supportive approach that prioritizes professional development and improvement. By providing guidance, training, and resources, regulatory bodies can help individuals and organizations address shortcomings, enhance their skills, and ensure regulatory compliance. This approach fosters an environment of continuous improvement and encourages open communication, collaboration, and trust between the regulatory body and the regulated entities.

- **Disciplinary Actions and Follow-up**: If the investigation uncovers a violation, and technical assistance is not deemed suitable, the state EMS office may impose disciplinary actions. These may include issuing warnings, reprimands, fines, suspensions, restrictions, or revocations of EMS practitioner's licenses or certifications. The office may also monitor the progress of recommended corrective actions and ensure compliance with established standards and regulations.
- **Appeals and Due Process**: EMS practitioners have the right to appeal the investigation's findings and disciplinary actions through established due process procedures. These procedures may involve hearings, reviews, and other legal mechanisms. It is crucial that the state EMS office ensures that the appeal process is equitable, transparent, and consistent with established regulations and due process rights.
- **Reporting and Documentation**: The state EMS office should maintain accurate and complete documentation of the investigation, including all evidence collected, statements obtained, conclusions reached, disciplinary actions taken, and appeals processed. This documentation may be used for future reference, quality assurance, and reporting purposes.

While investigation processes can vary across states, best practices should emphasize fairness, thoroughness, transparency, and adherence to established guidelines and due process rights. The goal is to ensure that complaints are addressed objectively and promptly, with appropriate actions taken to uphold professionalism, integrity, and consumer protections within the EMS system.

TECHNIQUES FOR ACCOUNTABILITY AND TRANSPARENCY

In the process of managing Emergency Medical Services (EMS), leaders often encounter a variety of challenges when executing disciplinary proceedings or investigations. A notable issue is the propensity of some EMS practitioners to attempt to evade the accountability process by relinquishing their state-issued EMS license before an investigation concludes and a decision is rendered. It's essential that EMS leaders understand the implications of this tactic and exercise caution in such situations.

The preemptive relinquishment of a license can serve as an escape route for EMS practitioners aiming to circumvent disciplinary actions or the potential negative outcomes of an investigation. This strategy opens the possibility for these providers to "jump-states", seeking an unrestricted license in another state and effectively evading the consequences of their actions.

Therefore, it is imperative that EMS leaders and state officials are aware of this tactic and are prepared to respond appropriately. Rather than accepting a license relinquishment to terminate an ongoing investigation, EMS leaders have several alternative options:

- **Refuse to accept the relinquishment**: If state laws allow, refusing to accept a license relinquishment during an ongoing investigation maintains the integrity of the process and discourages evasion of accountability.
- **Propose a legal stipulation agreement**: This agreement would formally outline the complaint and stipulate that both the state and the provider agree to the license relinquishment. However, the agreement should explicitly state that the relinquishment will be reported to the National Practitioner Data Bank (NPDB), the National EMS Coordinated Database (NEMSCD), and other necessary parties as required by law, thus ensuring appropriate reporting, and maintaining transparency.
- **Complete the investigation**: Regardless of the provider's attempt to relinquish their license, if possible, the investigation should proceed to its conclusion. This approach upholds the principle of accountability, ensuring that any potential misconduct is thoroughly examined and appropriately addressed.

By adopting these strategies, EMS leaders can ensure the integrity and efficacy of their disciplinary procedures and investigations. Maintaining these high standards in the face of evasive tactics not only serves the immediate needs of EMS management but also supports the broader objective of upholding public trust and accountability within the EMS profession.

NATIONAL PRACTITIONER DATA BANK (NPDB)

Under the mandate of the *Health Care Quality Improvement Act*[154] of 1986 (HCQIA) and its subsequent amendments, state Emergency Medical Services offices are obligated by federal law to report any disciplinary actions taken against EMS practitioners to the National Practitioner Data Bank (NPDB). The NPDB is a nationwide repository that gathers and preserves information regarding adverse actions against healthcare providers, including EMS practitioners, to foster transparency, accountability, and patient safety.

The reporting requirements to the NPDB typically involve the following:

- **Adverse Actions**: State EMS offices are required to report adverse actions taken against EMS practitioners, which may include disciplinary actions such as revocations, suspensions, restrictions, or other actions that impact the EMS practitioner's ability to practice. Adverse actions may also include settlements or judgments related to malpractice or negligence, as well as other legal or administrative actions that result in adverse consequences for the EMS practitioner's practice.

- **Timely Reporting**: State EMS offices are required to report adverse actions to the NPDB in a timely manner, typically within 30 days of the action being taken. Timely reporting is essential to ensure that accurate and up-to-date information is available to healthcare entities, employers, and the public for decision-making purposes.
- **Completeness and Accuracy**: State EMS offices are responsible for ensuring that the information reported to the NPDB is complete, accurate, and consistent with the requirements of the HCQIA and its amendments. This includes providing details of the adverse action, the reasons for the action, and any relevant supporting documentation or evidence.

The NPDB serves as a national repository of information on adverse actions taken against healthcare providers, including EMS practitioners, and is used by various entities for decision-making purposes. This includes healthcare entities, employers, licensing boards, credentialing agencies, and the public, who can access the NPDB to obtain information on the disciplinary history of healthcare providers, including EMS practitioners. The NPDB helps to promote transparency, accountability, and patient safety by providing a centralized and standardized source of information on adverse actions taken against healthcare providers and facilitating informed decision-making in the healthcare field.

In addition to the reporting requirements, the NPDB also serves as a resource for state EMS offices in conducting background checks and verifying the disciplinary history of EMS practitioners during the licensure or certification process. State EMS offices can access the NPDB to obtain information on adverse actions reported by other states or healthcare entities, which can help in evaluating the fitness of an EMS practitioner to practice in their state.

When a state submits a report to the NPDB, the report will contain, at minimum, an action and one or more basis code(s). While there are many possible codes, the following are the most relevant to EMS:

State License Action Codes

Code	Description
1110	Revocation of License
1125	Probation of License
1135	Suspension of License
1140	Reprimand or Censure
1148	Denial of License Renewal
1149	Denial of Initial License
1150	Interim Action - Voluntary Agreement to Refrain from Practice or to Suspend License Pending Completion of an Investigation
1151	Cease and Desist

1310	Revocation of Multi-State Licensure Privilege
1325	Probation of Multi-State Licensure Privilege
1335	Suspension of Multi-State Licensure Privilege
1338	Summary or Emergency Limitation or Restriction of Multi-State Licensure Privilege
1339	Summary or Emergency Suspension of Multi-State Licensure Privilege
1340	Reprimand or Censure of Multi-State Licensure Privilege
1345	Voluntary Surrender of Multi-State Licensure Privilege
1346	Voluntary Limitation or Restriction on Practice Authorized by Multi-State Licensure Privilege
1347	Limitation or Restriction on Multi-State Licensure Privilege
1351	Cease and Desist – Multi-State Licensing Privilege

In addition to the Action Code, the state will submit one or more Basis Code(s). A Basis Code is the reason(s) the action was taken. While there are many Basis Codes, the most common and relevant to EMS providers include:

Code	**Description**
19	Criminal Conviction
29	Practicing Beyond the Scope of Practice
AB	Practicing Beyond the Scope of Privileges
24	Practicing With an Expired License
A4	Practicing Without a Valid License
H6	Inappropriate Acquisition or Diversion of Controlled Substance
F9	Patient Abandonment
14	Patient Abuse
F6	Substandard Care or Inadequate Skill Level

The goals of reporting adverse actions to the NPDB and conducting investigations by state EMS offices are multifaceted and encompass several important aspects:

- **System Integrity**: The reporting of adverse actions to the NPDB and conducting investigations by state EMS offices are not only legal requirements, but also contribute to maintaining the integrity of the EMS system by ensuring that only qualified and competent EMS practitioners are allowed to practice. Adverse actions and investigations are mechanisms for identifying and addressing instances of professional misconduct, negligence, or incompetence among EMS practitioners, which can pose risks to patient safety and public health. By holding EMS practitioners accountable for their actions and maintaining a robust disciplinary process, state EMS offices help to preserve the integrity and reputation of the EMS system.

- **Professionalism**: Adverse actions and investigations by state EMS offices promote professionalism among EMS practitioners by upholding standards of conduct, competence, and ethics. EMS practitioners are expected to adhere to the highest standards of professionalism in their practice, which includes maintaining appropriate licensure or certification, adhering to regulations and protocols, and providing safe and quality care to patients. Adverse actions and investigations serve as a deterrent against unprofessional behavior and misconduct among EMS practitioners and help to maintain a culture of professionalism within the EMS field.

- **Consumer Protections**: Reporting adverse actions to the NPDB and conducting investigations by state EMS offices also serve as a means of protecting consumers, including patients, healthcare entities, and the public, from unsafe or incompetent EMS practitioners. Adverse actions and investigations help to identify and address instances of substandard care, negligence, or misconduct by EMS practitioners, which can pose risks to patient safety and public health. By taking appropriate disciplinary actions, state EMS offices help to safeguard the well-being of consumers and maintain public trust in the EMS system.

The role and purpose of state EMS offices in conducting investigations and taking disciplinary actions against EMS practitioners are multifaceted and encompass system integrity, professionalism, and consumer protections. Reporting adverse actions to the NPDB and conducting investigations are important mechanisms for identifying and addressing instances of professional misconduct, negligence, or incompetence among EMS practitioners, and promoting safe and quality care in the EMS system.

MEDICARE EXCLUSION DATABASE

The Medicare Exclusion Database, maintained by the Department of Health and Human Services (HHS), is a comprehensive record of individuals and entities barred from partaking in federally funded healthcare programs like Medicare, Medicaid, and other HHS programs. These entities primarily comprise healthcare providers convicted of offenses related to these federal programs.

Exclusion from participation in Medicare can be either mandatory or permissive. Mandatory exclusions are enforced by law for individuals and entities convicted of crimes including Medicare or Medicaid fraud, patient abuse or neglect, felony convictions for health care-related theft or financial misconduct, and felony convictions relating to the unlawful manufacture or distribution of controlled substances.

Permissive exclusions give the Office of the Inspector General (OIG) the discretion to exclude individuals and entities on several grounds. These grounds may include misdemeanor convictions related to healthcare fraud outside Medicare or a state health program, fraud in a program funded by any Federal, State, or local government agency, misdemeanor convictions related to the illegal manufacture or distribution of controlled substances, and other issues impacting professional competence or financial integrity.

The OIG maintains the List of Excluded Individuals/Entities (LEIE) — a current record of all excluded entities. Importantly, anyone who employs an individual or entity listed on the LEIE could face civil monetary penalties (CMP). As such, all healthcare entities – including Emergency Medical Service providers - are encouraged to check the list routinely to ensure their employees, both current and prospective, are not listed.

As vital components of the healthcare system, EMS agencies are also subject to these exclusion rules. These exclusions could have a severe impact on their financial viability due to the high proportion of patients that are insured by these federal programs.

Moreover, the Medicare Exclusion Database offers an essential reference for EMS leaders and government officials to ensure regulatory compliance within their operations. Regular cross-checking against this database can prevent EMS agencies from employing or collaborating with excluded individuals or entities, thereby avoiding substantial legal and financial penalties. By using this database, EMS leaders can also maintain public trust by demonstrating their commitment to high standards of care and ethical conduct.

Professionalism and Complaints

As the field of emergency medical services continues to evolve and expand, the importance of professionalism among EMS practitioners cannot be overstated. Professionalism is not only a vital component in the delivery of high-quality patient care but also plays a crucial role in shaping the public's perception and trust in EMS practitioners. This section aims to discuss the core professional attributes that EMS practitioners should embody to uphold the highest standards of practice and to minimize complaints.

In the ever-changing and demanding landscape of emergency medical care, professionalism envelops a broad range of traits, behaviors, and attitudes crucial for successful practice. These traits comprise clinical competency, effective communication, ethical decision-making, empathy, and cultural sensitivity, among others. By cultivating a culture of professionalism and consistently exhibiting these fundamental attributes, EMS practitioners can bolster their credibility, foster trust among patients and colleagues, and ultimately contribute to better patient outcomes. Here are some fundamental principles of EMS professionalism:

- **Treat every patient with respect**: It should be a priority for EMS personnel to treat every patient, irrespective of their age, race, gender, religion, socioeconomic status, or any other characteristic, with respect and dignity. This encompasses active listening to patients and their families, considering their concerns, involving them in decision-making, and addressing their needs and preferences to the utmost of their ability.

- **Maintain a professional demeanor:** EMS personnel should always maintain a professional demeanor, manifesting in both their appearance and behavior. This includes wearing the uniform properly, exhibiting appropriate identification, and utilizing suitable language and communication skills. EMS personnel should also be punctual, reliable, and take responsibility for their actions, adhering to established protocols, guidelines, and regulations.

- **Perform comprehensive patient assessments**: EMS personnel should carry out meticulous and systematic patient assessments – *on every patient* - to collect relevant information about the patient's condition, medical history, allergies, medications, and other significant details. This information is crucial to guide proper treatment decisions and ensures no potential issues are missed.

- **Show compassion to all patients**: EMS personnel should interact with patients with empathy, understanding, and compassion. Many patients might be experiencing physical or emotional pain, distress, or anxiety, and EMS personnel should strive to provide comfort and reassurance. This involves practicing good communication skills, being attentive to patients' emotional needs, and exhibiting empathy and kindness in their interactions.

- **Document meticulously**: Documentation is an essential aspect of EMS practice, serving as a legal and professional record of patient care. EMS personnel should document all aspects of their patient encounters accurately, thoroughly, and promptly. This involves documenting patient information, assessment findings, treatments administered, and other relevant details following established documentation guidelines and protocols.

- **Be mindful of video recording**: With the prevalent use of various recording devices today, EMS personnel should be cognizant that they might be recorded on video during patient encounters. This includes body cameras, dash cameras, surveillance cameras, and other devices. EMS personnel should always be mindful of their actions, words, and behaviors, as they may be recorded and reviewed in case of complaints or investigations.

- **Seek feedback and continuous improvement**: EMS personnel should be open to feedback from peers, supervisors, and patients, viewing it as an opportunity for self-reflection and improvement. This involves learning from mistakes, actively seeking feedback on their performance, and engaging in continual professional development to stay current with best practices and advancements in EMS care.

- **Maintain patient confidentiality**: EMS personnel should respect and protect the privacy of their patients by adhering to all applicable confidentiality laws, regulations, and guidelines. This involves not disclosing patient information without proper authorization and ensuring that sensitive information is stored and transmitted securely.

- **Collaborate effectively with other healthcare professionals**: EMS practitioners often collaborate closely with other healthcare professionals like physicians, nurses, and emergency department staff. Fostering and maintaining robust collaborative relationships with these colleagues is essential for providing optimal patient care. This includes sharing information, cooperating on treatment plans, and respecting the expertise of each team member.

- **Cultivate cultural competence**: EMS personnel should endeavor to develop cultural competence, which is the capability to understand, communicate, and effectively interact with people from diverse backgrounds. This requires acknowledging one's own biases and prejudices, striving to learn about different cultures, and tailoring care to meet the unique needs and preferences of patients from different cultural backgrounds.

- **Practice ethical decision-making**: EMS personnel should make decisions based on a strong ethical foundation, considering the best interests of the patient, the values of the profession, and the applicable laws and guidelines. This involves recognizing and addressing potential ethical dilemmas, engaging in ethical discussions with colleagues, and seeking guidance when faced with difficult decisions.

By adhering to these principles, EMS personnel can provide the highest level of patient care, maintain professionalism, and reduce the risk of complaints, investigations, and disciplinary actions. It is crucial for EMS practitioners to continually strive for excellence in their practice, exhibit integrity, and actively contribute to the positive image of the EMS profession.

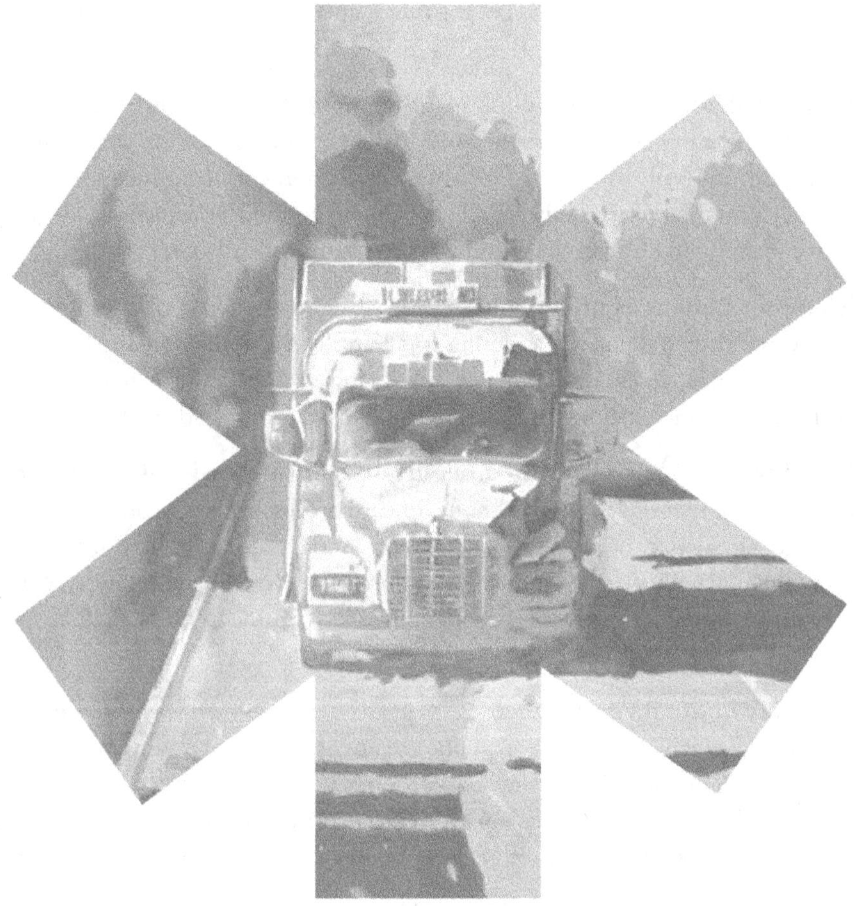

28

PUBLIC PROTECTION & BACKGROUND CHECKS

"The legitimate object of government is to do for a community of people whatever they need to have done but cannot do at all or cannot so well do for themselves in their separate and individual capacities."
- President Abraham Lincoln

THE LANDMARK DECISION SET FORTH BY THE U.S. SUPREME COURT in the 19th century case of *Hawker v. New York*[155] established the essential role of character in obtaining a medical license. This key verdict underscored the fact that state licensing processes are obligated to evaluate not only an applicant's medical knowledge but also their moral character and integrity. The court asserted that public trust in medical practitioners relies as much on their ethical conduct as it does their professional competence.

States, therefore, have an undeniable duty to assess the character qualifications of applicants before granting a license to practice. This responsibility goes beyond merely meeting public expectations; it is a core aspect of a state's licensing function. Confirming the ethical and moral integrity of EMS practitioners is as crucial as verifying their medical competence. This dual evaluation is vital to maintaining public trust and confidence in healthcare services.

Given this context, it is imperative that all states mandate fingerprinting as an integral part of assessing the character qualifications of EMS license applicants. Fingerprinting is a crucial tool that assists states in ensuring that only individuals of good moral character and high ethical standards are authorized to provide emergency medical care. The implementation of such measures demonstrates a state's commitment to protecting the public and maintaining the integrity of the EMS system.

- **Criminal Background Checks**: Fingerprinting is used as a means of conducting criminal background checks on EMS license applicants. Criminal background checks are essential for identifying any past criminal history or convictions that may pose a risk to public safety. This can include offenses such as assault, theft, fraud, drug-related offenses, or other crimes that could impact an individual's ability to provide emergency medical care safely and responsibly to patients. By conducting fingerprint-based criminal background checks, states can identify any potential red flags in an applicant's criminal history and take appropriate measures to protect the public from individuals who may pose a risk to patient safety.
- **Regulatory Compliance**: Fingerprinting of EMS license applicants is also done to ensure compliance with state and federal regulations. Many states have specific requirements for EMS practitioners, including background checks, as mandated by state laws or regulations. Additionally, state licensing board requirements and the EMS Compact's model legislation may require fingerprint-based background checks as part of the licensing process for EMS practitioners. Fingerprinting helps states ensure that they are following these regulations, which are in place to protect the public and maintain system integrity.
- **System Integrity**: Fingerprinting of EMS license applicants is crucial for maintaining the integrity of the EMS system. It helps prevent individuals with a history of criminal behavior, misconduct, or fraudulent activities from obtaining EMS licensure and potentially entering the EMS workforce. This helps to safeguard the reputation and credibility of the EMS system by ensuring that only qualified and suitable individuals are granted EMS licensure and allowed to provide emergency medical care to patients. Fingerprinting serves as a vital tool in identifying any potential risks to system integrity and taking appropriate measures to mitigate those risks.
- **Public Trust**: Fingerprinting of EMS license applicants also helps to build and maintain public trust in the EMS system. By conducting thorough background checks, including fingerprinting, states demonstrate their commitment to ensuring the safety and welfare of the public. It gives the public confidence that EMS practitioners have been thoroughly screened for any past criminal history or misconduct and are competent and trustworthy in their role as emergency medical care providers. This promotes public trust in the EMS system and enhances the credibility and professionalism of the EMS workforce.

Fingerprinting individuals pursuing a state EMS license is of paramount importance for public safety and the preservation of the EMS system's integrity. This measure not only facilitates comprehensive criminal background checks but also serves as a primary source verification of an individual's arrest records and convictions. It thereby aids states in complying with regulations, ensuring system integrity, and fostering public trust in the EMS system.

The incorporation of fingerprinting into the licensing process affords state EMS licensing officials an indispensable tool. When used in conjunction with license application form questions, it aids in the assessment of an applicant's character and integrity. The ability to unveil any potential risks within an applicant's criminal history is vital to ensure that only suitable and qualified individuals are awarded EMS licensure and thereby authorized to deliver emergency medical care to patients.

The minimum standard for ensuring public health, safety, and welfare is to require all medical professionals seeking state licensure to complete a biometric (fingerprint) background check. This is particularly crucial for EMS personnel, who frequently work in patients' homes, and frequently work alone while caring for vulnerable patients. To strengthen this vital accountability, the profession must self-regulate and uphold the highest standards for everyone seeking to be an EMS practitioner. Simultaneously, state EMS offices must actively monitor for any new criminal convictions, demonstrating an unwavering commitment to preserving the well-being of all those they serve.

The EMS profession demands an extraordinarily high level of public trust. Uniquely, many EMS personnel operate one-on-one with highly vulnerable patients for extended periods of time, often in isolation. This distinct context renders thorough background checks imperative. It is critical to ensure that those entrusted with providing medical care in these sensitive circumstances are individuals of high character, impeccable integrity, and who have been vetted rigorously for past criminal activity. By fulfilling this obligation, the EMS profession ensures the safety and well-being of the public, while upholding the credibility and trustworthiness that are integral to its role in healthcare.

Fingerprints and the Compact

The EMS Compact represents a formal interstate compact agreement that enhances the collective ability of states to protect public health and safety. As an agreement, it ensures standardized processes and procedures for EMS personnel across state lines, promoting consistency and reliability in the delivery of emergency medical services.

At the time of this publication, 24 states are members of the EMS Compact. These Member States have willingly committed to a common set of standards and procedures to promote uniformity in licensing EMS personnel. Included within these shared standards is the requirement for fingerprint-based background checks for all EMS license applicants.

It is important to clarify that this fingerprinting prerequisite for EMS personnel is a mandatory minimum standard that every Member State has codified in state law and committed to enforcing. This means that regardless of the specific state in which an EMS professional applies for an initial license, a fingerprint background check is now a universal requirement, strictly adhered to as a condition of being a compact Member State.

This uniform standard serves multiple critical roles. Firstly, it safeguards public safety by ensuring that individuals with a criminal history are appropriately identified and assessed before they are entrusted with public health responsibilities. Secondly, it reinforces the integrity of the EMS profession by creating a consistent licensure process across all member states. Finally, it enhances the public's trust in EMS agencies, as they can be assured that the EMS professionals serving them have met rigorous, standardized criteria before obtaining their license.

By requiring fingerprint background checks, the EMS Compact Member States demonstrate their unwavering commitment to uphold public safety and professional integrity. This requirement is a testament to the dedication of these states to maintain high standards in EMS licensure, aligning with their collective responsibility to protect and serve their communities effectively.

The EMS Compact serves as a symbol of interstate cooperation in advancing EMS agencies across the nation. The fingerprinting prerequisite for EMS licensure is a fundamental piece of this agreement, bolstering a unified, reliable, and trustworthy EMS system that serves the public effectively and efficiently. (More information about the EMS Compact is in Chapter 24.)

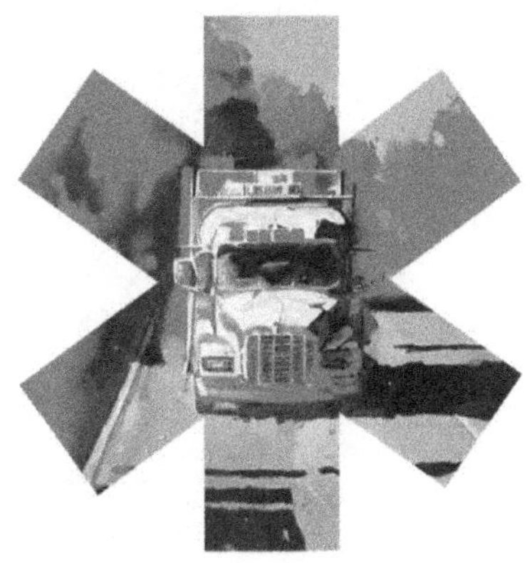

Section 5

LEADERSHIP & MANAGEMENT

"Leadership is the capacity to translate vision into reality."
-Warren Bennis

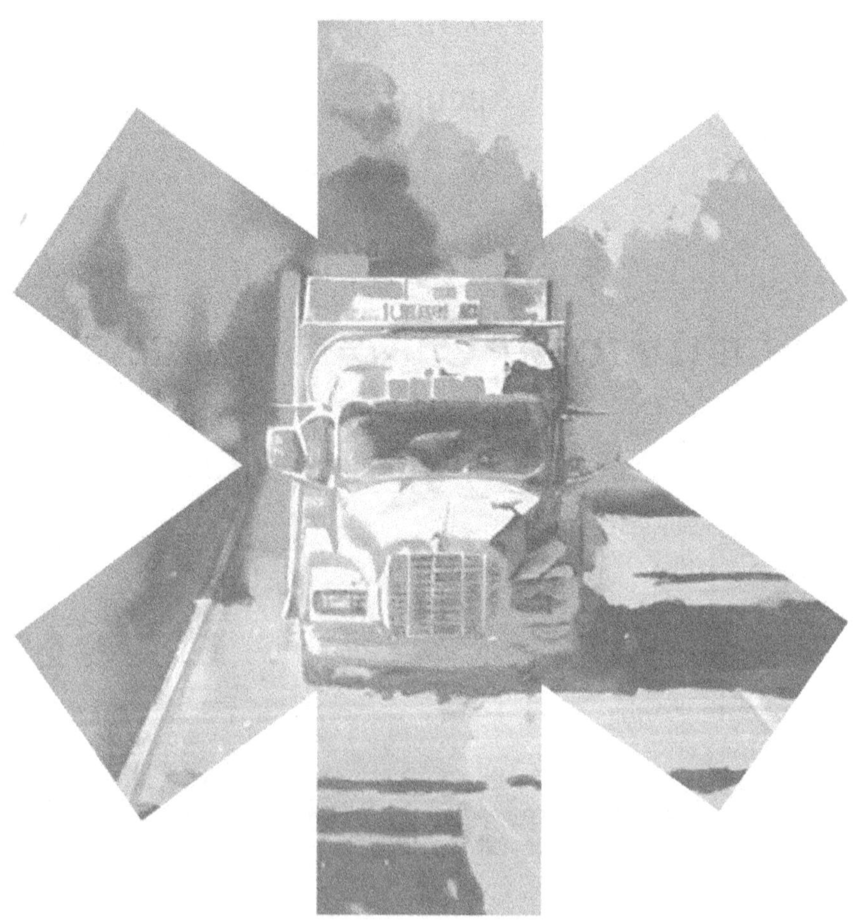

29

VISIONARY LEADERSHIP

"A leader has the vision and conviction that a dream can be achieved. He inspires the power and energy to get it done."

EMS LEADERS AND MANAGERS ARE CRUCIAL TO THE DELIVERY OF high-quality emergency medical services, providing oversight, guidance, and support to providers and staff in often challenging and rapidly changing environments. To be effective in their roles, EMS leaders must possess a unique combination of skills, knowledge, and vision that allows them to navigate the complexities of the industry and deliver optimal patient care. These skills and knowledge include a deep understanding of medical protocols and best practices, effective communication and collaboration skills, strategic planning and decision-making abilities, and a commitment to ongoing learning and improvement.

At the heart of effective EMS leadership is visionary leadership, which involves the ability to see beyond the present challenges and constraints and envision a better future for an organization or industry. In the context of EMS, visionary leadership has been essential in shaping the current state of the industry and driving its ongoing evolution. The contributions of past visionaries such as Rocco Morando, J.D. Farrington, MD, Peter Safar, MD, and James O. Page cannot be overstated. These individuals occupied pivotal positions in the development and implementation of the EMS systems relied upon today, and their enduring legacy serves as a source of inspiration and guidance for EMS leaders and managers across all levels.

VISIONARY LEADERSHIP IN EMS

Visionary leadership in EMS requires the capacity to foresee upcoming trends, difficulties, and opportunities, and to devise and put into action strategies that allow the agency to adapt effectively. This demands a blend of skills, expertise, and perspective that empowers the leader to look beyond the immediate demands and limitations of the field and envisage a superior future for their agency or the industry.

An essential aspect of visionary leadership in EMS involves maintaining a delicate equilibrium between immediate objectives and long-term vision and planning. While addressing pressing needs and demands is vital, these leaders also maintain a forward-looking view, readying themselves for future hurdles and possibilities. This necessitates the bravery to undertake measured risks, scrutinize assumptions, and fully welcome change and innovation.

Being a visionary requires an in-depth understanding of the field, encompassing current trends, regulations, and best practices. This calls for a pledge to perpetual learning and development, as well as the readiness to stay abreast of the field's latest advancements. This engagement can be cultivated by attending industry events, networking with fellow EMS leaders, keeping current with industry publications, and participating in ongoing education and training.

In addition to extensive industry knowledge, EMS leaders should have an array of leadership abilities and traits that empower them to inspire and lead their teams. This encompasses potent communication skills, the capacity to establish strong relationships and collaborate effectively, and an unwavering commitment to patient care and their team's wellbeing. Trailblazing leaders should also have the insight to recognize and develop talent within their organization, fostering a culture that values innovation, continuous enhancement, and excellence.

Visionary leadership in EMS involves envisioning a brighter future for both the industry and the patients it serves. It requires a deep understanding of recent trends and developments, along with the courage to take calculated risks and challenge established norms. By embracing these qualities, EMS leaders can ignite positive change and foster innovation, leading to enhanced patient care quality and increased organizational effectiveness.

Furthermore, visionary leaders in EMS need to actively advocate for their agency, team, and patients. This means effectively communicating the needs and achievements of the EMS community to external stakeholders, such as government officials, funding bodies, and the public. Advocacy can help attract necessary resources, influence policy changes, and enhance public perception and understanding of the EMS field.

Finally, visionary EMS leaders must be resilient. The nature of emergency medical services is unpredictable, often stressful, and regularly presents complex challenges. By demonstrating resilience, leaders can navigate these difficulties effectively, inspiring their team and maintaining high standards of patient care. Resilience also involves the ability to learn from setbacks and adapt strategies accordingly, a critical aspect of continual improvement and success in EMS leadership.

Traits of Visionary Leaders

Visionary leadership is a critical part of effective EMS management, demanding a distinct blend of skills, knowledge, and personality traits. Visionary leaders in EMS are those who have the capacity to look beyond the immediate industry demands and constraints, envisioning a more prosperous future for their organization and the sector at large. A visionary leader possesses several indispensable characteristics, including creativity and innovation, strategic foresight, unwavering passion and commitment, adept communication skills, adaptability and resilience, and a strong commitment to lifelong learning.

Curiosity and Exploration

Visionary leaders are driven by an insatiable curiosity that propels them beyond the typical. This curiosity is not limited to their specific field; it spans across disciplines, sectors, and even borders. They are constantly on a quest for deeper learning, better understanding, and further exploration. This thirst for knowledge and comprehension fuels their desire to pose challenging questions, investigate new theories, and venture into uncharted realms.

This curiosity is not merely a passive interest but an active, persistent, and systematic exploration of their surroundings. They're not content with merely understanding what's happening; they want to know why it's happening and how it can be improved. This curiosity encourages them to scrutinize problems from diverse perspectives, consider alternative solutions, and strive for continuous improvement.

Moreover, they understand the importance of cultivating a culture of curiosity within their teams and organizations. They foster an environment where questions, exploration, and experimentation are encouraged, recognizing this as key to innovation and growth. They appreciate that each team member, irrespective of their role or position, has unique insights and ideas that can contribute to the organization's overall success.

This curiosity also shapes their approach to risk. Visionary leaders are not reckless, but they understand that progress often requires stepping outside comfort zones and venturing into the unknown. They are willing to take calculated risks, and most importantly, they are prepared to learn from both their triumphs and failures. They see every experience as an opportunity for learning, adapting, and growing. It fuels their drive to innovate, adapt, and excel. It enables them to envision a better future and inspire others to participate in realizing that vision. It's a potent force for change and a crucial element in their success formula.

Strategic Thinking

Visionary EMS leaders anticipate and prepare for future trends and challenges, creating long-term strategies that allow their organization to adapt and respond effectively. They adeptly balance immediate needs with a long-term vision, making difficult choices to achieve their goals. This requires a deep understanding of the industry, coupled with a keen ability to stay up to date with the latest trends, regulations, and best practices. Visionary EMS leaders also develop and implement strategic plans that cater to their organization's needs and the wider community's needs, skillfully adjusting their strategies as situations evolve.

Drive and Dedication

At the core of visionary EMS leaders is a deeply rooted commitment to their organization's mission and an unrelenting passion for improving patient care and outcomes. They are the spark that motivates their teams, guiding them towards a shared vision of success and fostering an environment that breeds excellence and innovation. This demands more than just passion—it requires a deep sense of purpose and unwavering dedication to the values and objectives that underpin the organization. By leading by example, these leaders create a work environment that not only facilitates creativity and collaboration but also instills a deep commitment to patient care. In this way, they nurture a culture that goes beyond the ordinary, inspiring everyone in their organization to strive for extraordinary levels of service and care.

Effective Communication Skills

Visionary leaders possess strong communication skills and effectively articulate their vision and goals to their team, stakeholders, and the wider community. They prioritize building robust relationships and collaborations with other organizations and stakeholders. They tailor their communication styles to suit different audiences and contexts. This requires effective listening skills, the ability to articulate complex ideas clearly and concisely, and the capability to inspire and motivate others through persuasive communication.

Flexibility and Resilience

Visionary leaders in EMS exhibit remarkable adeptness at navigating shifting circumstances, demonstrating unyielding tenacity and resilience in the face of trials and challenges. They show an exceptional ability to adapt, alter their course when necessary, and stay steadfast when adversity strikes. They remain focused on their vision and goals, even when confronted with the most formidable obstacles.

This unwavering determination allows them to guide their teams through times of uncertainty and difficulties. A visionary leader provides consistent direction for their teams, inspiring them to persevere on their journey, irrespective of the challenges they encounter. In the face of adversity, these leaders don't just endure; they rise, they inspire, and they lead.

Such resilience stems from a mindset that is not just flexible but also adaptable. They understand that change is an integral part of growth and are always prepared to evolve as circumstances demand. They are skilled at maintaining composure and staying focused under intense pressure, providing a stable leadership presence that can weather any storm.

These visionary leaders also exhibit a remarkable ability to learn from failures and setbacks. They view these not as defeats, but as opportunities for learning and growth. They use these experiences to fuel continuous improvement within their organizations, transforming every challenge into opportunities for success. They instill this resilience within their teams, fostering a culture that embraces teamwork, celebrates success, and acknowledges failure as an integral part of the journey towards excellence.

The resilience and adaptability of visionary leaders are key to their success. They are not deterred by adversity; instead, they embrace it, learn from it, and use it as a catalyst for growth and improvement. Resilience and adaptability are not just traits; they are the driving forces that enable them to lead their organizations towards success, no matter the challenges they face.

Lifelong Learning

Visionary EMS leaders display a deep commitment to lifelong learning and development, staying abreast of the latest trends, technologies, and best practices within the field. They actively seek out opportunities for education and professional enhancement, fostering a culture of continuous growth and refinement within their organizations. This commitment to learning requires a growth mindset, a readiness to question assumptions, and an openness to adopting new ideas and methodologies. These visionary leaders stay informed of advancements in patient care, medical technologies, and regulatory changes, using this knowledge to catalyze innovation and progress within their organizations.

The essence of visionary leadership is a vital component of effective EMS management, demanding a unique amalgamation of skills, knowledge, and character traits. By nurturing these qualities, visionary EMS leaders have the power to inspire and propel their teams towards a collective vision of excellence in patient care and outcomes. Moreover, by staying attuned to the latest trends, technologies, and best practices in the field, visionary EMS leaders can stimulate continuous evolution and innovation within their organizations. Ultimately, by embracing and embodying visionary leadership, EMS managers can shape the trajectory of the industry, crafting a better world for patients, providers, and communities alike.

Innovation and Creativity

Innovation and creativity are the cornerstones of visionary leadership. Visionaries can think outside the box, exploring new ideas and approaches that can revolutionize the field. They foster an environment that encourages creative thinking and novel solutions, understanding that innovation is the pathway to progress.

Their creativity is not confined within the limits of their organization or the EMS industry. Visionary leaders have a broad perspective that spans across disciplines, sectors, and even borders. They draw insights from a range of fields, bringing a diverse array of ideas and strategies to their organization. They value and promote a culture of innovation, where everyone in the team feels empowered to share their ideas, thus fostering a fertile ground for breakthroughs.

Equally important is their ability to turn these creative ideas into actionable strategies. Visionary leaders in EMS possess the strategic acumen to translate innovative ideas into real-world solutions that enhance patient care and advance the EMS industry.

Emotional Intelligence

Emotional intelligence is another key trait of visionary leaders in EMS. They possess a deep understanding of their own emotions and those of others, allowing them to build strong relationships, manage conflicts, and inspire their teams. This emotional acumen enables them to navigate complex interpersonal dynamics effectively, fostering an environment of respect and collaboration.

Visionary leaders in EMS recognize the emotional demands of the field and strive to provide support to their teams. They exhibit empathy, understanding, and compassion, fostering an environment that acknowledges the emotional challenges that come with the job. This emotional intelligence is essential for nurturing a supportive and resilient team.

Empowerment and Delegation

Effective leaders empower and delegate. They understand the strengths and capabilities of their team members and are adept at delegating tasks in a manner that optimizes the talents within their team. They trust their team and encourage them to take on responsibilities and make decisions.

This empowering style of leadership fosters a sense of ownership and responsibility among team members, enhancing their motivation and engagement. It also promotes a culture of trust and respect, where everyone feels valued, and their contributions are recognized.

Visionary Leadership Strategies for Success

Visionary leaders harbor a distinct array of skills, knowledge, and character traits, allowing them to transcend immediate industry constraints and envisage a superior future for their organization or the field. For prosperity, visionary leaders in EMS should engage in pivotal activities that inspire their teams, formulate efficient strategies, and drive perpetual improvement and innovation. Here are specific tactics that visionary EMS leaders can employ to attain success:

- **Set a Clear Vision**: Crafting a precise and captivating vision for the organization is indispensable for success. Visionary leaders should understand the industry's challenges and opportunities in-depth, articulating a vision that propels the team towards a shared objective. This coherent vision aids in aligning efforts across the organization, from frontline staff to management, providing a blueprint for success.

- **Develop Effective Communication Strategies**: Proficient communication is vital for success in EMS management. Visionary EMS leaders should master communication techniques that allow them to lucidly convey their vision and goals to their team, stakeholders, and the broader community. The ability to build robust relationships and collaborations with various organizations and stakeholders, along with adapting their communication style to different audiences and situations, is paramount.

- **Foster a Culture of Innovation**: Cultivating an innovative atmosphere within the organization is crucial for success. Visionary EMS leaders should encourage staff to employ creative thinking and develop novel ideas and practices for patient care. They should equip teams with resources and support for experimenting and developing new technologies and procedures. Leaders should be ready to question traditional assumptions and embrace fresh approaches to patient care.

- **Build a Strong Team**: Forming a potent and efficient team is crucial for success in EMS management. Visionary leaders should recruit, educate, and develop staff, fostering a positive work environment that promotes creativity, collaboration, and a profound commitment to patient care. Clear and effective communication to the team is important, ensuring that all staff understand the organization's goals and their roles in realizing them.

- **Engage Proactively with Stakeholders:** Proactive engagement with stakeholders, including patients, families, community leaders, and other organizations, is crucial for success in EMS management. Visionary EMS leaders should forge strong relationships and collaborations with stakeholders, establishing trust and mutual understanding through effective communication. Engaging with stakeholders allows leaders to better grasp their community's needs and expectations and develop strategies that are responsive to these requirements.

- **Embrace Innovation and Opportunity**: Visionary leaders seize innovation and opportunity, understanding that the journey to success may entail mistakes. They see opportunities where others see failures and encourage their team to think unconventionally. A visionary leader should be receptive to fresh ideas and practices, unafraid to take calculated risks to achieve their objectives.

- **Prioritize Building Trust:** Establishing a strong foundation of trust is paramount for effective EMS management. Visionary leaders recognize the importance of building trust with their team, stakeholders, and the wider community. They achieve this by practicing transparency, consistency, and honesty in their communication and actions. It is crucial to note that leaders must demonstrate trust in their team members, particularly their direct reports, through their actions. Trust serves as a catalyst for fostering creativity, driving innovation, and enhancing productivity within the organization.

- **Embrace the Journey**: Visionary leaders not only appreciate the journey towards their vision, but they also prepare their team for the voyage. They recognize that the path to achieving their goals might not always be straightforward and will necessitate flexibility and adaptation. They maintain their focus on their vision while being open to new approaches and strategies.

- **Prepare your team**: Visionary leaders equip their teams for the journey by communicating the vision and goals clearly and honestly and building a strong foundation of trust within the team. They involve their team in strategizing and problem-solving, ensuring alignment and commitment to shared goals. Successful leaders are willing to pivot and adjust their strategies as needed, while staying true to their vision and purpose. They foster a culture of continuous improvement and innovation within their organization, encouraging their team to think creatively and adapt to new challenges and opportunities.

- **Embrace Learning Opportunities:** Visionary leaders see value in each learning opportunity. Understanding that growth often comes from challenges, they encourage their teams to embrace change, learn from mistakes, and continue striving for improvement. They also invest in professional development, demonstrating their commitment to learning not only for themselves but also for their team members.

- **Engage in Continuous Evaluation and Improvement**: Visionary leaders understand the importance of regular assessment and strive for continual betterment in their operations. They solicit feedback from team members and stakeholders to identify areas for improvement and implement strategies to address these areas. They not only accept constructive criticism but also see it as an opportunity to learn, grow, and strengthen their leadership capabilities.

By adopting these visionary leadership tactics for prosperity, EMS leaders have the potential to shape the future of the industry, creating a more effective world for patients, providers, and communities. Through setting a precise vision, mastering effective communication techniques, cultivating an atmosphere of innovation, assembling a robust team, and engaging proactively with stakeholders, visionary leaders can inspire and motivate their teams towards a collective vision of excellence in patient care and outcomes. They continually embrace learning opportunities, engage in regular evaluation and improvement, and strive to elevate standards of service and care to ensure the organization's continued success and growth.

BALANCING VISION & CHALLENGES

In the field of EMS management, visionary leadership is crucial for success. However, the art of visionary leadership is often a demanding and intricate task. Visionary leaders wield a distinctive blend of skills and traits that empower them to transcend the immediate challenges and constraints of the industry, envisaging a more effective future for their organization or the entire industry. Yet, it is imperative to remember that not all visions, objectives, or aspirations will materialize as planned, and failure is an inherent part of the journey.

Visionary leaders embrace humility, self-awareness, and an openness to learn from errors.

Visionary leaders should cultivate the ability to acknowledge when the initial goal or objective was misguided and adapt their direction and strategies accordingly. This necessitates humility, self-awareness, and an openness to learn from errors. Failure is a natural element of the visionary process and can indeed be a significant learning opportunity. Leaders who can embrace failure, learning from it to inform future decisions, are more likely to achieve long-term success.

Visionary leaders often have foresight that can appear to others as mere dreams or impossibilities. Consider Dr. Peter Safar, who in 1969 foresaw that EMS patient care reports would one day be standardized across the nation and analyzed by computers. In his time, this vision seemed improbable, given that many ambulance services of the era still had untrained personnel who weren't providing patient care, let alone writing medical reports. Visionary leaders, thus, must balance their aspirations with the practicalities of the industry and the complexities of implementation.

Visionary leaders should also inspire and invigorate their team while recognizing and addressing existing obstacles and limitations. They should proficiently communicate their vision, but also display receptiveness to feedback and critique from their team and other stakeholders. This demands a profound comprehension of the industry, a readiness to adopt novel technologies and procedures, and an unwavering commitment to perpetual learning and refinement.

Moreover, visionary leaders should balance the demands of their organization with the needs of the broader community. They need to comprehend the expectations and apprehensions of their stakeholders and balance these with their personal goals and objectives. This necessitates a deep understanding of the community and industry, coupled with adept communication and collaboration skills.

While visionary leadership is indispensable for success in EMS management, it certainly doesn't come easily. By seeing failure as a crucial learning opportunity, aligning their vision with the realities of the industry and the needs of their stakeholders, and by engaging in continuous learning and improvement, visionary leaders can stimulate continual enhancement and innovation within their organizations. In doing so, they ultimately bolster the quality of patient care and the overall efficacy of the EMS industry.

Implications of Visionary Leadership for EMS

The important role of visionary leadership in EMS management cannot be overstated. As the complexity and challenges of providing emergency medical services continue to evolve, so too must the leadership guiding these vital efforts. Effective visionary leadership has implications that reach far beyond the immediate team or organization; it can shape the entire industry and improve outcomes for patients and communities alike.

Visionary leaders who can balance their ambitious goals with the practical realities of the EMS field can drive much-needed innovation. Their readiness to experiment, to learn from mistakes, and to continuously adapt helps create an environment that encourages growth and evolution. This flexibility can propel improvements in technologies, processes, and even industry standards, leading to more effective patient care and better overall community health outcomes.

Further, visionary leaders serve as beacons of inspiration, not just for their teams, but for the entire EMS community. Their clear vision and commitment to achieving it can inspire others in the field to aim higher and strive for continuous improvement. This type of leadership can cultivate a collective spirit of resilience and innovation that is instrumental in overcoming industry-wide challenges and obstacles.

Lastly, visionary leaders who effectively balance organizational needs, patient needs, and the expectations of the wider community, can foster stronger, more trusting relationships between EMS practitioners and the populations they serve. Through open communication, transparency, and a clear commitment to serving community needs, these leaders can enhance public trust and cooperation, facilitating more effective EMS operations and better health outcomes.

Navigating the complexity of visionary leadership in EMS is no small feat, yet the potential benefits are profound. By embracing learning opportunities, balancing ambitious visions with practical realities, and fostering open, trust-based relationships, visionary leaders have the potential to guide the EMS industry into a future of increased effectiveness, efficiency, and excellence in patient care.

HIDDEN OPPORTUNITIES IN POOR LEADERSHIP

Leadership, an essential component of all organizations, often proves to be a challenging concept. Ironically, in many cases, employees do not have the privilege of selecting their leaders. Consequently, they may occasionally find themselves under the helm of a leader whose management style or decision-making abilities fall short of expectations. While such a scenario absolutely causes frustration and discontent, it also presents an unexpected avenue for professional growth and personal enrichment.

There is considerable value in scrutinizing the actions and behaviors of less-than-ideal leaders. A failing leader's traits, decision-making processes (or the lack thereof), and general attributes provide crucial lessons that can – ironically – be beneficial for employees. Observing poor leaders can serve as a powerful "what not to do" guide, helping aspiring leaders recognize ineffective leadership traits and avoid adopting these patterns in their own leadership journey.

However, the emotional toll of working under a poor leader should not be understated. It is important for employees to remember their feelings of discontent, frustration, confusion, or even helplessness. These emotional responses are potent reminders of the impact of poor leadership on morale and productivity. By reflecting on these feelings, future leaders can develop a deeper understanding of the psychological aspects of leadership and the importance of empathy, emotional intelligence, and effective communication in managerial roles.

One might argue that the knowledge gained from experiencing poor leadership is just as significant as learning from exceptional leaders. When subjected to substandard leadership, employees are provided with a unique perspective that allows them to identify the deficiencies within the system, as well as the opportunity to contemplate how they would alter the course if given a chance. By turning frustration into motivation, these circumstances can fuel one's desire to grow into a better leader, to prevent others from experiencing similar disappointments.

Understanding and acknowledging the paradox of poor leadership is an invaluable tool for those aspiring to EMS leadership or management positions. Rather than perceiving it solely as a negative experience, consider it a transformative opportunity to learn, grow, and ultimately become the leader you wished you had. In the realm of EMS, where every decision matters and every second counts, the importance of effective leadership cannot be overemphasized. By learning from the missteps of others, future EMS leaders can cultivate a leadership style that is both efficient and compassionate, ensuring a productive and harmonious work environment for their teams.

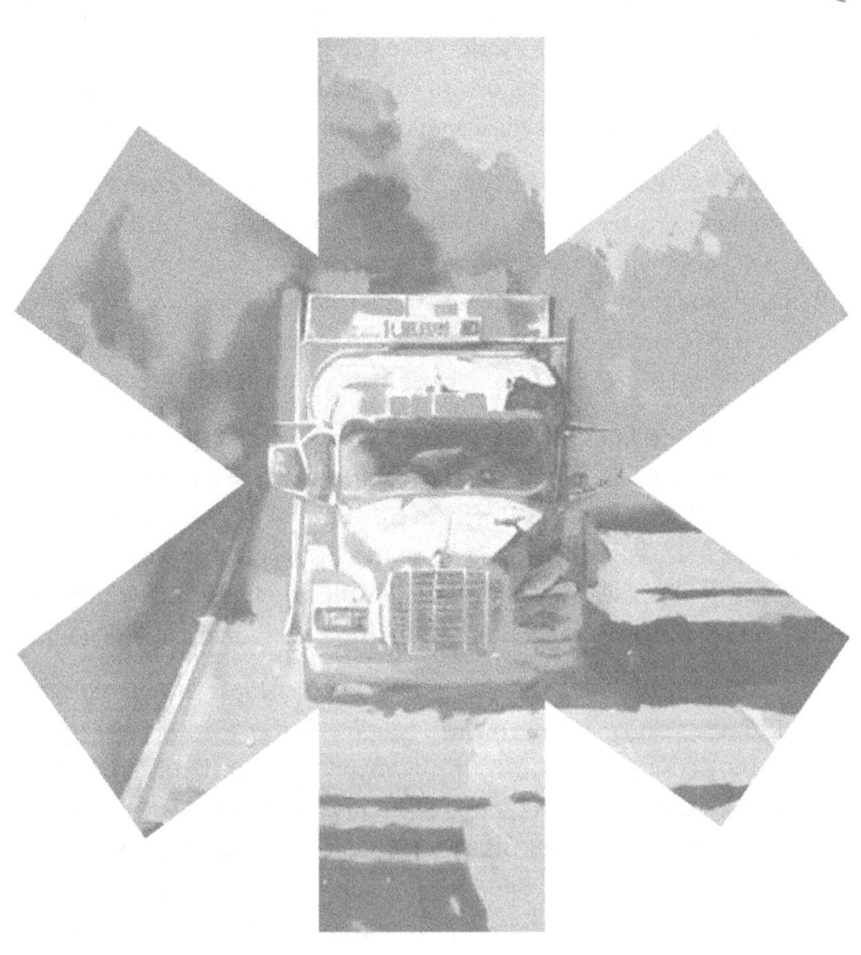

30

STAKEHOLDER ENGAGEMENT

"Engage your stakeholders in the dialogue that matters most to them. When you focus on what your stakeholders care about, they will talk back to you, and that's where the magic happens."

PROGRESSIVE EMS LEADERS ACKNOWLEDGE THE POWER OF ENGAGING with a wide spectrum of stakeholders. Defined as individuals or groups affected by or interested in the operations and outcomes of an organization, stakeholders may comprise patients, healthcare providers, EMS personnel, government bodies, and community members, among others. Effective stakeholder engagement is pivotal for EMS organizations across all strata; it equips leaders to comprehend the necessities and expectations of stakeholders, foster solid relationships, and collaborate towards realizing common objectives.

This chapter delves into the relevance of stakeholder engagement within EMS leadership, presents strategies for identifying, prioritizing, and involving stakeholders at local, state, and national echelons. It also sheds light on common slip-ups to evade during stakeholder interactions and imparts useful guidelines and best practices for efficient communication and negotiation when stakeholder interests are at odds.

IDENTIFYING STAKEHOLDERS

Accomplished EMS leaders pinpoint their stakeholders, who are individuals or entities influenced by the organization's actions and outcomes, and understand their interests and concerns. Stakeholders represent a diverse collection of entities: patients, healthcare providers, EMS personnel, government bodies, community organizations, and advocacy groups.

The method of identification can differ, however, seeking perspectives from industry-savvy associates and other internal or external stakeholders proves beneficial. Collecting feedback through surveys, focus groups, or interviews can help gauge the requirements and expectations of stakeholders and identify crucial contributors to the organization's goals. This information aids in compiling a comprehensive list of stakeholders and their interests.

Upon identification, stakeholders should be scrutinized based on their level of influence and interest in the organization, thereby allowing prioritization. Tools such as stakeholder maps provide a visual organization, categorizing stakeholders from key players (high influence and interest) to peripheral entities (low influence and interest).

ENGAGING STAKEHOLDERS IN EMS LEADERSHIP

The bedrock of cultivating relationships, securing support, and achieving fruitful outcomes is stakeholder engagement. This involves integrating stakeholders into the decision-making process, which augments understanding, engenders trust, and propels superior outcomes. Regular, transparent communication and soliciting feedback are essential for relationship building and ensuring stakeholders remain abreast of relevant issues and decisions.

Engagement can also involve collaboration on shared objectives or projects. This nurtures trust, bolsters support, and eventually leads to more successful results. For example, alliances with community organizations to escalate public awareness, upgrading patient care in collaboration with healthcare providers, or lobbying for favorable EMS policies with government agencies are instances of such collaborative efforts.

CHALLENGES IN STAKEHOLDER ENGAGEMENT

Despite the advantages of stakeholder engagement, certain hurdles exist. These include restricted resources, competing priorities, and stakeholder resistance. Limited time, staff, or funds may make stakeholder engagement challenging, particularly for smaller organizations. At the same time, balancing various priorities, such as patient care, staff training, and organizational development, can prove difficult, and conflicts might surface with stakeholders who have their own priorities and interests. Also, certain stakeholders may resist change or have interests contrasting the organization's goals, adding complexity to engagement and garnering support.

To overcome these obstacles, EMS leaders must accord priority to stakeholder engagement and allocate resources appropriately. This might involve setting aside staff time and budget for engagement activities and incorporating stakeholder engagement into regular procedures and strategic plans. Moreover, establishing relationships with stakeholders through consistent communication, collaboration, and addressing their needs and priorities can overcome resistance and stimulate support for organizational initiatives. Despite best efforts, oversights like a lack of transparency, excluding stakeholders from decision-making, and ineffective communication can occur. By proactively engaging stakeholders and avoiding these pitfalls, EMS leaders can forge strong relationships, inspire support, and achieve desirable outcomes.

Strategic Approach: Embracing Compromise for Mutual Benefit

A vital aspect of successful stakeholder engagement in EMS leadership lies in the readiness to find common ground. For matters involving budgetary or financial discussions with stakeholders, EMS leaders could consider proposing a higher, yet judiciously calculated, figure than strictly required. This approach enables the organization to negotiate based on stakeholder feedback and strike a balance that is favorable to all involved parties.

Presenting a realistic figure slightly above the bare necessity should not be misconstrued as financial imprudence or misuse of resources. On the contrary, by proposing a rational request that factors in potential unforeseen costs and contingencies, EMS leaders showcase their commitment to fiscal accountability. At the same time, they express a willingness to collaborate with stakeholders to reach a mutually agreeable consensus.

In discussions with various stakeholders, including community members, local officials, and healthcare providers, EMS leaders can collect valuable feedback and input. Armed with this information, the organization can negotiate with stakeholders to achieve a solution that is beneficial to everyone. This may involve modifying the initial budget request to prioritize the most crucial items for patient care or identifying alternative funding resources. By proposing an initially higher yet justifiable figure and being open to adjustment based on stakeholder feedback, EMS leaders can cultivate trust, foster stakeholder commitment, and ensure the organization is equipped to provide top-quality patient care.

However, this approach to stakeholder engagement must be grounded in sincerity and integrity. Offering a slightly higher request or opening negotiations from a more inclusive standpoint should not be viewed as a manipulative tactic. Instead, it's a strategic move to strengthen relationships and discover solutions that benefit all parties involved. EMS leaders must consistently place patient safety and quality care at the forefront of their decisions, underpinned by a commitment to transparency and honesty in all stakeholder interactions. By tackling stakeholder engagement with honesty, a genuine willingness to collaborate, and the goal of finding mutually beneficial solutions, EMS leaders can establish robust relationships and pave the way for successful outcomes.

TIPS FOR SUCCESSFUL STAKEHOLDER ENGAGEMENT

Effective stakeholder engagement in EMS leadership demands a strategic blend of methodologies and tactics to cultivate relationships, gather support, and attain successful results. Here are some key principles for successful stakeholder engagement in EMS leadership:

- **Identify and prioritize stakeholders**: As discussed earlier in this chapter, identifying and prioritizing stakeholders is a critical first step in effective stakeholder engagement. By understanding who the stakeholders are and their interests and priorities, EMS leaders can focus their efforts and resources on engaging those stakeholders who have the greatest impact on the organization's goals and objectives.

- **Be proactive in engagement**: Effective stakeholder engagement requires proactive efforts to build relationships, communicate regularly, and involve stakeholders in decision-making processes. By being proactive in engagement, EMS leaders can demonstrate a commitment to stakeholder needs and priorities and build trust and support.

- **Be transparent and honest**: Effective communication is essential to successful stakeholder engagement. EMS leaders should be transparent and honest in their communication with stakeholders, providing regular updates on organizational activities, responding to questions and concerns, and seeking feedback from stakeholders.

- **Collaborate on shared goals**: Collaborative initiatives are an effective way to engage stakeholders and achieve shared goals and objectives. By working collaboratively with stakeholders, EMS leaders can build strong relationships and generate support for organizational initiatives.

- **Be aware of cultural and diversity factors**: EMS leaders should be aware of cultural and diversity factors when engaging stakeholders. This includes understanding the cultural norms and values of different stakeholder groups, and adapting engagement strategies accordingly to build stronger relationships and generate support.

- **Measure and evaluate engagement**: Effective stakeholder engagement requires ongoing measurement and evaluation to assess the effectiveness of engagement strategies and identify areas for improvement. EMS leaders should establish clear metrics for measuring engagement and use this data to refine and improve their engagement strategies over time.

EMS leaders can build strong relationships with stakeholders, generate support for organizational initiatives, and achieve successful outcomes. However, despite best efforts, there are common mistakes and pitfalls that EMS leaders can fall into when engaging stakeholders. These mistakes can lead to strained relationships, resistance to organizational initiatives, and ultimately, unsuccessful outcomes. Here are some common mistakes and pitfalls to avoid in stakeholder engagement in EMS leadership:

- **Not listening to stakeholder concerns**: Effective stakeholder engagement requires active listening to stakeholder concerns and feedback. EMS leaders should avoid dismissing stakeholder concerns or feedback, as this can lead to resentment and resistance to organizational initiatives.

- **Failing to communicate effectively**: Effective communication is essential to successful stakeholder engagement. EMS leaders should avoid being unresponsive to stakeholder inquiries or concerns or failing to communicate regularly and transparently with stakeholders.

- **Not prioritizing stakeholder engagement**: Stakeholder engagement should be a priority for EMS leaders. Failing to prioritize stakeholder engagement in the organization's strategic plan can lead to missed opportunities and strained relationships with stakeholders.

- **Lack of transparency**: Stakeholders expect transparency in organizational decision-making processes. EMS leaders should avoid being secretive or withholding information, as this can lead to mistrust and resistance to organizational initiatives.

- **Not recognizing cultural or diversity factors**: EMS leaders should be aware of cultural and diversity factors when engaging stakeholders. Failure to recognize these factors can lead to misunderstandings and strained relationships with stakeholder groups.

- **Ignoring stakeholder feedback**: Stakeholder feedback should be taken seriously and incorporated into organizational decision-making processes. EMS leaders should avoid ignoring stakeholder feedback, as this can lead to stakeholder resistance and a lack of support for organizational initiatives.

- **Poor Relationship Building**: Strong relationships form the core of successful stakeholder engagement. Neglecting to invest time in building and maintaining these relationships can lead to mistrust and lack of cooperation from stakeholders.

- **Lack of Continual Engagement**: Stakeholder engagement is not a one-time event but a continuous process. It requires ongoing dialogue, feedback, and collaboration. Failure to maintain this continual engagement can result in stakeholders feeling neglected or undervalued, leading to decreased support and collaboration.

- **Inconsistency in Engagement Efforts**: Consistency is key in successful stakeholder engagement. This includes consistent messaging, consistent efforts at collaboration, and consistent follow-through on commitments. Inconsistency can lead to confusion, mistrust, and lack of faith in leadership.

- **Limited Perspective Sharing**: Stakeholders come from diverse backgrounds and bring a variety of perspectives. Failure to allow for and encourage the sharing of these different perspectives can lead to a lack of creativity and innovation. Ultimately this will limit the effectiveness of engagement efforts.

- **Not Aligning Stakeholder Interests with Organizational Goals**: Aligning stakeholder interests with organizational goals not only aids in achieving those goals, but also ensures stakeholder buy-in and support. Ignoring this alignment can lead to conflict, resistance, and lack of progress towards goals.

By avoiding these common pitfalls and following the key principles outlined, EMS leaders can successfully engage stakeholders, build strong relationships, gain support for organizational initiatives, and ultimately achieve successful outcomes. The importance of stakeholder engagement cannot be overstated; it is vital for effective EMS leadership and the success of the organization.

THE DELICATE BALANCING ACT

Effective EMS leadership demands a nuanced ability to harmoniously balance the diverse interests and priorities of stakeholders. This necessitates an in-depth understanding of the needs, goals, and expectations of each stakeholder group, and the aptitude to construct strategies that accommodate these varied interests to yield successful results.

One of the central challenges lies in comprehending and reconciling the legitimate, albeit occasionally opposing needs and priorities of different stakeholder groups. Stakeholders range from patients, healthcare providers, government agencies, to community organizations, each with their distinctive needs and objectives. For instance, while patients may emphasize timely, high-quality care, healthcare providers may focus on efficient resource utilization and cost control. Government agencies might be more concerned with regulatory compliance and accountability, whereas community organizations could stress community engagement and involvement.

To adeptly balance these interests, EMS leaders must thoroughly grasp the perspectives and priorities of each stakeholder group. This understanding is best cultivated through active stakeholder engagement and communication, alongside the collection and analysis of data and feedback. Having a profound awareness of each group's needs and priorities allows EMS leaders to formulate strategies that balance these interests and produce successful outcomes.

One such strategy involves prioritizing the needs of the most critical stakeholders. This concept, like triage in mass casualty situations, implies that the needs and priorities of certain stakeholder groups may supersede those of others. By centering on the needs of vital stakeholders, EMS leaders can ensure resources are judiciously allocated for maximum effect.

Another strategy includes identifying commonalities and areas of agreement among different groups. For example, both healthcare providers and government agencies might prioritize cost control and resource efficiency. Recognizing these overlapping areas allows EMS leaders to conceive strategies that simultaneously cater to the needs and priorities of multiple stakeholder groups. Facilitating open communication and fostering collaboration are also effective strategies, serving to build trust, mutual understanding, and develop solutions addressing multiple groups' needs simultaneously.

While assembling stakeholder groups, EMS leaders should establish a clear set of guiding principles or values that shape decision-making. These principles might encompass ethical considerations such as prioritizing patient safety and well-being, alongside organizational values like fostering innovation, collaboration, and accountability. Decision-making, guided by these principles and values, ensures consistency and fairness across diverse stakeholder groups.

Effectively engaging stakeholders and balancing their interests is seldom straightforward. It calls for a commitment to continuous learning and improvement. EMS leaders should be receptive to feedback, willing to tweak their strategies, and strive to better accommodate stakeholder needs and priorities. This may entail gathering and analyzing data, seeking diverse perspectives, and pursuing continuous education and professional development. Conflicts and challenges are inevitable, requiring difficult decisions. However, by adhering to the principles and strategies of effective stakeholder engagement, EMS leaders can navigate these challenges and realize successful outcomes.

Balancing stakeholder interests is a crucial facet of successful EMS leadership, often distinguishing success from failure. Leaders committed to understanding the needs, goals, and expectations of each stakeholder group, along with the aptitude to formulate strategies that balance these interests, are poised for success. Proactive leaders who seek balance among stakeholder interests can build resilient relationships, foster support, and achieve positive results for patients, providers, and communities.

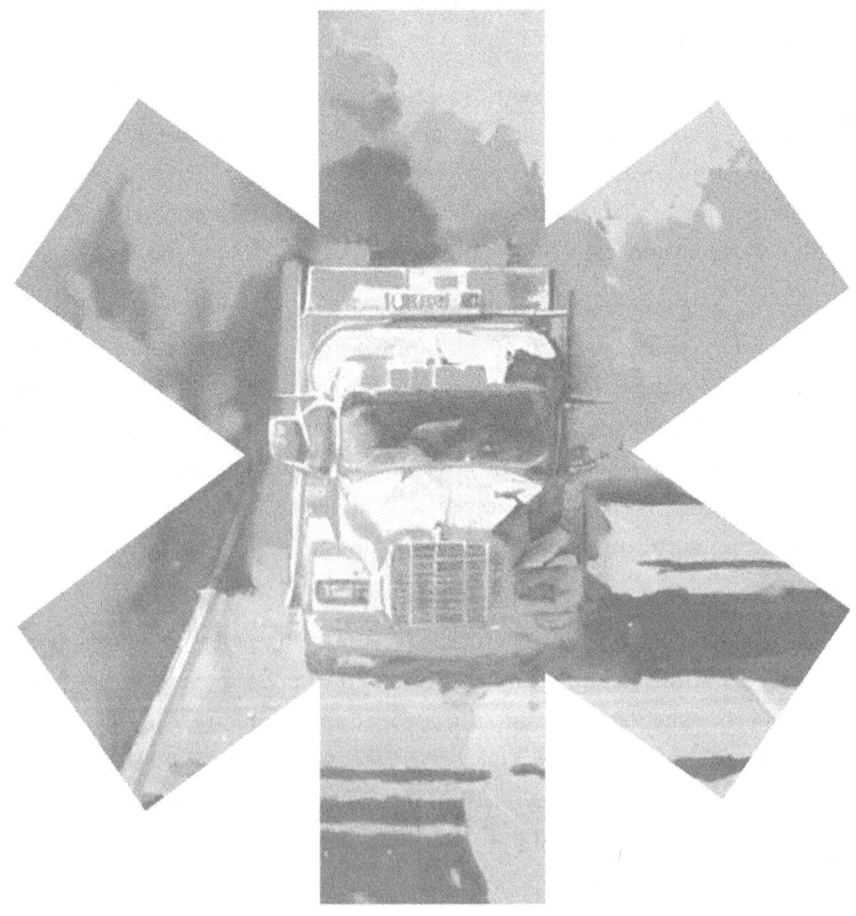

31

LEADING CHANGE MANAGEMENT

"Change is the law of life. And those who look only to the past or present are certain to miss the future."
- President John F. Kennedy

AS THE EMS INDUSTRY CONTINUES TO EVOLVE AND GROW, CHANGE is inevitable. With new regulations, guidelines, technological advancements, and techniques emerging, EMS leaders must possess the ability to navigate their organizations through transformative periods effectively. Change is crucial to maintain relevance and deliver the highest standard of patient care. However, leading change in any industry, particularly in EMS, can present complex and formidable challenges. The EMS field often experiences resistance to change, as local pride and ownership frequently clash with national standards and initiatives. Despite these hurdles, proficient change management is vital for the long-term prosperity of EMS organizations. This chapter delves into the concept of leading change in EMS, emphasizing the significance of change management, identifying common obstacles to change, and offering strategies to successfully navigate transformative periods in the EMS realm. By comprehending and implementing these strategies, EMS leaders can contribute to the ongoing growth and triumph of their organizations.

UNDERSTANDING CHANGE IN EMS

The EMS industry is constantly evolving, driven by advancements in technology, changes in treatment protocols, and evolving patient needs. As EMS leaders, it is essential to effectively manage change to maintain organizational relevance, efficiency, and effectiveness. However, leading change in EMS is challenging due to the unique characteristics of the industry, such as the decentralized nature of the EMS system, the need to balance patient care with fiscal responsibility, and the inherent resistance to change that is common in the EMS culture.

To effectively lead change, EMS leaders need to have a clear understanding of what change is and how it impacts organizations and individuals within those organizations. Change can take many forms, such as implementing new technology, adopting new treatment protocols, or restructuring organizational systems. Regardless of the specific nature of the change, it generally has positive and negative impacts on individuals and organizations.

Managing change in EMS is particularly challenging due to the deeply ingrained culture of the industry. The history of EMS has roots in community-based systems that are deeply rooted in local pride and ownership. The highly personal nature of EMS creates some inherent resistance to change, as providers and stakeholders may view new processes or systems as a threat to their established way of doing things. If not addressed effectively, this resistance can manifest in various forms and derail change initiatives.

EMS leaders must have a thorough understanding of the change process and the factors that influence it. They must be able to identify and address resistance to change and develop strategies to engage stakeholders in the process. By taking a proactive approach to change management, EMS leaders can ensure that their organizations are well-positioned to adapt to changes and remain competitive in the industry. Regardless of the origin, change is a challenging process for EMS leaders to navigate, especially when met with resistance from stakeholders who are invested in maintaining the status quo. By understanding the change process and the factors that influence it, EMS leaders can navigate change with confidence and ensure that their organizations are well-prepared to adapt to the evolving needs of their patients and communities.

PREPARING FOR CHANGE

Preparing for change is an essential step in leading change. Effective preparation requires a thorough understanding of the change that is being proposed, as well as the impact that the change will have on the organization and its stakeholders. It also involves developing a plan to effectively communicate the need for change, gain buy-in from stakeholders, and manage resistance to the change.

One of the first steps in preparing for change is to clearly define the change that is being proposed. This involves identifying the problem or opportunity that is driving the need for change, as well as the specific changes that will be made to address the issue or opportunity. It is important to involve key stakeholders in this process, as they can provide valuable insights and perspectives that will help to shape the proposed changes.

Once the changes have been identified, it is important to assess the impact that they will have on the organization and its stakeholders. This includes considering the operational and financial implications of the change, as well as the potential impact on patient care and outcomes. It is also important to consider the impact of the change on stakeholders such as employees, patients, and community partners.

In addition to assessing the impact of the change, it is important to develop a plan to effectively communicate the need for change and gain buy-in from stakeholders. This involves identifying key messages and messengers, as well as developing a communication strategy that is tailored to the needs of different stakeholders. It is important to be transparent and honest about the reasons for the change, and to clearly articulate the benefits of the change for all stakeholders.

Managing resistance to change is another critical component of preparing for change. Resistance to change is a natural human response, and EMS leaders must be prepared to address this resistance in a constructive and effective way. This involves identifying the sources of resistance and developing strategies to address them. It may also involve providing training and support to employees and stakeholders to help them adapt to the change.

Another key aspect of preparing for change is developing a plan to monitor and evaluate the change. This involves setting clear goals and objectives for the change, as well as developing metrics to track progress and evaluate the success of the change. By monitoring and evaluating the change, EMS leaders can identify areas for improvement and adjust as needed.

Preparing for change is a critical step in leading change in EMS. It involves clearly defining the change that is being proposed, assessing the impact of the change on the organization and its stakeholders, developing a communication strategy to gain buy-in from stakeholders, managing resistance to change, and monitoring and evaluating the change. By effectively preparing for change, EMS leaders can position their organizations for success and ensure that they are well-equipped to adapt and evolve in response to the changing needs of their patients and communities.

COMMUNICATING CHANGE

Effective communication is a critical aspect of successful change management in EMS. Communication should be a strategic priority throughout the change process, from the initial announcement of the change through implementation and evaluation. EMS leaders must develop a comprehensive communication plan that includes messaging, methods, and timing that is tailored to the specific stakeholders and their needs.

One of the most important aspects of communicating change is transparency. EMS leaders must be transparent about the reason for the change, the process that will be followed, and the expected outcomes. This helps to build trust with stakeholders and ensures that they are invested in the success of the change initiative.

Communication methods should be carefully selected based on the audience and the message. For example, email or a memo may be appropriate for announcing the change, while a town hall meeting or one-on-one meetings may be better for addressing questions and concerns from stakeholders. It is important to use multiple methods of communication to ensure that stakeholders receive the message and have an opportunity to provide feedback.

In addition to being transparent and using appropriate communication methods, EMS leaders must also be proactive in addressing resistance to change. Resistance to change is a natural response to uncertainty and can manifest in various forms, including skepticism, denial, and active resistance. EMS leaders must be prepared to address these responses and provide reassurance and support to stakeholders.

It is also important to acknowledge the impact that change can have on individuals and teams. Change can create uncertainty and anxiety, and EMS leaders must be prepared to provide resources and support to help stakeholders manage these emotions. This can include providing training and education, offering counseling services, or creating support groups.

Finally, it is important to evaluate the effectiveness of the communication plan and adjust as needed. EMS leaders should seek feedback from stakeholders throughout the change process to ensure that their communication needs are being met and that they are adequately informed and supported.

Effective communication is a critical component of successful change management in EMS. EMS leaders must be transparent, use appropriate communication methods, address resistance to change, acknowledge the impact of change on stakeholders, and evaluate the effectiveness of their communication plan. By following these guidelines, EMS leaders can ensure that their change initiatives are well-received and effectively implemented.

Implementing Change

Implementing change is often the most challenging phase of the change process, as it requires a significant amount of coordination and effort to ensure that the change is implemented successfully. The foundation of implementing change is to ensure that all stakeholders have the necessary resources to implement the change effectively. This includes providing training, updating policies and procedures, and ensuring that necessary equipment or technology is in place. EMS leaders must also be prepared to provide ongoing support and guidance to stakeholders throughout the implementation process.

Remaining flexible and adaptable is important during the implementation phase. Unexpected issues or challenges frequently arise during the implementation process, and EMS leaders must be prepared to adjust their plans and strategies as needed to ensure that the change is implemented successfully. This involves adjusting timelines, processes, or resource allocation.

As changes are implemented, effective strategies to monitor the progress are required. This should include clear metrics and goals for the implementation process. By monitoring progress and collecting data, EMS leaders can identify areas where additional support or resources may be needed and adjust accordingly.

Finally, celebrating successes and acknowledging the efforts of those involved in the change process is not only a component of good leadership, but this will help set a strong foundation for the next project. This will build momentum and support for future change initiatives and can help to foster a positive organizational culture that values continuous improvement and innovation. Implementing change requires a significant amount of effort and coordination, but with proper planning, communication, and support, EMS leaders can ensure that the change is implemented successfully and that their organizations are well-positioned for continued success and growth.

Leading Continuous Change in EMS

Change is a continuous process, and leaders must be prepared to lead continuous change initiatives because it allows organizations to remain relevant, efficient, and effective in an ever-changing healthcare landscape. However, leading continuous change requires a culture committed to ongoing improvement, and leaders must encourage their teams to embrace change as an opportunity for growth and development. Here are some strategies that EMS leaders can employ to lead continuous change:

- **Develop a Culture of Continuous Improvement**: EMS leaders must create a culture of continuous improvement within their organizations. This involves encouraging employees to identify areas for improvement and providing them with the resources and support they need to implement changes. Leaders should also promote a growth mindset that encourages employees to view change as an opportunity for growth and development.
- **Emphasize Data-Driven Decision Making**: To drive continuous improvement, EMS leaders must rely on data to inform decision making. Leaders should collect and analyze data on key performance indicators to identify areas for improvement and track progress over time. This data should be used to inform ongoing change initiatives and to measure the effectiveness of those initiatives.
- **Encourage Collaboration and Innovation**: Continuous change requires collaboration and innovation. EMS leaders should encourage their teams to work together to identify creative solutions to problems and to share ideas and best practices. Leaders should also provide opportunities for professional development and training to support ongoing innovation and growth.
- **Foster a Balanced Sense of Urgency**: While continuous change necessitates a sense of urgency, it's essential to balance this with careful and considered action. Leaders should communicate the need for change and the potential benefits of that change to stakeholders in a manner that motivates, rather than panics. The adage "slow is fast and fast is slow" should be kept in mind, ensuring that change is implemented in a methodical, measured manner, which in the long run often proves quicker and more effective.
- **Celebrate Success**: Finally, it is important for EMS leaders to celebrate the successes that come with continuous change. By recognizing and celebrating the accomplishments of their teams, leaders can build momentum for ongoing improvement and inspire their teams to continue driving change initiatives.

Leading continuous change in EMS requires a commitment to ongoing improvement, collaboration, innovation, and data-driven decision making. By creating a culture of continuous improvement, emphasizing the importance of data, encouraging collaboration and innovation, fostering a sense of urgency, and celebrating successes, EMS leaders can position their organizations for ongoing success and growth.

32

LEADERSHIP LESSONS

"I believe that truth is the glue that holds government together, not only our Government, but civilization itself." - President Gerald R. Ford, August 9, 1974

ACROSS THE UNITED STATES, EMERGENCY MEDICAL SERVICES GRAPPLE with significant recruitment and retention issues. This intricate issue has roots in various factors, one of the most cited in research and surveys being deficiencies in appropriate leadership and management. As such, the role of effective leadership has never been more critical. Leaders in EMS are tasked with not only managing daily operations and navigating crisis situations, but also creating a working environment that encourages growth, fosters resilience, and cultivates job satisfaction. This section, "Leadership Lessons," offers some practical advice leaders should consider. From nurturing growth and emotional intelligence to promoting continuous learning and balancing work-life demands, these insights serve as a guide towards establishing an effective, efficient, and harmonious working environment that aids in recruitment, advancement, and retention.

- **Authentic Leadership: Staying True** – True leadership lies in authenticity, the ability to stay true to oneself and one's values. An authentic leader learns from others, but they do not imitate; they chart their unique course, drawing upon their distinctive abilities to inspire and influence their teams.

- **Balancing Work and Life: Nurturing Wellness** – Leaders in the high-stress EMS field must emphasize the importance of balancing work with personal life for themselves and their team members. Promoting wellness and allowing time for rest, rejuvenation, and personal pursuits help prevent burnout and foster a more engaged and productive team.

- **Building on Strengths: Enriching Teams Through Diversity** – Effective leaders understand that an impactful team thrives on a mix of diverse skills and perspectives. Therefore, when hiring, leaders look for individuals whose strengths can fill the gaps within the team, ensuring a wide range of expertise that enhances the team's resilience and adaptability in managing the diverse challenges that arise in emergency care.

- **Continuous Learning: Cultivating Personal and Professional Growth** – True leadership embodies a commitment to lifelong learning. Leaders who actively seek new knowledge, embrace changes in the EMS field, and continuously reflect on their own practices can inspire similar attitudes in their teams, fostering an environment where learning and growth become the norm.

- **Demanding Professional Accountability** – Effective leaders hold their teams to high standards and demand professional accountability. They set clear expectations, ensure everyone understands their roles and responsibilities, and address issues promptly and fairly when performance falls short.

- **Embracing Emotional Intelligence** – Emotional intelligence, or the capacity to understand and manage one's emotions and empathize with others, is a crucial aspect of effective leadership, especially in the emotionally charged environment of EMS. Leaders who display emotional intelligence can foster strong, trusting relationships within their teams, navigating the emotional complexities of emergency care with compassion, and understanding.

- **Embracing Technical Assistance: Acknowledging and Learning from Mistakes** – Effective leaders acknowledge that mistakes are inevitable and create an environment where errors become opportunities for learning and growth. They leverage technical assistance, re-training, and education to prevent the recurrence of errors, turning mistakes into valuable lessons and enhancing team performance and resilience.

- **Empowering and Trusting Your Team** – Micromanagement can inhibit creativity and foster resentment. In contrast, leaders who empower their team members and trust them to make decisions and perform their roles effectively foster an environment of increased job satisfaction, enhanced productivity, and stronger teamwork. Providing guidance when needed without taking over fosters a culture of mutual trust.

- **Encouraging Innovation** – Effective leaders encourage their team members to think creatively, offering them the space and support to innovate. A culture of innovation fuels the development of new ideas and solutions, contributing to the growth and success of the team and the organization.

- **Leading by Example: Inspiring through Action** – A leader's actions often speak louder than words. Leaders who model the values and behaviors they wish to see in their teams, such as integrity, empathy, dedication, and resilience, can inspire their teams to strive for the same.
- **Listening: An Essential Leadership Skill** – Effective leaders are good listeners, particularly to their direct reports and team members. The role of senior leaders is not necessarily to solve issues deep in the organization, but rather to listen to their direct reports, offer advice and wisdom as appropriate, and empower them to resolve problems. Listening helps leaders understand the nuances of their team's experiences and encourages open communication and trust.
- **Nurturing Growth: The Heart of Leadership** – Effective leadership involves cultivating a growth-oriented environment that allows each team member to reach their full potential. It's less about exercising authority and more about providing service to the team.
- **Recognizing Unique Skills:** Leadership abilities and clinical skills are not one and the same. It is essential to recognize that a team member's proficiency as an EMT or paramedic does not inherently equip them with the capabilities to manage a team, devise strategic plans, or make high-level decisions. This understanding helps create a leadership structure that's both effective and sustainable.
- **Saying "Thank You" Often: Recognizing Individual Contributions** – One of the most powerful phrases a leader can say is "Thank You." Regularly expressing gratitude for team members' contributions boosts morale and fosters a culture of mutual respect and teamwork, making everyone feel valued for their unique contributions.
- **Sharing Leadership: The Power of Empowerment** – Empowering others to take on leadership roles can boost a team's collective capacity to handle challenges and make decisions. This strategy builds trust within the team and aids in developing future leaders.

Leadership is multifaceted, challenging, and essential. It requires emotional intelligence, authenticity, continuous learning, empathy, resilience, and the ability to balance work and personal life, among other skills. Commitment to the growth of individuals, the team, and the organization at large is key. Recognizing and practicing these leadership lessons is a crucial step toward addressing the recruitment and retention challenges facing the EMS field today.

CONSEQUENCES OF OVER-PROMOTION INTO LEADERSHIP ROLES

Choose leaders carefully. Promoting an individual beyond their capabilities into a leadership role has severe negative implications for both the person and the organization. This scenario often results in a leader who cannot delegate effectively, leading to a myriad of challenges.

- **Ineffective Delegation and Macro-level Neglect**: Effective leaders understand the importance of delegation, empowering their team and freeing up time for more strategic decision-making. When leaders fail to delegate and instead get stuck in performing menial tasks, they are communicating a lack of trust in the team. This preoccupation with the minutiae often couples with neglecting macro-level responsibilities. Leaders steer the organization's overall direction, and losing sight of this results in a lack of vision and a misguided trajectory for the organization.
- **Time Mismanagement and Stifled Professional Growth**: Overpromoted leaders often struggle with time management due to their disproportionate focus on trivial tasks. Such mismanagement results in missed opportunities for strategic initiatives and addressing significant challenges. Furthermore, this leadership failure denies team members the chance to grow professionally and develop new skills by refusing to delegate, resulting in a stagnant and demotivated workforce.
- **Frustration, Burnout, and Innovation Deficit**: Overpromoted leaders frequently experience disproportionate stress levels, leading to frustration and burnout. Exhausted leaders become less effective in decision-making, stifling innovation within the organization. When leaders get caught up in routine tasks, they leave little room for creativity and innovation, hindering the organization's adaptability and competitiveness.
- **Poor Strategic Planning and Short-Sightedness**: Ineffective leaders excessively focus on minor issues and often neglect strategic thinking and planning – a critical component for the long-term success of an organization. Furthermore, they fail to see the broader implications of their decisions and actions, leading to short-sighted decisions that can obstruct the organization's growth and progress.
- **Reduced Visibility and Resistance to Change**: Overpromoted leaders that are constantly occupied with low-level tasks often become less visible and accessible to their teams. This lack of visibility breaks down communication, harms organizational dynamics, and often results in the leader being disconnected from the organization. These failing leaders resist delegating tasks or adapting to changes; this results in a rigid organizational culture that is resistant to innovation and improvement.

Promoting individuals into leadership positions beyond their abilities can have far-reaching and detrimental consequences for the organization's success. Organizations should exercise caution to avoid overpromoting leaders into roles they are not qualified for. Similarly, leaders must actively prioritize effectively and work on improving delegation, time management, and strategic focus as these are fundamental to effective leadership. Enhancing these skills significantly improves a leader's ability to guide the organization towards success.

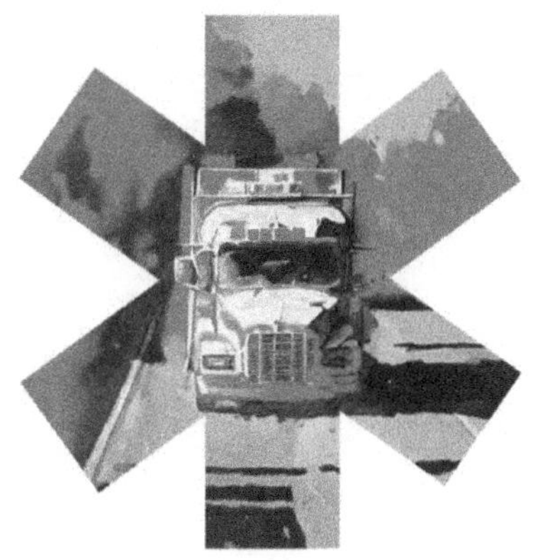

Section 6

EMERGING ISSUES

"The future rewards those who press on. I don't have time to feel sorry for myself. I don't have time to complain. I'm going to press on."
- President Barack Obama

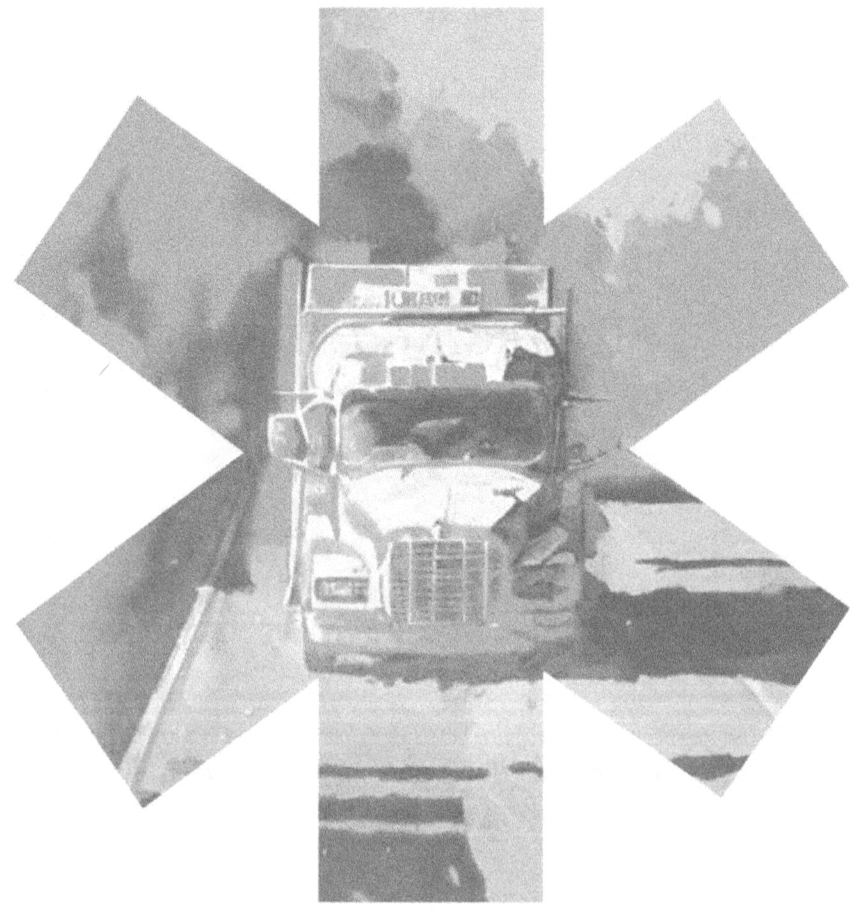

33

HEALTH EQUITY AND SOCIAL DETERMINANTS OF HEALTH

"Health equity means that everyone has a fair and just opportunity to be as healthy as possible. This requires removing obstacles to health such as poverty, discrimination, and their consequences, including powerlessness and lack of access to good jobs with fair pay, quality education and housing, safe environments, and health care." - Robert Wood Johnson Foundation

IN THE REALM OF PUBLIC HEALTH, THE CONCEPTS OF HEALTH EQUITY and social determinants of health have gained increasing recognition for the significant roles they play in shaping health outcomes. They are also pivotal in the operational landscape of Emergency Medical Services. Understanding their influence on access to EMS, service utilization, and health outcomes is crucial in informing policy decisions and formulating strategies for enhancing the quality of EMS delivery and overall population health.

Health equity is the principle underlying a commitment to reduce—and ultimately eliminate—disparities in health and its determinants that adversely affect marginalized or disadvantaged groups. It is closely intertwined with social determinants of health, which are the conditions in the environments where people are born, live, learn, work, play, worship, and age, that affect a wide range of health, functioning, and quality-of-life outcomes and risks.

Several considerations on how health equity and social determinants of health relate to EMS are discussed below.

- **Access to Healthcare and EMS agencies**: Access to healthcare is a fundamental determinant of health. However, not all populations have equitable access, especially those residing in rural and underserved areas. Limited access can affect EMS by increasing response times, delaying care, and intensifying demand for ambulance services. Health equity, which advocates for the just distribution of health resources, is essential for ensuring that everyone, regardless of their income, race, ethnicity, or geographic location, has access to EMS.
- **Socioeconomic Factors**: Socioeconomic status, encompassing income, education, and employment, can exert significant influence on ambulance service utilization. Lower-income populations may face barriers to accessing healthcare, including ambulance services, due to cost considerations, lack of insurance, or limited transportation options.
- **Demographic Factors**: Demographic factors, such as age, race, and ethnicity, can have profound effects on ambulance service demand. For instance, older adults may require more frequent use of ambulance services due to age-related health conditions, while racial and ethnic minorities may experience disparities in healthcare access and quality, affecting their utilization of these services.
- **Geographic Disparities**: Geographic location significantly impacts ambulance services. Rural and frontier communities often face unique challenges in accessing healthcare services, including ambulance services, due to long distances, limited resources, and challenging terrain.
- **Social Support Networks**: The presence or absence of social support networks can influence the demand for ambulance services. Lack of social support, such as caregivers or community resources, may result in increased reliance on ambulance services for non-emergency or social needs.
- **Health Literacy and Behaviors**: Health literacy—the ability to understand and navigate healthcare information and services—can impact ambulance service use. Limited health literacy may result in delayed or inappropriate use of ambulance services. Additionally, health behaviors can affect health outcomes and the utilization of ambulance services.
- **Health Outcomes and Population Health**: Social determinants of health can significantly impact health outcomes. Disparities in these determinants can contribute to disparities in health outcomes for different populations. Addressing health equity and social determinants of health is crucial for improving overall population health and reducing health disparities.

- **Equity in EMS Workforce**: Ensuring equity, diversity, and inclusion in the EMS workforce is essential for addressing health disparities and providing culturally competent care. Efforts to recruit and retain a diverse EMS workforce can improve the overall quality of care and reduce disparities in EMS agencies.
- **Health Equity and EMS Access**: The notion of health equity reverberates strongly within the EMS framework, as inadequate access to EMS agencies can result in delays in receiving timely medical care, potentially leading to adverse health outcomes or even death. Ensuring equitable access to EMS agencies can foster health equity, where everyone, regardless of socio-economic status, race, ethnicity, gender, or other demographics, can attain their highest level of health.
- **Disparities in Care**: Unfortunately, disparities exist in access to EMS agencies, especially among underserved and marginalized communities. These populations may face barriers to accessing EMS agencies due to factors such as lack of insurance coverage, limited transportation options, language barriers, or discriminatory practices. Addressing these disparities is a social justice issue, as it involves promoting equitable access to EMS agencies for all individuals, irrespective of their background or resources.
- **Social Determinants of Health and EMS Access**: The relationship between social determinants of health and access to EMS is integral to understanding health disparities. These determinants, which include the social, economic, and environmental factors that influence an individual's health status, often intersect with issues of social justice and health equity, highlighting the importance of ensuring equitable access to EMS agencies.
- **Workforce Diversity and Representation**: Diversity and representation within the EMS workforce can help reduce disparities in care and promote equitable access to EMS agencies. Cultivating diversity in the EMS workforce is not only a social justice issue but also a practical necessity to ensure that the EMS workforce reflects the communities it serves.

In view of the above, it becomes evident that the sustainability of the EMS system should prioritize health equity and social justice in its planning, delivery, and regulation. To ensure equal access to EMS agencies for all individuals, the system should be organized, funded, and managed in a way that addresses social determinants of health, promotes workforce diversity and representation, and delivers culturally competent care.

Such an approach to EMS systems will not only improve health outcomes and reduce health disparities but also promote overall population health. It calls for a holistic understanding of health, one that transcends the boundaries of traditional healthcare and integrates social determinants to provide a comprehensive, equitable, and high-quality EMS system.

Health equity and social determinants of health are more than just buzzwords in public health. They are integral components of an equitable EMS system, influencing its organization, delivery, and outcomes. Acknowledging their impact and integrating them into EMS policies and practices is vital for enhancing the quality of care, reducing health disparities, and promoting overall population health. Going forward, the task for EMS leaders, policymakers, and practitioners lies in transforming these principles from theoretical concepts into tangible realities in the everyday functioning of EMS systems.

Addressing social determinants of health is a complex and multifaceted task, presenting unique challenges for EMS leaders. Traditionally, the focus of EMS leadership has been on immediate, clinical needs, often leaving broader social determinants on the periphery of operational considerations. However, in an ever-evolving health system where health outcomes are increasingly recognized as the product of a multitude of interrelated factors, it is becoming critical for EMS leaders to broaden their focus. It is not sufficient for these leaders to merely be aware of the social determinants of health that affect their communities; they must proactively identify and act upon those elements that fall within their sphere of influence. The following table presents several key social determinants of health, their impacts on EMS, and practical steps that EMS leaders can take to address these disparities. By taking an active role in recognizing and mitigating the effects of these determinants, EMS leaders can contribute significantly to the improvement of health equity and overall community health.

Practical Steps for EMS Leaders		
Issue	**Impact on EMS**	**Practical Steps**
Access to Healthcare and EMS agencies	Limited access to healthcare, especially in rural areas, can result in longer EMS response times and increased demand for services.	• Advocate for policies that expand healthcare access in underserved areas. • Implement community paramedicine programs to provide non-emergency healthcare services in rural and underserved areas.
Socioeconomic Factors	Lower income, lack of education and unemployment can create barriers to accessing EMS agencies due to cost, lack of insurance, or transportation.	• Establish partnerships with social services to connect patients with resources. • Offer community education on the role of EMS and when to utilize it.
Demographic Factors	Age, race, and ethnicity can affect the demand for and utilization of EMS agencies due to health conditions and disparities in healthcare access.	• Provide culturally competent training to EMS personnel. • Engage community leaders in outreach and education efforts.
Geographic Disparities	Rural and frontier communities often face challenges in accessing EMS agencies due to long distances, limited resources, and challenging terrain.	• Invest in telemedicine and remote consultation technologies. • Advocate for increased funding for rural EMS agencies.
Social Support Networks	Lack of social support may result in increased reliance on EMS for non-emergency or social needs.	• Develop programs to connect patients with community resources. • Train EMS staff to identify and report social needs.
Health Literacy and Behaviors	Limited health literacy may result in inappropriate use of EMS agencies.	• Implement community education programs on health literacy. • Collaborate with public health agencies for health promotion initiatives.

Health Outcomes and Population Health	Social determinants can contribute to disparities in health outcomes, affecting the demand for EMS.	• Develop policies addressing social determinants of health. • Partner with public health and community organizations to improve population health.
Equity in EMS Workforce	Lack of diversity in the EMS workforce can affect the quality of care and contribute to disparities.	• Actively develop relationships with diverse populations • Develop recruitment strategies to attract a diverse EMS workforce.
Health Equity and EMS Access	Inadequate access to EMS can lead to adverse health outcomes.	• Create systems that ensure equitable access to EMS. • Implement strategies to reduce response times in underserved areas.
Disparities in Care	Certain populations may face barriers to accessing EMS due to lack of insurance, transportation, language barriers, or discrimination.	• Seek to identify barriers to accessing care in your service area, then work with the community to address the barrier.
Social Determinants and EMS Access	Social determinants can affect access to EMS and health outcomes.	• Establish policies addressing social determinants. • Partner with social service agencies to address social needs.
Workforce Diversity and Representation	Lack of diversity in the EMS workforce can contribute to disparities in care.	• Develop recruitment and retention strategies for a diverse workforce. • Provide cultural competency and implicit bias training for EMS staff.

34

AGING POPULATIONS & EMS SYSTEMS

*"Growing old is not an option. It is a fact of life.
And while some may try to fight it, to deny it,
or to ignore it, we should all embrace it."*

WITH THE AGING AMERICAN POPULATION, THE NATION'S EMS SYSTEM is facing a growing set of challenges. Older adults tend to have more chronic health conditions and are at higher risk for injuries, falls, and other medical emergencies, requiring increased demand for EMS agencies. Providing appropriate care for older adults may require additional skills, training, and specialized equipment for EMS practitioners to effectively manage their complex medical needs. Additionally, managing care transitions and allocating resources effectively to meet the growing demand for EMS agencies from the aging population can be challenging for the national EMS system. In this context, it is essential to understand and address the impacts of the aging population on the national EMS system to ensure that individuals receive timely and high-quality emergency medical care, regardless of their age or health status.

The impacts of the aging population are impacting multiple aspects of the national EMS system:

- **Increased Demand for EMS agencies**: With the aging population, there is an increased demand for EMS agencies. Older adults tend to have more chronic health conditions and are at higher risk for injuries, falls, and other medical emergencies, requiring the need for EMS agencies. This increased demand can strain the EMS system, including ambulance availability, response times, and overall capacity to meet the needs of the aging population.

- **Complexity of Care**: Older adults often have complex medical needs, including multiple chronic conditions, polypharmacy, and cognitive impairments. Providing appropriate care for older adults may require additional skills, education, and specialized equipment for EMS practitioners to effectively manage these complex cases. This can pose challenges for the EMS system, including the need for ongoing education and training for EMS practitioners to adequately care for the aging population.

- **Longer On-Scene Times**: Older adults may require more time for assessment, stabilization, and transport due to their complex medical needs. This can result in longer on-scene times for EMS practitioners, which can impact ambulance availability, response times, and system capacity. Managing longer on-scene times while maintaining efficient ambulance utilization is a challenge for the national EMS system, particularly in rural and remote areas.

- **Care Transitions**: Older adults may require frequent transitions between different healthcare settings, such as hospitals, long-term care facilities, and home care. Coordination and communication among different healthcare providers and settings are critical for safe and effective care transitions. EMS practitioners play a crucial role in facilitating these care transitions, including communication with hospitals and other healthcare facilities. Managing care transitions can pose challenges for the EMS system, particularly in rural and underserved areas with limited healthcare resources and coordination.

- **Education and Equipment Needs**: Providing care for older adults may require specialized training and equipment for EMS practitioners. Geriatric-specific training, such as geriatric assessment, communication with older adults, and management of common geriatric conditions, may be needed to effectively care for the aging population. Additionally, specialized equipment, such as equipment and tools to assist with lifting and moving older adults, may be necessary. Ensuring that EMS practitioners have the appropriate training and equipment to care for the unique needs of older adults is a challenge for the national EMS system.

- **Resource Allocation**: Meeting the increased demand for EMS agencies from the aging population may require additional resources, including personnel, ambulances, equipment, and funding. Allocating and managing these resources effectively to meet the growing demand for EMS agencies from the aging population is challenging for the national EMS system, particularly in rural and underserved areas with limited resources.

The aging American population will continue to impact the national EMS system, including increased demand for services, complexity of care, longer on-scene times, care transitions, training and equipment needs, and resource allocation. Addressing these challenges requires ongoing education and training for EMS practitioners, specialized care for older adults, coordination and communication among healthcare settings, and resource allocation strategies to ensure that the EMS system can effectively meet the needs of the aging population.

35

RESILIENCE, RELIABILITY, AND SUSTAINABILITY

"This is no time for ease and comfort. It is time to dare and endure."

RESILIENCE, RELIABILITY, AND SUSTAINABILITY ARE THREE ESSENTIAL qualities that define a successful EMS system. Resilience refers to the ability of an EMS system to adapt to changing circumstances, recover from disruptions or setbacks, and maintain its essential functions during times of crisis or emergencies. Reliability, on the other hand, is the consistent delivery of high-quality care, effective communication with other healthcare providers, and prompt response to emergencies. Finally, sustainability encompasses the long-term financial stability, environmental responsibility, and workforce development needed to ensure the continued provision of EMS agencies.

Developing a resilient, reliable, and sustainable statewide EMS system is crucial for providing timely, efficient, and effective pre-hospital care to communities. Such a system ensures that EMS practitioners are prepared to face various challenges, including public health emergencies, natural disasters, and evolving healthcare needs. A well-rounded EMS system enhances patient outcomes, reduces healthcare costs, and contributes to the overall health and well-being of the communities it serves. Moreover, a strong EMS system fosters collaboration and coordination among healthcare providers, public health agencies, and other stakeholders, improving the overall response to emergencies and promoting a seamless continuum of care for patients.

KEY COMPONENTS OF A SUCCESSFUL EMS SYSTEM

A successful EMS system is built on several key components that work together to ensure resilience, reliability, and sustainability. These components include:

- **Strong leadership and governance structure**: Effective EMS leaders and regulators provide clear vision and mission, ensure accountability and transparency, and foster collaboration among stakeholders.

- **Effective communication and information sharing**: Clear channels of communication and rapid information sharing, often facilitated by technology, are vital for coordinating EMS agencies and enhancing patient care.

- **Workforce development and retention**: A skilled and diverse workforce is essential for providing high-quality EMS agencies. Strategies for recruitment, training, and retention help maintain a dedicated and capable workforce.

- **Financial sustainability and resource management**: Sustainable funding models, efficient allocation of resources, and cost-saving measures ensure the long-term financial viability of EMS systems.

- **Integration with the broader healthcare system**: Strong partnerships with healthcare organizations and innovative care models, such as community paramedicine, contribute to a more comprehensive and effective healthcare system.

- **Quality improvement and performance measurement**: A culture of continuous quality improvement, data-driven decision-making, and regular evaluation of system performance helps maintain and enhance the quality of EMS agencies.

- **Preparedness and response planning for public health emergencies**: Developing robust protocols, stockpiling necessary supplies, and enhancing communication during emergencies improve the EMS system's ability to respond effectively to crises.

- **Community outreach and education**: Engaging with the community and fostering strong relationships with local organizations and stakeholders promote awareness of EMS agencies and enhance overall public health.

Developing a Strong Leadership and Governance Structure

Developing a robust leadership and governance structure forms the bedrock of a resilient, reliable, and sustainable statewide EMS system. It serves as the cornerstone for establishing a framework that can effectively guide and steer the entire EMS organization towards its goals and objectives. Effective leadership within the EMS system is crucial for ensuring smooth operations, efficient resource allocation, and seamless coordination among various stakeholders.

A strong leadership structure not only provides direction but also facilitates the ability to adapt to the ever-changing landscape of healthcare. EMS leaders must possess the vision and strategic acumen to anticipate emerging trends, technological advancements, and regulatory changes that can impact the delivery of prehospital care. By staying abreast of industry developments and fostering a culture of continuous improvement, leaders can proactively navigate these shifts and position their organizations for success.

Furthermore, a robust governance structure ensures accountability, transparency, and effective decision-making within the EMS system. Well-defined governance frameworks establish clear lines of authority and responsibility, promoting efficient resource allocation and strategic decision-making at all levels. This helps to minimize bureaucracy, streamline processes, and foster a culture of innovation and collaboration within the EMS organization.

In addition, effective leadership and governance structures enable seamless integration and coordination with other healthcare entities, such as hospitals, emergency departments, and public health agencies. By aligning with the broader healthcare landscape, EMS leaders can promote interdisciplinary collaboration, enhance patient outcomes, and contribute to the overall improvement of the healthcare system.

Roles and responsibilities of EMS leaders

EMS leaders play a pivotal role in shaping the direction, vision, and mission of the EMS system. Their responsibilities include:

- **Setting strategic goals and objectives**: EMS leaders are responsible for developing and communicating a clear vision for the future of the EMS system, along with specific goals and objectives that align with this vision.
- **Establishing policies and procedures**: EMS leaders create and implement policies and procedures that ensure the delivery of high-quality care and promote a culture of continuous improvement.
- **Allocating resources**: Leaders are responsible for making informed decisions about the allocation of resources, such as personnel, equipment, and funding, to support the efficient operation of the EMS system.
- **Promoting collaboration**: EMS leaders facilitate partnerships and coordination with other healthcare providers, public health agencies, and community organizations to enhance patient care and improve overall health outcomes.

- **Ensuring accountability and transparency**: Leaders must hold themselves and their teams accountable for the performance of the EMS system, regularly evaluating and reporting on key performance indicators and outcomes.

ESTABLISHING A CLEAR VISION AND MISSION

Establishing a clear vision and mission is a pivotal undertaking in shaping the trajectory and ultimate triumph of an EMS system, whether at the state or local level. A well-crafted vision and mission statement provide a solid framework for strategic planning, informed decision-making, and comprehensive performance evaluation. Recognizing the significance of a clear vision and mission for the EMS system, it becomes imperative to comprehend the process involved in developing these guiding principles, as well as exploring effective strategies for state EMS leaders and local EMS chiefs to communicate and successfully implement them within their respective organizations.

Crafting a compelling vision requires a deep understanding of the EMS system's purpose, values, and long-term aspirations. It involves envisioning the future state of the EMS organization and articulating a succinct yet inspiring description of what it seeks to achieve. The vision statement should encapsulate the desired outcomes, the impact the EMS system aims to make on the community, and the overarching goals that will guide its actions.

Similarly, formulating a mission statement involves clarifying the fundamental purpose and unique role of the EMS system. It outlines the specific objectives, services, and target population that the organization aims to serve. A well-crafted mission statement sets the direction for the EMS system's day-to-day operations, ensuring alignment with its broader vision.

The process of developing a clear vision and mission should involve collaboration and input from key stakeholders, including EMS personnel, healthcare providers, community members, and other relevant partners. Through a participatory approach, diverse perspectives can be considered, fostering a sense of ownership and buy-in among those involved.

Once the vision and mission statements are established, effective communication and implementation are essential. State EMS leaders and local EMS chiefs play a critical role in conveying the vision and mission to their teams and translating them into actionable strategies and goals. Regular communication, both through formal channels and informal interactions, helps to ensure that all EMS personnel understand and embrace the shared vision and mission.

To effectively implement the vision and mission, organizational structures, processes, and resources must be aligned with the stated goals. This may involve revisiting policies, procedures, and training programs to ensure they are in line with the desired outcomes. Ongoing monitoring and evaluation are also crucial to gauge progress and adjust as necessary.

Establishing a clear vision and mission is a foundational step in shaping the direction and success of an EMS system. By developing these guiding principles through a collaborative process and effectively communicating and implementing them, state EMS leaders and local EMS chiefs can inspire their organizations and foster a shared sense of purpose and commitment among EMS personnel. This, in turn, sets the stage for strategic planning, informed decision-making, and ultimately, the delivery of high-quality care to the community.

A clearly articulated vision and mission provides numerous benefits:

- **Direction and focus**: A well-defined vision and mission give EMS systems a sense of direction and focus, ensuring that all efforts at both state and local levels are aligned with the overall goals and objectives.
- **Motivation and inspiration**: A compelling vision and mission can inspire and motivate EMS personnel, fostering a sense of purpose and commitment to their work, whether they serve in state leadership roles or on the front lines of patient care.
- **Decision-making**: A clear vision and mission serve as a cornerstone for making decisions about resource allocation, priorities, and strategic initiatives across all levels of EMS. Importantly, it should be recognized that choosing not to decide is a decision, and almost always a detrimental one. Inaction or delayed decisions can have significant implications, often leading to negative outcomes.
- **Performance measurement**: A well-defined vision and mission provide a basis for evaluating the EMS system's progress and effectiveness at both state and local levels, allowing for continuous improvement and adaptation.

The process of developing a vision and mission for an EMS system involves several key steps, which should be applied at both state and local levels:

- **Assess the current state of the EMS system**: Begin by conducting a thorough SWOT assessment of your EMS system's current Strengths, Weaknesses, Opportunities, and Threats. This will provide a foundation for determining the desired future state of the system.
- **Engage stakeholders:** Engage a diverse group of stakeholders, including EMS personnel, healthcare partners, public health agencies, and community representatives, in the process of developing the vision and mission. This ensures that multiple perspectives are considered and helps build buy-in and support for the guiding principles across all levels of EMS.
- **Define the vision**: The vision should articulate the desired future state of the EMS system, describing what the organization aspires to achieve in the long term. The vision should be inspiring, ambitious, and clearly communicate the system's overarching goals for both state and local EMS organizations.

- **Define the mission**: The mission statement should outline the core purpose of the EMS system, describing its primary functions and objectives at both the state and local levels. The mission should be concise, clear, and focused on the system's commitment to providing high-quality care and improving community health.
- **Align the vision and mission with strategic goals and objectives**: Once the vision and mission are defined, ensure that they are integrated into the strategic planning processes at both state and local levels. This will help align all efforts and initiatives with the overarching guiding principles.

National, state, and local EMS leaders play a crucial role in effectively communicating and implementing the vision and mission within their organizations. Consider the following strategies for promoting understanding and commitment to these guiding principles across all levels of EMS:

- **Communicate the vision and mission clearly and consistently**: Regularly share the vision and mission with EMS personnel, partners, and stakeholders at both state and local levels, using a variety of communication channels (e.g., meetings, newsletters, websites).
- **Integrate the vision and mission into the organizational culture**: Embed the vision and mission into the EMS system's culture at both state and local levels by incorporating them into training programs, performance evaluations, and internal communications.
- **Set short-term and long-term goals aligned with the vision and mission**: Develop SMART goals (Specific, Measurable, Achievable, Relevant, and Time-bound) and objectives that align with the vision and mission at both state and local levels. Regularly review progress and adjust as needed to ensure continued alignment with the guiding principles.
- **Celebrate successes and recognize achievements**: Recognize and celebrate milestones and accomplishments that demonstrate progress toward the vision and mission at both state and local levels. This helps maintain momentum, motivate personnel, and reinforce the importance of the guiding principles.
- **Continuously reassess and refine the vision and mission**: Periodically review the vision and mission to ensure they remain relevant and aligned with the changing needs of the EMS system at both state and local levels. This allows for timely adjustments and ensures that the guiding principles continue to support the overall goals and objectives of the EMS system.

By applying these strategies, state EMS leaders and local EMS chiefs can work together to develop, communicate, and implement a clear vision and mission for their EMS system. This will ultimately result in a more resilient, reliable, and sustainable system that is better positioned and capable to serve the needs of their communities and improve overall public health.

Collaboration And Coordination Among Stakeholders

Collaboration and coordination among stakeholders are fundamental elements for the success of EMS systems. By establishing strong partnerships across various sectors, EMS organizations can enhance resource sharing, streamline communication, and ultimately achieve improved patient outcomes and community health.

Recognizing the interconnected nature of healthcare, collaboration among stakeholders is crucial. EMS systems do not operate in isolation; they interact with hospitals, healthcare providers, public health agencies, and other community organizations. Through collaborative efforts, stakeholders can combine their expertise, resources, and knowledge to deliver comprehensive and integrated care.

Effective collaboration requires clear communication channels and a shared understanding of goals and objectives. Regular meetings, joint planning sessions, and open dialogue are essential for establishing and maintaining effective partnerships. Building relationships based on trust, mutual respect, and a common commitment to patient-centered care fosters collaboration and coordination among stakeholders.

Creating mechanisms for resource sharing is another vital aspect of collaboration in EMS systems. This involves sharing data, best practices, and innovative approaches to care delivery. By leveraging the strengths and expertise of each stakeholder, EMS systems can enhance efficiency, optimize resource utilization, and ensure the most appropriate and timely response to emergencies.

EMS leaders play a pivotal role in fostering collaboration within their organizations and beyond. They can promote a culture of collaboration by encouraging teamwork, interdisciplinary education, and training opportunities. Recognizing and acknowledging the contributions of all stakeholders involved in the EMS system helps build trust and fosters a sense of shared responsibility.

Furthermore, EMS leaders can facilitate collaboration through the establishment of formal partnerships and agreements with key stakeholders. These agreements outline roles, responsibilities, and expectations, ensuring alignment and coordination of efforts. Collaborative initiatives, such as joint trainings, shared protocols, and information exchange platforms, further strengthen relationships and promote seamless coordination.

At the state level, EMS leaders can provide guidance and support to local EMS agencies, fostering collaboration across different regions. They can facilitate the sharing of best practices, encourage the adoption of standardized protocols, and promote the exchange of ideas and experiences.

By building effective partnerships, enhancing communication, and sharing resources, EMS systems can contribute to improved patient outcomes and community health. Through a culture of collaboration and working together at all levels, EMS leaders can drive the integration of services, enhance the effectiveness of care, and ultimately have a positive impact on the well-being of the community they serve.

EMS leaders can leverage the following strategies to foster collaboration and coordination among stakeholders in EMS systems:

- **Identify key stakeholders**: Start by identifying the stakeholders who play a crucial role in the EMS system, such as healthcare providers, public health agencies, emergency management organizations, community groups, and other public safety agencies.
- **Establish a shared vision and goals**: Work with stakeholders to develop a shared vision and set of goals for the EMS system, ensuring alignment between state and local EMS organizations and their partners.
- **Build trust and open communication**: Encourage open and honest communication among stakeholders, fostering an environment of trust and mutual respect. This will help create a strong foundation for collaboration and problem-solving.
- **Develop formal partnerships and agreements**: Create formal partnerships and agreements, such as memorandums of understanding or interagency agreements, to clarify roles and responsibilities, establish communication protocols, and facilitate resource sharing among stakeholders.
- **Engage in regular meetings and collaboration opportunities**: Schedule regular meetings and collaboration opportunities, such as workshops, conferences, and training sessions, to foster ongoing communication and partnership development among stakeholders.

Fostering collaboration at all levels of EMS systems takes work and commitment. Here are some strategies to help improve collaborations:

- **Model collaborative leadership**: Demonstrate a commitment to collaboration by actively engaging with stakeholders, sharing resources, and working together to address common challenges and goals.
- **Provide support and resources for collaboration**: Allocate resources and support for collaborative initiatives, such as training, technical assistance, and funding opportunities, to help strengthen partnerships among stakeholders.
- **Encourage cross-disciplinary training and education:** Support cross-disciplinary training and education opportunities that bring together EMS personnel and other stakeholders, fostering a better understanding of each other's roles and responsibilities and enhancing collaboration.
- **Monitor and evaluate collaborative efforts**: Regularly assess the effectiveness of collaborative efforts, identifying areas for improvement and adjusting strategies as needed to ensure that partnerships continue to meet the needs of the EMS system and its stakeholders.

By prioritizing collaboration and coordination among stakeholders, EMS leaders can help build more resilient, reliable, and sustainable EMS systems that are better equipped to meet the diverse needs of their communities and improve overall public health.

PROMOTING ACCOUNTABILITY & TRANSPARENCY

Accountability and transparency are critical components of successful EMS systems that provide emergency medical care to individuals in need. EMS leaders are responsible for upholding these principles and maintaining a culture of accountability and transparency within their organizations. A commitment to accountability and transparency promotes trust and confidence among the public, healthcare partners, and other stakeholders. These are also necessary for ethical and responsible decision-making related to patient care, resource allocation, and organizational management. Through transparency, EMS leaders will build trust with the public and promote a culture of continuous improvement. The benefits of accountability and transparency in EMS systems are numerous and include:

- **Public Trust**: Accountability and transparency help build and maintain public trust in EMS systems, ensuring that communities feel confident in their EMS practitioners' ability to deliver high-quality care and support.
- **Ethical and Responsible Decision-making**: By promoting accountability and transparency, EMS systems can demonstrate their commitment to making ethical and responsible decisions related to patient care, resource allocation, and organizational management.
- **Effective Oversight**: Accountability and transparency enable effective oversight of EMS systems, ensuring that state and local EMS organizations adhere to established standards, guidelines, and regulations.
- **Continuous Improvement**: Commitment to accountability and transparency allows EMS systems to identify areas for improvement, learn from mistakes, and continuously adapt and evolve to better serve their communities.

While the benefits of accountability and transparency are clear, implementing these principles is challenging for many EMS systems. Some of the challenges associated with implementing accountability and transparency include:

- **Complexity**: EMS systems are complex, and it is challenging to establish clear policies and procedures that promote accountability and transparency across all levels of the organization.
- **Resistance to Change**: Resistance to change is a common barrier to implementing accountability and transparency in EMS systems. Some EMS personnel may be hesitant to adopt new policies and procedures, and organizational culture may be resistant to change.

- **Lack of Resources**: Lack of resources is a significant barrier to implementing accountability and transparency in EMS systems. Resources such as time, funding, and technology are often necessary to establish effective accountability and transparency systems.

However, despite the challenges associated with implementing accountability and transparency in EMS systems, there are several strategies that EMS leaders can use to promote these principles. These strategies include:

- **Establish Clear Policies and Procedures**: Develop and implement clear policies and procedures that outline expectations for ethical behavior, responsible decision-making, and adherence to established standards and guidelines.

- **Implement Performance Measurement and Reporting Systems**: Use performance measurement and reporting systems to track progress, identify areas for improvement, and demonstrate accountability to stakeholders.

- **Encourage Open Communication and Feedback**: Foster an environment of open communication and feedback within the EMS system, allowing personnel and stakeholders to voice concerns, ask questions, and share ideas for improvement.

- **Engage in Regular Audits and Evaluations**: Conduct regular audits and evaluations of EMS system operations, finances, and performance to ensure compliance with established standards and guidelines, and to identify areas for improvement.

- **Share Information with Stakeholders**: Communicate openly with stakeholders, including the public, healthcare partners, and other agencies, about the EMS system's operations, performance, and decision-making processes.

EMS leaders play a critical role in promoting and maintaining accountability and transparency within their organizations. By modeling accountable and transparent leadership, providing training and support, monitoring compliance, and engaging with stakeholders, EMS leaders can ensure that their EMS systems operate in a manner that is transparent, ethical, and trustworthy. Some of the ways that EMS leaders can promote accountability and transparency in their organizations include:

- **Model Accountable and Transparent Leadership**: EMS leaders should demonstrate a commitment to accountability and transparency in all aspects of leadership, decision-making, and communication. They should lead by example and set the tone for the organization.

- **Provide Education and Support**: EMS leaders should offer education and support to EMS personnel on the importance of accountability and transparency, as well as the specific policies and procedures that support these principles. This can include training on data collection and analysis, communication techniques, and ethical decision-making.

- **Monitor and Enforce Compliance**: EMS leaders should regularly monitor compliance with policies and procedures related to accountability and transparency, taking corrective action when necessary to address issues and ensure adherence to established standards.

- **Engage with Stakeholders**: EMS leaders should actively engage with stakeholders, including the public, healthcare partners, and other agencies, to solicit feedback, share information, and foster trust and collaboration. This can include attending community meetings, participating in healthcare coalitions, and engaging with regulatory agencies.

Accountability and transparency are critical to maintaining public trust and confidence in EMS systems. By establishing clear policies and procedures, implementing performance measurement and reporting systems, encouraging open communication and feedback, engaging in regular audits and evaluations, and sharing information with stakeholders, EMS leaders can promote accountability and transparency at all levels of their organizations. These efforts will help to build more resilient, reliable, and sustainable EMS systems that are better equipped to meet the diverse needs of their communities and maintain the trust and confidence of the public and other stakeholders. While implementing accountability and transparency is challenging, it is essential for the long-term success of EMS systems and the patients they serve.

Characteristics of a Resilient EMS System

A resilient EMS system is one that can effectively adapt to and recover from challenges, crises, and changes in the operating environment. Resilience is a crucial characteristic of successful EMS systems, as it enables organizations to continue providing high-quality care and support to their communities during times of uncertainty and stress. Resilient EMS systems possess several key characteristics that enable them to adapt and respond effectively to challenges:

- **Flexibility and adaptability:** Resilient EMS systems are flexible and adaptable, able to modify their operations, protocols, and procedures in response to changing conditions and needs.

- **Robust infrastructure and resources**: Resilient EMS systems have a robust infrastructure and sufficient resources, including equipment, personnel, and funding, to ensure continued operations during times of crisis or change.

- **Strong leadership and governance**: Resilient EMS systems have effective leadership and governance structures in place that promote clear communication, sound decision-making, and coordinated action.

- **Collaborative relationships and partnerships**: Resilient EMS systems maintain strong relationships and partnerships with stakeholders, including healthcare providers, public health agencies, emergency management organizations, and community groups, to enhance resource sharing and coordination.

- **Continuous learning and improvement**: Resilient EMS systems are committed to continuous learning and improvement, regularly evaluating their performance, and adjusting their strategies to better meet the needs of their communities and stakeholders.

- **Proactive planning and preparedness**: Resilient EMS systems engage in proactive planning and preparedness activities to anticipate and address potential challenges and crises.

EMS leaders should consider the following strategies to build and maintain resilience within their EMS systems:

- **Invest in infrastructure and resources**: Allocate funding and resources to develop and maintain a robust infrastructure, including equipment, personnel, and technology, that can support EMS operations during times of crisis or change.

- **Foster a culture of flexibility and adaptability**: Encourage a culture of flexibility and adaptability within the EMS system, empowering personnel to adapt to changing conditions and needs while maintaining high standards of care.

- **Develop and implement robust policies and procedures**: Establish clear and comprehensive policies and procedures that promote resilience and guide decision-making during times of uncertainty or stress.

- **Strengthen partnerships and collaboration**: Build and maintain strong partnerships and collaborative relationships with stakeholders, leveraging their resources and expertise to enhance the EMS system's capacity to respond to challenges.

- **Engage in ongoing training and education**: Provide ongoing training and education opportunities for EMS personnel to ensure they have the skills, knowledge, and capabilities needed to adapt and respond effectively to challenges and crises.

- **Conduct regular evaluations and assessments**: Regularly evaluate and assess the EMS system's performance, infrastructure, and resources, using the findings to identify areas for improvement and inform strategic planning efforts.

By focusing on these strategies, EMS leaders can help build and maintain resilient EMS systems that are better equipped to meet the diverse needs of their communities and withstand the challenges and uncertainties that may arise in the future.

CHARACTERISTICS OF A RELIABLE SYSTEM

The reliability of an EMS system is a crucial aspect of its success. A reliable EMS system is characterized by its consistent and high-quality care provision to patients, seamless integration with the broader healthcare system, prompt response to emergencies, and ongoing measurement and improvement of its performance. In emergency situations, patients and their families rely on the swift and effective delivery of care, and reliable EMS systems play a pivotal role in ensuring that patients receive the necessary care in a timely manner. Reliable EMS systems have the capacity to consistently deliver high-quality care, integrate with the broader healthcare system, promptly respond to emergencies, and continuously measure and enhance their performance.

Consistent Delivery of High-Quality Care

Reliability in Emergency Medical Services refers to the consistent delivery of high-quality care to patients in a timely and effective manner. The reliability of an EMS system is critical because lives depend on the rapid and effective delivery of care. Reliable EMS systems have highly trained personnel who are competent in delivering high-quality care, adhering to established clinical protocols, and using the latest medical technologies and equipment. The goal of reliable EMS systems is to ensure that patients receive consistent care regardless of the time of day, day of the week, or location.

To achieve reliable delivery of high-quality care, EMS systems must have well-trained personnel who are competent in delivering patient care. Highly trained EMS personnel can effectively and efficiently respond to emergencies and provide life-saving interventions in a timely manner. To ensure the competence of EMS personnel, EMS systems must invest in training programs that provide ongoing education, clinical training, and skills development. The training should be based on the latest evidence-based guidelines, and personnel should receive regular updates and refresher training to ensure they remain competent and up to date with the latest medical technologies and techniques.

In addition to well-trained personnel, reliable EMS systems must also adhere to established clinical protocols that guide patient care. Clinical protocols are standardized sets of procedures and guidelines that define the appropriate care for specific medical conditions. Protocols ensure that EMS personnel provide consistent care to patients and reduce the risk of medical errors. Reliable EMS systems regularly review and update their protocols to ensure they are based on the latest evidence-based practices and are consistent with national standards.

The use of the latest medical technologies and equipment is also critical for the reliable delivery of high-quality care in EMS. Reliable EMS systems must invest in the latest medical technologies and equipment to ensure that personnel have the tools they need to deliver high-quality care. The latest medical technologies and equipment can help to reduce the time it takes to provide care, improve patient outcomes, and enhance the safety of EMS personnel and patients.

The reliable delivery of high-quality care is a critical component of successful EMS systems. Reliable EMS systems must have well-trained personnel, adhere to established clinical protocols, and invest in the latest medical technologies and equipment. By focusing on these key areas, EMS leaders can build and maintain reliable EMS systems that provide exceptional care to patients, improve patient outcomes, and ensure the long-term sustainability of EMS agencies in their communities.

INTEGRATION WITH THE BROADER HEALTHCARE SYSTEM

Integration with the broader healthcare system is an essential aspect of reliable EMS systems. These systems must seamlessly collaborate and coordinate with the larger healthcare network to provide patients with cohesive and well-coordinated care. Integration ensures that patients receive consistent and continuous care throughout their entire medical journey.

To achieve integration, reliable EMS systems require strong partnerships and collaboration with healthcare organizations and providers. Establishing robust relationships with hospitals, primary care physicians, and other healthcare providers ensures that patients receive coordinated and high-quality care. Information exchange plays a critical role in integration, as EMS practitioners need to share relevant patient information with healthcare providers to enable informed decision-making and appropriate follow-up care.

EMS leaders play a crucial role in promoting integration with the broader healthcare system. They need to develop protocols and systems that facilitate effective information exchange between EMS practitioners and healthcare providers. These protocols should align with national standards and guidelines, and EMS personnel should receive training on how to exchange information efficiently and in compliance with privacy regulations.

Furthermore, EMS leaders should explore innovative care models, such as community paramedicine, to provide appropriate care beyond the traditional EMS setting. By engaging in community paramedicine and similar programs, EMS personnel can deliver preventive care, chronic disease management, and follow-up services to patients, thereby enhancing integration and continuity of care.

Engagement of patients in their own care is also crucial for integration. EMS leaders should encourage patient involvement and provide them with information about their care. Empowering patients to participate in decision-making regarding their treatment not only improves patient outcomes but also helps reduce healthcare costs.

Moreover, EMS leaders must prioritize diversity and inclusion within the healthcare system. By cultivating a diverse and inclusive workforce, addressing healthcare disparities, and implementing strategies to reach underserved communities, EMS leaders can foster equitable access to care and enhance integration with all patient populations.

Integration with the broader healthcare system is paramount for reliable EMS systems. EMS leaders play a pivotal role in fostering collaboration, information exchange, and community engagement to ensure coordinated and high-quality care for patients. By promoting diversity and inclusion, EMS leaders contribute to reducing healthcare disparities and improving healthcare outcomes for all patients.

TIMELY RESPONSE TO EMERGENCIES AND EFFECTIVE COMMUNICATION

Emergency Medical Services play a crucial role in emergency situations, offering life-saving care to patients. The timeliness of response and effective communication are vital for improving patient outcomes and reducing mortality rates. In this context, modern public safety answering points (PSAPs) hold significant value as they provide pre-arrival instructions to callers, guiding them through critical life-saving procedures prior to EMS arrival. This discussion will focus on the key elements of efficient emergency response and effective communication in EMS systems.

The prompt response to emergencies necessitates efficient and effective dispatch systems. PSAPs, or EMS dispatchers, must have the necessary skills and knowledge to prioritize emergency calls and allocate appropriate resources promptly. Reliable EMS systems should incorporate modern communication technologies, enabling swift and effective information exchange between dispatchers, EMS personnel, and other relevant parties. These technologies might comprise computer-aided dispatch systems, two-way radios, and/or mobile data terminals, among others.

Effective communication plays a critical role in emergency response and the delivery of high-quality care. Reliable EMS systems should have robust communication infrastructures to ensure all stakeholders stay updated about the patient's condition and treatment plan. Clear, concise, and timely communication is crucial to ensure all parties understand the situation and can respond appropriately.

Moreover, reliable EMS systems should employ well-trained personnel who can respond rapidly and provide appropriate care. EMS personnel should have the skills, knowledge, and resources to offer effective care during emergencies. Continuous training and education are essential to keep personnel competent and current with the latest medical technologies and techniques. They should also demonstrate excellent communication skills with patients and their families, providing necessary information and support during crises.

In addition to a prompt response and effective communication, EMS systems should have efficient transport systems. This ensures that patients are transported quickly and safely to appropriate healthcare facilities. Reliable EMS systems should have transport protocols outlining the most suitable transport method based on the patient's condition and medical needs. Access to reliable and updated information about healthcare facilities is also crucial to ensure patients are transported to the most suitable locations.

A timely response to emergencies and effective communication, including vital pre-arrival instructions from modern PSAPs, are integral components of reliable EMS systems. EMS leaders should focus on establishing efficient dispatch systems, implementing effective communication technologies, and training competent personnel. By emphasizing these areas, they can build and maintain reliable EMS systems that deliver exceptional care to patients and ensure the long-term sustainability of EMS agencies within their communities.

Continuous Quality Improvement and Performance Measurement

Continuous quality improvement (CQI) and performance measurement are integral aspects of reliable Emergency Medical Services (EMS) systems. These processes involve the ongoing assessment and enhancement of EMS system performance, aiming to ensure the delivery of high-quality care to patients. Performance measurement involves the collection and analysis of data to monitor EMS system performance and identify areas for improvement. In this regard, EMS leaders play a crucial role in implementing strategies to achieve these goals.

CQI entails the continuous evaluation and improvement of EMS system performance. Reliable EMS systems foster a culture of continuous improvement, constantly seeking ways to enhance patient care. This involves utilizing data to identify areas in need of improvement and developing strategies to address them. EMS leaders are responsible for establishing comprehensive CQI programs that encompass regular assessments of EMS system performance, data analysis, and the development and implementation of improvement strategies.

Performance measurement is a vital component of CQI. Reliable EMS systems must have robust performance measurement systems in place to effectively monitor and evaluate their performance. Performance measures should be aligned with national standards and guidelines, and EMS leaders must ensure that EMS personnel receive adequate training to collect and analyze data accurately. Regular review of performance data is essential, allowing EMS leaders to use the insights gained to promote improvement strategies.

EMS leaders must foster a culture of continuous learning and improvement within their organizations. Encouraging EMS personnel to pursue new knowledge and skills and apply them to their practice is crucial. Providing ongoing training and education opportunities ensures that EMS personnel possess the necessary skills and knowledge to deliver high-quality care.

Moreover, EMS leaders should prioritize the development and implementation of evidence-based practices. These practices are supported by research and evaluation, demonstrating their effectiveness. EMS leaders must establish processes for evaluating new technologies and techniques, adopting those that have proven to be effective through rigorous evaluation.

Sharing best practices with other EMS systems is another important responsibility of EMS leaders. Active participation in national and regional EMS organizations enables learning from other systems' experiences and the exchange of insights. This facilitates the identification of new strategies for improvement and enhances the overall quality of care provided to patients.

CQI and performance measurement are vital components of reliable EMS systems. EMS leaders are instrumental in fostering a culture of continuous improvement, establishing performance measurement systems, implementing evidence-based practices, and sharing best practices with other EMS systems. By prioritizing these key areas, EMS leaders can ensure that patients receive high-quality care, while simultaneously maintaining the reliability and sustainability of EMS systems in the long run.

36

TELEHEALTH: A NEW FRONTIER

"Prediction is very difficult, especially about the future." - Danish proverb, often attributed to Niels Bohr

IN THE NOT-TOO-DISTANT FUTURE, A NEW DAWN FOR EMERGENCY Medical Services is imminent, one where the power of technology combined with telehealth fundamentally redefines emergency care. Envision a new kind of EMS practitioner: a Tele-Medic, not just skilled in conventional emergency medical services, but also credentialed in the advanced delivery of telehealth. This future is quickly taking shape and holds the potential to transform EMS, particularly in the rural and frontier expanses of the United States.

Picture a patient residing in an isolated location; the nearest critical access hospital is an hour's journey away, while the closest with a comprehensive range of specialties, is nearly 3.5 hours distant. Traditionally, the patient would face a tiresome journey to one, if not both, of these facilities. But in this future, the dynamics of distance and time in healthcare delivery are revolutionized.

Equipped with groundbreaking technology such as the Microsoft HoloLens or a comparable augmented reality device, the Tele-Medic is a hub within a network of national medical expertise. The remote geographical location poses no obstacle, as the Tele-Medic is connected virtually to a host of medical specialists scattered across the nation.

When the call for help arrives, it pertains to a known case of diabetes and congestive heart failure (CHF) presenting with weakness and a recent change in medication. The Tele-Medic promptly arrives, performs an initial assessment, and point of care blood work, swiftly gathering vital data. In a seamless transition, the Tele-Medic initiates a virtual consultation with the patient's primary care physician's office and the on-call endocrinologist and cardiologist.

Rather than an exhausting transfer of the patient hundreds of miles to a regional medical center, only for them to be discharged days, or even hours, later with a referral back to their primary care physician, a more efficient and patient-centered approach is adopted. The Tele-Medic, backed by the virtual presence of the specialists, identifies the impact of the medication change. The endocrinologist, in conjunction with the patient's medical team, adjusts the prescriptions, using the EKG and point of care labs provided by you, the Tele-Medic, for informed decision-making.

This new approach brings about an additional benefit. The EMS service can bill the patient's insurance for the home care visit, which is reimbursed at a premium rate, recognizing the comprehensive care provided in the patient's home, thus avoiding unnecessary ambulance transport and hospital admissions. The once financially struggling community ambulance service is now, for the first time in 40 years, financially solvent.

The prospect of such a transformation within a decade is not merely wishful thinking. It's an impending reality powered by the fusion of telehealth into EMS. The era of the Tele-Medic is on the horizon, promising a future where high-quality, comprehensive emergency care is accessible to all, regardless of their geographic location. This is the dawn of a new era where the delivery of emergency medical services is not constrained by distance but empowered by technology.

FUTURE OF TELEHEALTH AND EMS

Integration of telehealth into EMS promises enhanced coordination among healthcare providers, potentially improving patient outcomes. Real-time communication and data sharing enabled by telehealth, involving EMS practitioners, emergency department staff, and remote specialists, is expected to facilitate more efficient care transitions, reducing the risk of medical errors, and boosting patient satisfaction.

Telehealth also shows promise in increasing the capacity of EMS to treat a greater number of patients at home, thus eliminating the need for transport. This transformation could potentially redefine the financial model of EMS, paving the way for novel revenue sharing models beneficial to patients, EMS practitioners, remote specialists, and the healthcare system.

An exciting prospect for telehealth application in EMS is the potential development of a specialized Telehealth Emergency Medical Technician (Tele-Medic) role. Tele-Medics, with specific training and credentials, could fully harness the potential of telehealth technologies, thus improving emergency medical care delivery. This unique skill set would include advanced telecommunication abilities, remote medical assessments, remote-guided procedures, tele-triage, and collaboration with remote specialists and other healthcare providers.

The Tele-Medic role could help tackle real-world challenges by enhancing access to care, reducing healthcare costs, and promoting superior coordination among healthcare providers. With specialized training in telehealth technologies and remote care delivery, Tele-Medics could deliver an elevated level of care to patients, ensuring they receive the most suitable and prompt care possible.

Incorporation of telehealth into EMS promises various benefits, including improved access to healthcare resources, better patient outcomes, and more efficient resource utilization. Research indicates that telehealth can reduce unnecessary transports, increase EMS efficiency, maintain patient satisfaction and outcomes, and contribute to the evolution of EMS, fostering a more patient-centered emergency care system. As telehealth technologies continue to evolve, their integration into EMS and the resulting transformation of emergency medical care is anticipated to proliferate. With the implementation of these innovative solutions, EMS practitioners and healthcare systems may be better equipped to meet the diverse needs of patients, ultimately improving overall health outcomes.

Future Career Pathways

The fusion of telehealth and Emergency Medical Services may again offer a unique opportunity not only to reshape the delivery of emergency care but also to create advanced educational pathways that culminate in lucrative professional careers. If carefully navigated and embraced, telehealth could provide new opportunities for EMS professionals to create a new career pathway.

The evolution of the Tele-Medic role is a significant innovation in EMS, tackling current challenges in system financing, personnel recruitment, and critically, retention. When Dr. Farrington called upon the AMA to recognize EMT-Paramedic as an Allied Health Profession in 1975, Paramedics were in the same category as Physician Assistants, Physical Therapists, Occupational Therapists, and others. However, over the ensuing decades, many of these professions morphed into independent medical practitioners, most with Master's or Doctorate level degrees. Telehealth offers EMS an opportunity to carve out a new career path that demands advanced education and, in return, provides significantly higher remuneration.

The Tele-Medic role enhances the core competencies of traditional EMS professionals, combining specialized training in telehealth technologies, advanced diagnostics, laboratory testing, and imaging. Equipped with cutting-edge tools and techniques, Tele-Medics would work seamlessly with medical specialists to provide patient-centered care tailored to individual needs, a level of care previously unavailable outside of specialized healthcare facilities.

The Tele-Medic role within the EMS profession offers an attractive career pathway, marrying advanced training with the potential for higher compensation. This specialized role, capitalizing on technological advancements and the growing demand for remote healthcare, presents a compelling proposition for aspiring and practicing healthcare professionals. The allure of pioneering medical innovation, the opportunity for continual skill and knowledge enhancement, and the chance to work alongside a diverse team of healthcare providers add to the appeal.

The Tele-Medic role could also introduce new opportunities for financial sustainability into the EMS system. By reducing hospital transports, Tele-Medics can alleviate the strain on emergency departments and optimize the utilization of existing EMS resources. The potential cost savings could facilitate the development and implementation of innovative revenue-sharing models that would benefit patients, EMS practitioners, remote specialists, and the broader healthcare system.

Moreover, the introduction of the Tele-Medic role can positively impact population health outcomes, particularly in rural or underserved areas, by providing more accessible, specialized care at home. By ensuring timely intervention and management of medical conditions, complications and the need for more costly interventions later can be prevented, leading to overall healthcare cost reduction.

The advent of the Tele-Medic role signifies a crucial opportunity for growth within the EMS profession. It opens doors to advanced education and rewarding careers, thereby attracting, and retaining top talent while addressing the challenges of system financing and resource allocation. The Tele-Medic role, in essence, has the potential to revolutionize healthcare delivery, leading to a more patient-centered, efficient, and equitable system, with EMS professionals playing an integral role in its evolution.

Challenges and Considerations: Embracing Telehealth in EMS

As the Emergency Medical Services industry contemplates incorporating telehealth as a new frontier of medicine, it faces several obstacles and considerations that must be addressed to ensure a successful transition. This transformation is akin to the evolution of EMS in the 1960s when ambulances primarily served for patient transportation, with minimal focus on pre-hospital care. The introduction of telehealth is another paradigm shift that will require comprehensive adjustments to traditional operational models, training programs, technological infrastructures, and regulatory standards.

One of the most significant challenges in integrating telehealth into EMS is the need for a robust, reliable technological infrastructure. The adoption of telehealth requires reliable, high-speed internet access and state-of-the-art telecommunication devices capable of real-time, high-definition audio-visual communication, digital data transmission, and integration with electronic health records. While rural areas may lack the necessary broadband capabilities, thus inhibiting the reach of telehealth services and exacerbating existing healthcare disparities, satellite-based internet services are now a viable alternative to cable or cellular technology.

Moreover, comprehensive training and education will be essential for EMS professionals transitioning into the Tele-Medic role. This training should encompass not only the technical aspects of using telehealth technologies but also the nuances of telehealth etiquette, communication, and patient privacy considerations. Additionally, Tele-Medics will require advanced training in diagnostics and treatment procedures, as they will be expected to manage a broader range of medical conditions than traditional EMS professionals.

Legislation and regulation will certainly pose a challenge, as current laws were not designed to fully accommodate the practice of telehealth within EMS. Issues such as licensure, reimbursement, and patient privacy laws will need to be reviewed and revised to provide an effective and secure framework for the delivery of telehealth services. However, navigating the required political and regulatory changes will require a unified voice from the profession. Tele-Medics and EMS organizations must navigate a complex web of local, state, and federal regulations, all of which may have different requirements and limitations.

The acceptance and adaptation of patients and communities will be crucial for the success of telehealth in EMS. While the convenience and potential cost savings of telehealth are appealing, some patients may be hesitant to engage with remote healthcare providers, particularly for complex or urgent medical conditions. Therefore, patient education, transparency, and continual feedback mechanisms will be critical to gaining public trust and acceptance.

Financially, transitioning to a telehealth-based model will present additional challenges. Initial investments in technology, training, and infrastructure are substantial. Moreover, changes in reimbursement models from a transportation benefit or fee-for-service model to value-based care models will require careful planning and collaboration with insurance companies and other healthcare providers.

Despite these challenges, the benefits and potential of incorporating telehealth into EMS are undeniable. By addressing these hurdles head-on, EMS organizations can transform the delivery of emergency care, enhancing access to specialized care, improving patient outcomes, and revolutionizing the EMS profession. The path forward will require foresight, creativity, and collaboration among a diverse array of stakeholders, but the potential rewards – for patients, EMS professionals, and the healthcare system as a whole – make the journey worth the effort.

New Horizons: Telemedicine and EMS

Looking into the future of EMS, telehealth emerges as a significant factor with transformative potential. By integrating telehealth into their operations, EMS practitioners can expand their traditional role as transporters and actively provide comprehensive healthcare. The introduction of the Tele-Medic role offers a significant opportunity to broaden the scope of EMS, delivering advanced care in patients' homes and reducing the need for hospital transports.

However, realizing this future vision will require substantial efforts and investments. It will be crucial to establish the necessary infrastructure, develop new regulatory and reimbursement frameworks, provide training for Tele-Medics, and promote public acceptance of telehealth. Despite the challenges, the potential benefits, such as improved patient outcomes and enhanced professional development opportunities for EMS practitioners, make it worthwhile to tackle these obstacles.

The development of the Tele-Medic role can also address the retention of experienced EMS practitioners seeking alternatives to ambulance transports while attracting new talent to the EMS profession. This specialized career path, combining medical expertise with advanced technology, can nurture a new generation of EMS professionals who are ready to meet the evolving demands of the healthcare landscape.

From a financial perspective, integrating telehealth into EMS may offer a sustainable solution to the perennial challenges of EMS funding. By reducing unnecessary hospital transports and optimizing resource utilization, telehealth can contribute to a more resilient and adaptable EMS system. This could open doors to new financing models, such as subscription-based services or partnerships with health insurers, hospitals, and other healthcare providers, creating a more sustainable EMS system for the future.

Importantly, telehealth has the potential to improve healthcare equity, particularly in underserved or rural areas where traditional EMS agencies may face limitations. By providing remote care, Tele-Medics can overcome geographical barriers, ensuring that every patient receives timely care regardless of their location.

As the integration of telehealth into EMS approaches, it is important to acknowledge that there is still much to learn and explore. This journey of incorporating telehealth into EMS will require ongoing research, evaluation, and adaptation. Moving forward, it will be crucial to gather data and insights that shed light on the impacts of telehealth on patient outcomes, healthcare costs, and the EMS profession. This knowledge will enable continuous refinement and improvement of telehealth practices, ensuring the best possible outcomes for patients and the healthcare system.

The future of EMS is on the brink of transformation through the integration of telehealth. This integration offers a promising pathway to address the current challenges faced by EMS and to reshape the delivery of emergency medical care. Embracing this new frontier will undoubtedly be complex, requiring significant effort, collaboration, and innovation. However, by fully embracing this new horizon, the EMS community envisions a future where EMS practitioners, including Tele-Medics, play a central and vital role in a patient-centered, efficient, and equitable healthcare system. The integration of telehealth into EMS holds the potential to ensure that high-quality emergency care is accessible to all individuals, regardless of their geographic location, thereby contributing to a healthier and more resilient society.

37

WE ARE EMS

"Unity is strength... when there is teamwork and collaboration, wonderful things can be achieved."
- Mattie Stepanek

WITHIN THE EMERGENCY MEDICAL SERVICES COMMUNITY, THERE are many challenges that must be acknowledged and addressed, but prominent among these is the fragmented professional identity. EMS professionals often grapple with associating themselves with the larger EMS profession, choosing instead to identify with specialized roles within the industry or their employer's profile: Private EMS practitioners, firefighter-EMT or firefighter-medic, flight-medic, community paramedic, etc. Charting the path towards the future necessitates all EMS professionals also unify at a macro level as EMS professionals. Perhaps the simple phrase "We Are EMS" balances the varied employers and work environments with a shared commitment, resilience, and passion that binds all EMS professionals, regardless of their specialized roles.

The EMS Agenda 2050[156], published in 2019, offers a compelling vision for the future of EMS. This ambitious blueprint necessitates collaboration among every EMS practitioner, leader, manager, and policymaker to overcome the distinctive challenges that the profession faces. By pledging allegiance to and embodying the foundational principles of the EMS Agenda 2050, the future of EMS as a vital element of public health and safety can be assured.

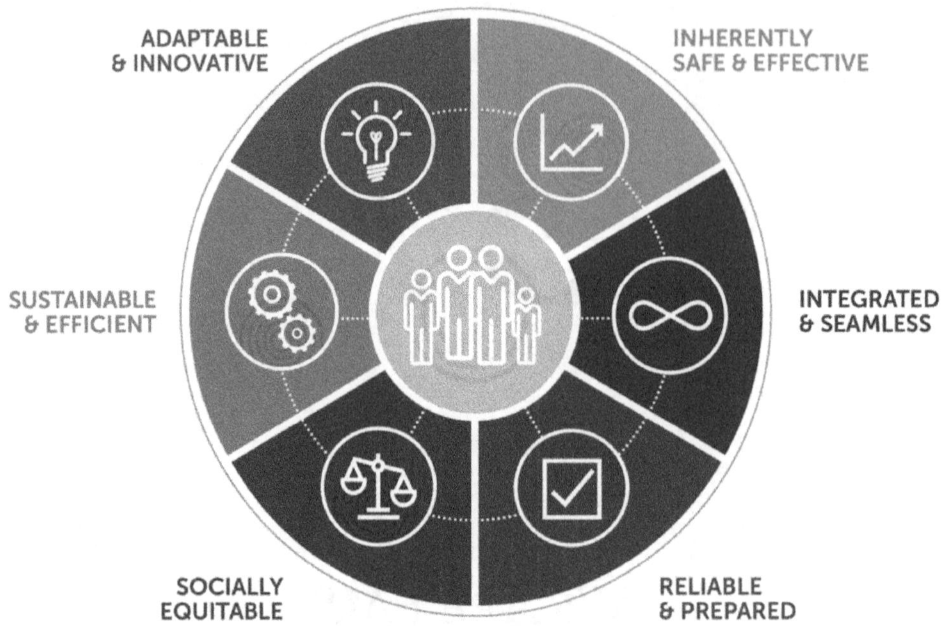

157

The EMS Agenda 2050 is underpinned by six key pillars:

1. **Inherent Safety and Effectiveness**: This principle ensures that safety and effectiveness are at the heart of every EMS operation. It's not only about executing the job but doing so excellently and securely.

2. **Integrated and Seamless operations**: This aspires to create a unified EMS system that transcends traditional barriers, facilitating seamless coordination and communication among diverse units and specialties.

3. **Reliability and Preparedness**: EMS should be poised to respond efficiently and effectively to any emergency, routine, or catastrophic. Dependability should be a hallmark of EMS.

4. **Social Equity**: EMS is tasked with guaranteeing access to quality emergency medical care for all, irrespective of socioeconomic status, race, gender, age, or geographical location.

5. **Sustainability and Efficiency**: The future of EMS lies in sustainable and efficient practices that strike a balance between delivering high-quality care and managing costs and resources effectively.

6. **Adaptability and Innovation**: Given the fast pace of medical technology and practice evolution, EMS must be adaptable and innovative, staying abreast with changes and continually enhancing services.

The multifaceted nature of EMS is a testament to the resilience of this emergent profession, exemplifying the sacrifices made to ensure its survival. However, it is not merely desirable, but an absolute necessity for all EMS professionals to cultivate a robust, unified voice. This is a critical requirement for the profession's continuous evolution, effective representation at local, state, and federal levels, and to formulate substantial solutions addressing concerns of EMS funding, sustainability, and reliability.

The EMS Agenda 2050 projects a vision and presents a comprehensive platform for all EMS stakeholders. Regardless of their individual roles, each member must contribute to the transformation of the EMS industry. Under the unifying banner, "We Are EMS," a collaborative unity must be cultivated that transcends the barriers of employers, operational models, remuneration, and geography. Through such a unified macro-identity, both the public and policy makers will gain a better understanding of EMS's indispensable contributions at community, state, and national levels.

Sidestepping minor differences, the phrase "We Are EMS" serves as a potent statement that educates, unifies, and reminds stakeholders of the value, role, and importance of EMS. Every EMS professional must uphold their professional responsibility to remember their unique and vital role in molding EMS into a cohesive, unified entity, poised to meet the dynamic needs of the communities they serve.

The challenge of unification must not only be accepted, but also wholly embraced. A shared commitment must be manifest as we unite to shape the future of EMS. Today's EMS leaders must translate the conceptual EMS 2050 Vision into tangible reality, thereby solidifying EMS's standing as a pillar of strength and resilience. The phrase "We Are EMS" must be more than just a slogan; it must epitomize our collective dedication, unity, and aspiration for a brighter, more resilient future.

#WeAreEMS

Private
Tactictal
Wilderness
Military
Public
Community
Hospital
Flight
Volunteer
Interfacility
Industrial
Fire
Federal

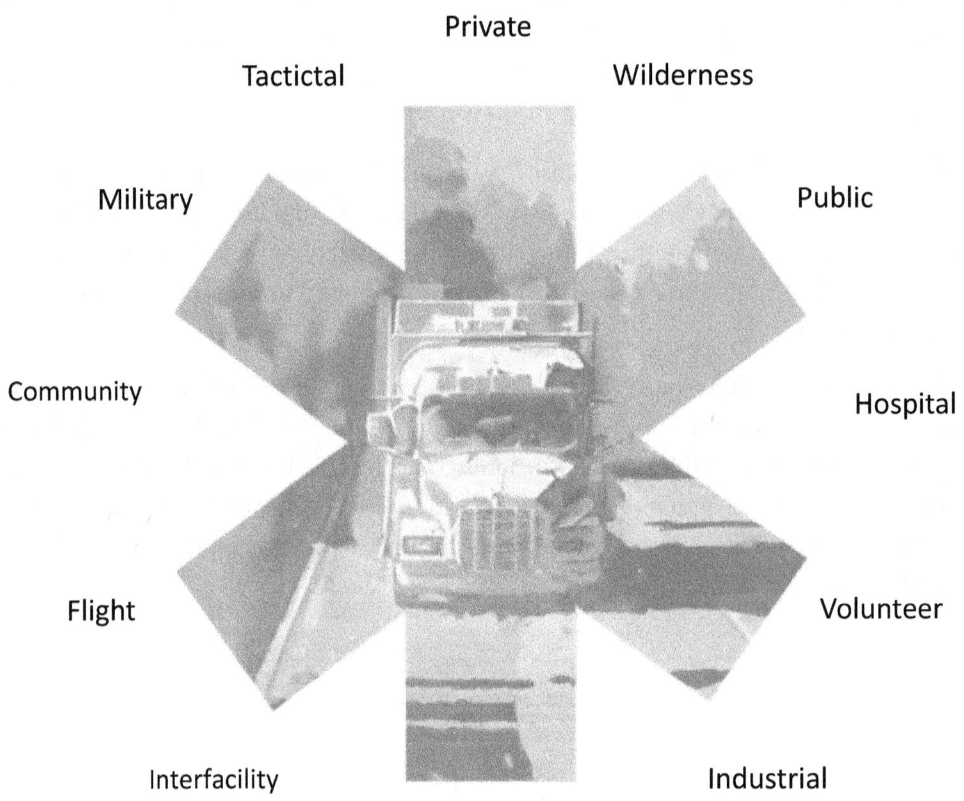

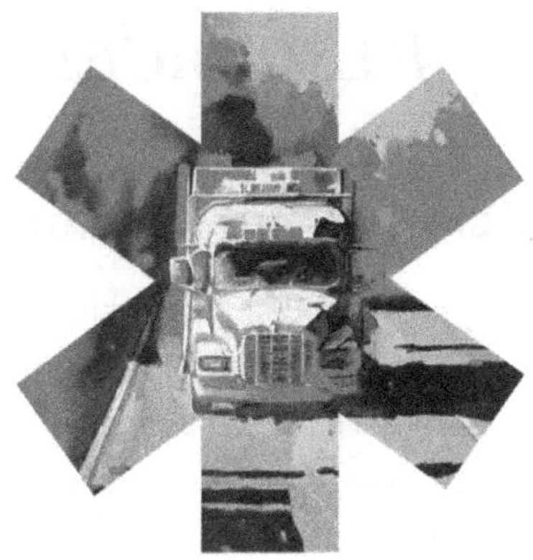

APPENDIX

RESOURCES

PETER'S LAWS FOR THE NAVIGATION OF LIFE

In 2002, Dr. Peter Safar's colleagues compiled a collection of his frequently used quotes and idioms, titling it "Peter's Laws for the Navigation of Life," and subtitling it "The Creed of the Sociopathic Obsessive Compulsive."[158] This collection has since been widely disseminated, with reproductions appearing on posters hung in medical schools and hospital staff break rooms. Additionally, it has gained significant traction on social media, further extending its reach and impact.

- If anything can go wrong, fix it!
- When given a choice, take both.
- Multiple projects lead to multiple successes.
- Start at the top and work your way up.
- Do it by the book… but be the author.
- When forced to compromise, ask for more.
- If you can't beat them, join them, and then beat them.
- If it's worth doing, it's got to be done now!
- If you can't win, change the rules.
- If you can't change the rules, then ignore them.
- Perfection is not optional.
- When faced without a challenge, make one.
- "No" simply means begin again at one level higher.
- Don't walk when you can run.
- Bureaucracy is a challenge to be conquered with a righteous attitude, a tolerance for stupidity, and a bulldozer when necessary.
- When in doubt, THINK!
- Patience is a virtue, but persistence to the point of success is a blessing.
- The squeaky wheel gets replaced.
- The faster you move, the slower time passes, the longer you live!
- Death is not the enemy but occasionally needs help with timing.
- When on thin ice, dance.
- It's up to us to save the world.

1976 ABSTRACTS[159]

The following abstracts were compiled by the Department of Health, Education and Welfare following a 1976 conference on Emergency Medical Services.

BY NORMAN MCSWAIN, MD: PARAMEDIC TRAINING

PARAMEDIC TRAINING IN JUNIOR COLLEGES

The University of Kansas Medical Center has been training paramedics since 1973 utilizing facilities of the School of Medicine and equipment of the Emergency Medical Training Program. In addition to conducting its own paramedic training classes, the University acts as the authorizing agency for all training programs within the state of Kansas. This authority to review and approve or disapprove all training program proposals was given to the University by the Kansas Legislature.

Several junior colleges in the State have approached the University and asked for assistance in starting a training program. The University forwards its teaching objectives to the college where they are reviewed by the college's administration and faculty. These groups make what revisions they feel necessary in order to fit the objectives into their particular teaching situation. These revisions are returned to the University for evaluation by the staff of the Emergency Medical Training Program. If the objectives, as formulated by the junior college, are found to be satisfactory, they are given approval by the University.

In addition to reviewing teaching objectives, staff members of the University make on-site visits to the junior college to evaluate clinical facilities of the area hospitals. The University then assists the junior college in drawing up clinical schedules that will give the students adequate experience.

Each junior college has incorporated the paramedic training program, which is spread over a full years time span, into an Associate of Arts Degree program. The students spend their first year at the college taking courses such as English, life sciences, and business administration. Adding these courses to their paramedic training enables the students to receive an Associate of Arts Degree thus, starting them on a career ladder.

Pers.

Norman E. McSwain, Jr., M.D.
University of Kansas Medical Center
39th & Rainbow Boulevard
Kansas City, Kansas 66103

1976 Abstract By Nancy Caroline, MD: National Standard Curriculum

USDOT Curriculum for Advanced
Emergency Medical Technicians

A curriculum for the training of emergency medical technicians to the level of Paramedic has been developed at the University of Pittsburgh under the auspices of the United States Department of Transportation. This curriculum was based upon a review of all major curricula currently in use in this country as well as the standards set down by the National Research Council of the National Academy of Sciences.

The curriculum consists of three major documents:

(1) a Course Guide, which provides resource material on administration of the course to the individual charged with course coordination;

(2) Instructor Lesson Plans, which furnish instructional materials for each unit of the course;

(3) a Student Study Guide, which serves as a textbook and reference volume for the student.

Each of these documents will be described in detail.

The course is organized into 15 modules and arranged in such a way that each module can be taught independently of the others-- to enable flexibility of scheduling and take into account the special constraints of rural and volunteer services. Each module is further subdivided into units, each of which contains objectives, content outlines, guides to demonstration and practice sessions, and skill evaluation sheets.

The curriculum will be generally available by early summer, 1976 through regional offices of the National Highway Traffic Safety Administration.

Pers.

Nancy L. Caroline, M.D.
Assistant Professor of Clinical/
Anesthesiology Critical Care Medicine
University of Pittsburgh

1976 Abstract: Innovations in Distance Education

ROCKY MOUNTAIN EMT SATELLITE REFRESHER COURSE

During the spring of 1975 Colorado EMT's shared with EMT's from seven other Rocky Mountain states, the unique experience of participating in a satellite communications EMT refresher course. One hundred EMT's from Colorado, some travelling up to four hours, attended the seven Saturday morning classes. The NASA ATS-6 satellite had been originally utilized to broadcast educational programming in eight mountain states to 56 rural isolated communities and 11 Public Broadcasting Stations. The EMT refresher course piggybacked onto the existing system and was able to provide quality EMT refresher instruction to Colorado EMT's in dire need of this supplemental training. The achievement of the satellite program was the utilization of top level EMS people from around the Rocky Mountain region. These experts were brought to Denver where the program was broadcasted and videotaped. Rural mountain towns in remote locations were able to share the knowledge and experience of known experts directly in their own small communities. The potential for training health personnel by satellite is infinite. This was only a demonstration project, but the concept of broadcasting EMS training programs via satellite to small isolated communities in Colorado, as well as other Rocky Mountain states, holds a brilliant promise and hopefully a future for this region.

Pers., Comm.,

James C. McShane, Dr. H., M.P.H.
Acting Chief
Emergency Health Services Section
Colorado Department of Health
4210 East 11th Avenue
Denver, Colorado 80220

USE OF THE TELEPHONE CONFERENCE IN EMERGENCY MEDICAL TRAINING

One of the most pressing problems in the rural areas is education for members of the health team. Distance, availability of personnel, and travel and per diem expenses are major considerations for the rural community hospitals.

Valley View Hospital in Ada, Oklahoma has provided one solution - the use of the telephone conference network for EMT-A instruction for both basic and refresher training. The present network has grown from seven, originally funded under the Regional Medical Program, to 96 hospitals state wide.

To date, more than 150 EMT's have been trained by the teleconference method in southeast and south central Oklahoma. The only restriction in expanding instruction is the number of training kits available, the present seven having come from HEW funding for emergency medical services. Pushing one button could make the programs available to the remainder of the state.

Dr. David Ramsay, FACS, is in charge of all EMT-A instruction, based on the 81 hour Dunlap course. A local physician is present at each of the six or seven sites receiving the teleconference simultaneously. Each physician is assisted by either a Registered EMT or RN. Cooperative assistance has been provided by the Oklahoma Trauma Research Society in testing for national or state registry.

The teleconference has also been used in conjunction with seminars to provide a 24 hour course in emergency room nursing on a state wide basis. After 16 hours of initial instruction by teleconference, instructional teams visited the following population centers in Oklahoma: Bartlesville, Lawton, Enid, Oklahoma City and Ada to provide eight hours of seminar instruction. More than 1,000 nurses profited from this opportunity.

In short, the teleconference method of emergency medical personnel instruction has met with highly favorable results. It has made instruction available to remote areas, it has reduced time for both students and instructors away from the job; it has reduced the costs of travel and per diem; and most importantly, it has attracted the interest and allowed the direct involvement of the physicians.

Pers., Comm.

John M. White, Jr.
Billie Frank Turner
Oklahoma State Department of Health
Northeast 10th Street & Stonewall
Post Office Box 53551
Oklahoma City, Oklahoma 73105

1976 Abstract: National Registry

THE NATIONAL REGISTRY OF EMERGENCY MEDICAL TECHNICIANS

The National Registry of Emergency Medical Technicians was conceived in 1966 as a direct result of the recommendations of the President's Committee on Traffic Safety as it related to the care and transportation of the sick and injured.

Accepting the recommendation that there be a national accreditation agency to establish uniform standards for training and personnel, and realizing that a national registry is essential for improved ambulance services, the Commission on Emergency Medical Services of the American Medical Association on January 21, 1970 called together a task force consisting of representatives of all National organizations involved in the delivery of emergency care, including representatives of the many concerned and involved medical societies and associations.

On June 4, 1970 at the A.M.A. headquarters in Chicago, the National Registry was born. Organizational funds were provided by the American Medical Association and Employer's Insurance of Wausau, Wisconsin. The first examinations were administered on October 29-30, 1971 to 1,520 Emergency Medical Technicians simultaneously at 51 sites throughout the U. S. To date, the National Registry has accepted and processed 75,000 applications from EMTs representing all 50 states and the military. The Registry examinations are in two parts, a written and a practical. The reliability of the written examination is continuously monitored by way of a computerized item analysis.

The National Registry of Emergency Medical Technicians headquartered in Columbus, Ohio continues to grow in numbers and stature. Working in concert with the Department of Health, Education, and Welfare - Department of Transportation and the medical community the Registry is fulfilling its purposes relative to the Emergency Medical Technicians.

Org.

Rocco V. Morando
P. O. Box 29233
Columbus, Ohio 43229

1976 EMS Development Progress Report

EMERGENCY MEDICAL SERVICES PROGRESS REPORT FOR THE UNITED STATES OF AMERICA WITH FUTURE PROGRAM PROJECTION

The appreciated need for improved emergency medical services in this country started in 1966 with the National Research Countil's white paper entitled, "Trauma, the Neglected Disease of Modern Society." This document reflected much of the professional concern for the lack of a comprehensive approach to the accident victim and called for most of the essential components that now exist in the Emergency Medical Services System Act of 1973. Prior to this, the National Highway Safety Act of 1966 has provided support to Local governments for elements of Emergency Transportation Care and other Health an Public Safety agencies have provided some support for certain elements of an Emergency Medical Services System.

In 1972 the then Assistant Secretary for Health Merlin K. DuVal stated, "Nowhere is this lack of accessibility more crucial and yet more widespread...than in the area of emergency care. Any description of our current emergency medical services becomes a litany of inadequacy and neglect." Subsequently in 1972 a special Presidential initiative provided some $15 million to demonstrate the feasibility of the EMS systems approach. The five demonstration projects (States of Arkansas, Illinois and regions of Jacksonville, Florida, San Diego, California and Southeast Ohio) have been completed and significant lessons have been gained: (1) EMS systems can be developed so they will be locally continued; (2) When developed, EMS systems do have a significant impact on patient care services including morbidity and mortality; (3) That regions need at least 4 to 5 years for development and stabilization (BLS and ALS), (4) Successful EMS systems require the involvement of the health authority and medical leadership; (5) EMS systems need initial Federal support for organizational and program development to coordinate other Federal health initiatives and to develop a base for local support; (6) EMS systems development are difficult and frustrating enterprises that must involve the community, the medical provider, governmental and political interests.

The Robert Wood Johnson Foundation, in 1973, established a national grant competition for the development of Regional EMS systems by emphasizing access, communications and regionalization of emergency medical care. Enactment of the Emergency Medical Services Systems Act of 1973 (P.L. 93-154) was a major effort on the part of Congress to meet the demand and need for coordinating the development of Regional Emergency Medical Care delivery systems and providing $100 million authorization. The major provisions of the EMSS Act may be outlined as follows: A. <u>Grants and Contracts</u>; (1) Feasibility Studies and Planning (Section 1202); (2) Establishment and Initial Operations (Section 1203); (3) Expansion and Improvement (Section 1204); (4) Research (Section 1205); (5) Training (Title VII of the PHS Act) B. <u>EMS Systems Requirements (Section 1206(b)(4)(c)</u>. In order to

establish an EMS system that will provide improved emergency medical care to any and all emergency patients within a region, a sound integration of the fifteen mandatory Congressional components is required as stated in the EMSS Act. The EMSS Act requires that where plans are developed and systems established, expanded and improved, the following components of a system must exist: (1) the provision of manpower; (2) training of personnel; (3) communications; (4) transportation; (5) facilities; (6) critical care units; (7) use of public safety agencies; (8) consumer participation; (9) accessibility to care; (10) transfer of patients; (11) standard medical record keeping; (12) consumer information and education; (13) independent review and evaluation; (14) disaster linkage; and (15) mutual aid agreements.
C. Technical Assistance (Section 1206(b)(5), D. Administrative Unit (Section 1208), E. Interagency Committee on Emergency Medical Service EMS (Section 1209), F. Annual Report to Congress (Section 1210)

Last November, on the anniversary of the passage of the EMSS Act, President Ford reaffirmed that emergency medical care was of a high National priority and this January he attended a special White House Conference on EMS systems.

The DEMS reports that of 235 nationally possible EMS systems 125 are planning EMSS under section 1202; 83 are initiating EMSS under section 1203; and 27 are expanding EMSS under section 1204.

Fed.,Leg. Fed.$

David R. Boyd, M.D.C.M.
Director, Division of
Emergency Medical Services
6525 Belcrest Rd., Rm. 320
W. Hyattsville, Md. 20782

EMS COMPACT MODEL LEGISLATION

Compacts require all member states to enact substantially the same legislation, and to facilitate this, Model Legislation is provided. The Model Legislation for the Recognition of EMS Personnel Licensure Interstate Compact, as drafted in 2013, is included for reference.

RECOGNITION OF EMERGENCY MEDICAL SERVICES PERSONNEL LICENSURE INTERSTATE COMPACT ("REPLICA")

EMS PERSONNEL LICENSURE INTERSTATE COMPACT
SECTION 1. PURPOSE

In order to protect the public through verification of competency and ensure accountability for patient care related activities all states license emergency medical services personnel, such as emergency medical technicians (EMTs), advanced EMTs and paramedics. This Compact is intended to facilitate the day-to-day movement of EMS personnel across state boundaries in the performance of their EMS duties as assigned by an appropriate authority and authorize state EMS offices to afford immediate legal recognition to EMS personnel licensed in a member state. This Compact recognizes that states have a vested interest in protecting the public's health and safety through their licensing and regulation of EMS personnel and that such state regulation shared among the member states will best protect public health and safety.

This Compact is designed to achieve the following purposes and objectives:

1. Increase public access to EMS personnel;
2. Enhance the states' ability to protect the public's health and safety, especially patient safety;
3. Encourage the cooperation of member states in the areas of EMS personnel licensure and regulation;
4. Support licensing of military members who are separating from an active duty tour and their spouses;
5. Facilitate the exchange of information between member states regarding EMS personnel licensure, adverse action and significant investigatory information;
6. Promote compliance with the laws governing EMS personnel practice in each member state; and
7. Invest all member states with the authority to hold EMS personnel accountable through the mutual recognition of member state licenses.

SECTION 2. DEFINITIONS

In this compact:

A. "Advanced Emergency Medical Technician (AEMT)" means: an individual licensed with cognitive knowledge and a scope of practice that corresponds to that level in the National EMS Education Standards and National EMS Scope of Practice Model.

B. "Adverse Action" means: any administrative, civil, equitable or criminal action permitted by a state's laws which may be imposed against licensed EMS personnel by a state EMS authority or state court, including, but not limited to, actions against an individual's license such as revocation, suspension, probation, consent agreement, monitoring or other limitation or encumbrance on the individual's practice, letters of reprimand or admonition, fines, criminal convictions and state court judgments enforcing adverse actions by the state EMS authority.

C. "Alternative program" means: a voluntary, non-disciplinary substance abuse recovery program approved by a state EMS authority.

D. "Certification" means: the successful verification of entry-level cognitive and psychomotor competency using a reliable, validated, and legally defensible examination.

E. "Commission" means: the national administrative body of which all states that have enacted the compact are members.

F. "Emergency Medical Technician (EMT)" means: an individual licensed with cognitive knowledge and a scope of practice that corresponds to that level in the National EMS Education Standards and National EMS Scope of Practice Model.

G. "Home State" means: a member state where an individual is licensed to practice emergency medical services.

H. "License" means: the authorization by a state for an individual to practice as an EMT, AEMT, paramedic, or a level in between EMT and paramedic.

I. "Medical Director" means: a physician licensed in a member state who is accountable for the care delivered by EMS personnel.

J. "Member State" means: a state that has enacted this compact.

K. "Privilege to Practice" means: an individual's authority to deliver emergency medical services in remote states as authorized under this compact.

L. "Paramedic" means: an individual licensed with cognitive knowledge and a scope of practice that corresponds to that level in the National EMS Education Standards and National EMS Scope of Practice Model.

M. "Remote State" means: a member state in which an individual is not licensed.

N. "Restricted" means: the outcome of an adverse action that limits a license or the privilege to practice.

O. "Rule" means: a written statement by the interstate Commission promulgated pursuant to Section 12 of this compact that is of general applicability; implements, interprets, or prescribes a policy or provision of the compact; or is an organizational, procedural, or practice requirement of the Commission and has the force and effect of statutory law in a member state and includes the amendment, repeal, or suspension of an existing rule.

P. "Scope of Practice" means: defined parameters of various duties or services that may be provided by an individual with specific credentials. Whether regulated by rule, statute, or court decision, it tends to represent the limits of services an individual may perform.

Q. "Significant Investigatory Information" means:

   1. investigative information that a state EMS authority, after a preliminary inquiry that includes notification and an opportunity to respond if required by state law, has reason to believe, if proved true, would result in the imposition of an adverse action on a license or privilege to practice; or
   2. investigative information that indicates that the individual represents an immediate threat to public health and safety regardless of whether the individual has been notified and had an opportunity to respond.
      a. "State" means: any state, commonwealth, district, or territory of the United States.
      b. "State EMS Authority" means: the board, office, or other agency with the legislative mandate to license EMS personnel.

SECTION 3. HOME STATE LICENSURE

A. Any member state in which an individual holds a current license shall be deemed a home state for purposes of this compact.

B. Any member state may require an individual to obtain and retain a license to be authorized to practice in the member state under circumstances not authorized by the privilege to practice under the terms of this compact.

C. A home state's license authorizes an individual to practice in a remote state under the privilege to practice only if the home state:

1. Currently requires the use of the National Registry of Emergency Medical Technicians (NREMT) examination as a condition of issuing initial licenses at the EMT and paramedic levels;
2. Has a mechanism in place for receiving and investigating complaints about individuals;
3. Notifies the Commission, in compliance with the terms herein, of any adverse action or significant investigatory information regarding an individual;
4. No later than five years after activation of the Compact, requires a criminal background check of all applicants for initial licensure, including the use of the results of fingerprint or other biometric data checks compliant with the requirements of the Federal Bureau of Investigation with the exception of federal employees who have suitability determination in accordance with U.S. CFR §731.202 and submit documentation of such as promulgated in the rules of the Commission; and
5. Complies with the rules of the Commission.

SECTION 4. COMPACT PRIVILEGE TO PRACTICE

A. Member states shall recognize the privilege to practice of an individual licensed in another member state that is in conformance with Section 3.

B. To exercise the privilege to practice under the terms and provisions of this compact, an individual must:

1. Be at least 18 years of age;
2. Possess a current unrestricted license in a member state as an EMT, AEMT, paramedic, or state recognized and licensed level with a scope of practice and authority between EMT and paramedic; and
3. Practice under the supervision of a medical director.
    a. An individual providing patient care in a remote state under the privilege to practice shall function within the scope of practice authorized by the home state unless and until modified by an appropriate authority in the remote state as may be defined in the rules of the commission.
    b. Except as provided in Section 4 subsection C, an individual practicing in a remote state will be subject to the remote state's authority and laws. A remote state may, in accordance with due process and that state's laws, restrict, suspend, or revoke an individual's privilege to practice in the remote state and may take any other necessary actions to protect the health and safety of its citizens. If a remote state takes action it shall promptly notify the home state and the Commission.

C. If an individual's license in any home state is restricted or suspended, the individual shall not be eligible to practice in a remote state under the privilege to practice until the individual's home state license is restored.

D. If an individual's privilege to practice in any remote state is restricted, suspended, or revoked the individual shall not be eligible to practice in any remote state until the individual's privilege to practice is restored.

SECTION 5. CONDITIONS OF PRACTICE IN A REMOTE STATE

An individual may practice in a remote state under a privilege to practice only in the performance of the individual's EMS duties as assigned by an appropriate authority, as defined in the rules of the Commission, and under the following circumstances:

1. The individual originates a patient transport in a home state and transports the patient to a remote state;
2. The individual originates in the home state and enters a remote state to pick up a patient and provide care and transport of the patient to the home state;
3. The individual enters a remote state to provide patient care and/or transport within that remote state;
4. The individual enters a remote state to pick up a patient and provide care and transport to a third member state;
5. Other conditions as determined by rules promulgated by the commission.

SECTION 6. RELATIONSHIP TO EMERGENCY MANAGEMENT ASSISTANCE COMPACT

Upon a member state's governor's declaration of a state of emergency or disaster that activates the Emergency Management Assistance Compact (EMAC), all relevant terms and provisions of EMAC shall apply and to the extent any terms or provisions of this Compact conflict with EMAC, the terms of EMAC shall prevail with respect to any individual practicing in the remote state in response to such declaration.

SECTION 7. VETERANS, SERVICE MEMBERS SEPARATING FROM ACTIVE DUTY MILITARY, AND THEIR SPOUSES

A. Member states shall consider a veteran, active military service member, and member of the National Guard and Reserves separating from an active duty tour, and a spouse thereof, who holds a current valid and unrestricted NREMT certification at or above the level of the state license being sought as satisfying the minimum training and examination requirements for such licensure.

B. Member states shall expedite the processing of licensure applications submitted by veterans, active military service members, and members of the National Guard and Reserves separating from an active duty tour, and their spouses.

C. All individuals functioning with a privilege to practice under this Section remain subject to the Adverse Actions provisions of Section VIII.

SECTION 8. ADVERSE ACTIONS

A. A home state shall have exclusive power to impose adverse action against an individual's license issued by the home state.

B. If an individual's license in any home state is restricted or suspended, the individual shall not be eligible to practice in a remote state under the privilege to practice until the individual's home state license is restored.

   1. All home state adverse action orders shall include a statement that the individual's compact privileges are inactive. The order may allow the individual to practice in remote states with prior written authorization from both the home state and remote state's EMS authority.
   2. An individual currently subject to adverse action in the home state shall not practice in any remote state without prior written authorization from both the home state and remote state's EMS authority.

C. A member state shall report adverse actions and any occurrences that the individual's compact privileges are restricted, suspended, or revoked to the Commission in accordance with the rules of the Commission.

D. A remote state may take adverse action on an individual's privilege to practice within that state.

E. Any member state may take adverse action against an individual's privilege to practice in that state based on the factual findings of another member state, so long as each state follows its own procedures for imposing such adverse action.
F. A home state's EMS authority shall investigate and take appropriate action with respect to reported conduct in a remote state as it would if such conduct had occurred within the home state. In such cases, the home state's law shall control in determining the appropriate adverse action.
G. Nothing in this Compact shall override a member state's decision that participation in an alternative program may be used in lieu of adverse action and that such participation shall remain non-public if required by the member state's laws. Member states must require individuals who enter any alternative programs to agree not to practice in any other member state during the term of the alternative program without prior authorization from such other member state.

SECTION 9. ADDITIONAL POWERS INVESTED IN A MEMBER STATE'S EMS AUTHORITY

A member state's EMS authority, in addition to any other powers granted under state law, is authorized under this compact to:

1. Issue subpoenas for both hearings and investigations that require the attendance and testimony of witnesses and the production of evidence. Subpoenas issued by a member state's EMS authority for the attendance and testimony of witnesses, and/or the production of evidence from another member state, shall be enforced in the remote state by any court of competent jurisdiction, according to that court's practice and procedure in considering subpoenas issued in its own proceedings. The issuing state EMS authority shall pay any witness fees, travel expenses, mileage, and other fees required by the service statutes of the state where the witnesses and/or evidence are located; and
2. Issue cease and desist orders to restrict, suspend, or revoke an individual's privilege to practice in the state.

SECTION 10. ESTABLISHMENT OF THE INTERSTATE COMMISSION FOR EMS PERSONNEL PRACTICE

A. The Compact states hereby create and establish a joint public agency known as the Interstate Commission for EMS Personnel Practice.
    1. The Commission is a body politic and an instrumentality of the Compact states.
    2. Venue is proper and judicial proceedings by or against the Commission shall be brought solely and exclusively in a court of competent jurisdiction where the principal office of the Commission is located. The Commission may waive venue and jurisdictional defenses to the extent it adopts or consents to participate in alternative dispute resolution proceedings.
    3. Nothing in this Compact shall be construed to be a waiver of sovereign immunity.
B. Membership, Voting, and Meetings
    1. Each member state shall have and be limited to one (1) delegate. The responsible official of the state EMS authority or his designee shall be the delegate to this Compact for each member state. Any delegate may be removed or suspended from office as provided by the law of the state from which the delegate is appointed. Any vacancy occurring in the Commission shall be filled in accordance with the laws of the member state in which the vacancy exists. In the event that more than one board, office, or other agency with the legislative mandate to license EMS personnel at and above the level of EMT exists, the Governor of the state will determine which entity will be responsible for assigning the delegate.
    2. Each delegate shall be entitled to one (1) vote with regard to the promulgation of rules and creation of bylaws and shall otherwise have an opportunity to participate in the business and affairs of the Commission. A delegate shall vote in person or by such other means as provided

in the bylaws. The bylaws may provide for delegates' participation in meetings by telephone or other means of communication.

3. The Commission shall meet at least once during each calendar year. Additional meetings shall be held as set forth in the bylaws.
4. All meetings shall be open to the public, and public notice of meetings shall be given in the same manner as required under the rulemaking provisions in Section XII.
5. The Commission may convene in a closed, non-public meeting if the Commission must discuss:
    a. Non-compliance of a member state with its obligations under the Compact;
    b. The employment, compensation, discipline or other personnel matters, practices or procedures related to specific employees or other matters related to the Commission's internal personnel practices and procedures;
    c. Current, threatened, or reasonably anticipated litigation;
    d. Negotiation of contracts for the purchase or sale of goods, services, or real estate;
    e. Accusing any person of a crime or formally censuring any person;
    f. Disclosure of trade secrets or commercial or financial information that is privileged or confidential;
    g. Disclosure of information of a personal nature where disclosure would constitute a clearly unwarranted invasion of personal privacy;
    h. Disclosure of investigatory records compiled for law enforcement purposes;
    i. Disclosure of information related to any investigatory reports prepared by or on behalf of or for use of the Commission or other committee charged with responsibility of investigation or determination of compliance issues pursuant to the compact; or
    j. Matters specifically exempted from disclosure by federal or member state statute.
6. If a meeting, or portion of a meeting, is closed pursuant to this provision, the Commission's legal counsel or designee shall certify that the meeting may be closed and shall reference each relevant exempting provision. The Commission shall keep minutes that fully and clearly describe all matters discussed in a meeting and shall provide a full and accurate summary of actions taken, and the reasons therefore, including a description of the views expressed. All documents considered in connection with an action shall be identified in such minutes. All minutes and documents of a closed meeting shall remain under seal, subject to release by a majority vote of the Commission or order of a court of competent jurisdiction.

C. The Commission shall, by a majority vote of the delegates, prescribe bylaws and/or rules to govern its conduct as may be necessary or appropriate to carry out the purposes and exercise the powers of the compact, including but not limited to:

1. Establishing the fiscal year of the Commission;
2. Providing reasonable standards and procedures:
    a. for the establishment and meetings of other committees; and
    b. governing any general or specific delegation of any authority or function of the Commission;
3. Providing reasonable procedures for calling and conducting meetings of the Commission, ensuring reasonable advance notice of all meetings, and providing an opportunity for attendance of such meetings by interested parties, with enumerated exceptions designed to protect the public's interest, the privacy of individuals, and proprietary information, including trade secrets. The Commission may meet in closed session only after a majority of the membership votes to close a meeting in whole or in part. As soon as practicable, the Commission must make public a copy of the vote to close the meeting revealing the vote of each member with no proxy votes allowed;

4. Establishing the titles, duties and authority, and reasonable procedures for the election of the officers of the Commission;
5. Providing reasonable standards and procedures for the establishment of the personnel policies and programs of the Commission. Notwithstanding any civil service or other similar laws of any member state, the bylaws shall exclusively govern the personnel policies and programs of the Commission;
6. Promulgating a code of ethics to address permissible and prohibited activities of Commission members and employees;
7. Providing a mechanism for winding up the operations of the Commission and the equitable disposition of any surplus funds that may exist after the termination of the Compact after the payment and/or reserving of all of its debts and obligations;
8. The Commission shall publish its bylaws and file a copy thereof, and a copy of any amendment thereto, with the appropriate agency or officer in each of the member states, if any.
9. The Commission shall maintain its financial records in accordance with the bylaws.
10. The Commission shall meet and take such actions as are consistent with the provisions of this Compact and the bylaws.

D. The Commission shall have the following powers:
1. The authority to promulgate uniform rules to facilitate and coordinate implementation and administration of this Compact. The rules shall have the force and effect of law and shall be binding in all member states;
2. To bring and prosecute legal proceedings or actions in the name of the Commission, provided that the standing of any state EMS authority or other regulatory body responsible for EMS personnel licensure to sue or be sued under applicable law shall not be affected;
3. To purchase and maintain insurance and bonds;
4. To borrow, accept, or contract for services of personnel, including, but not limited to, employees of a member state;
5. To hire employees, elect or appoint officers, fix compensation, define duties, grant such individuals appropriate authority to carry out the purposes of the compact, and to establish the Commission's personnel policies and programs relating to conflicts of interest, qualifications of personnel, and other related personnel matters;
6. To accept any and all appropriate donations and grants of money, equipment, supplies, materials and services, and to receive, utilize and dispose of the same; provided that at all times the Commission shall strive to avoid any appearance of impropriety and/or conflict of interest;
7. To lease, purchase, accept appropriate gifts or donations of, or otherwise to own, hold, improve or use, any property, real, personal or mixed; provided that at all times the Commission shall strive to avoid any appearance of impropriety;
8. To sell, convey, mortgage, pledge, lease, exchange, abandon, or otherwise dispose of any property real, personal, or mixed;
9. To establish a budget and make expenditures;
10. To borrow money;
11. To appoint committees, including advisory committees comprised of members, state regulators, state legislators or their representatives, and consumer representatives, and such other interested persons as may be designated in this compact and the bylaws;
12. To provide and receive information from, and to cooperate with, law enforcement agencies;
13. To adopt and use an official seal; and
14. To perform such other functions as may be necessary or appropriate to achieve the purposes of this Compact consistent with the state regulation of EMS personnel licensure and practice.

E. Financing of the Commission
   1. The Commission shall pay, or provide for the payment of, the reasonable expenses of its establishment, organization, and ongoing activities.
   2. The Commission may accept any and all appropriate revenue sources, donations, and grants of money, equipment, supplies, materials, and services.
   3. The Commission may levy on and collect an annual assessment from each member state or impose fees on other parties to cover the cost of the operations and activities of the Commission and its staff, which must be in a total amount sufficient to cover its annual budget as approved each year for which revenue is not provided by other sources. The aggregate annual assessment amount shall be allocated based upon a formula to be determined by the Commission, which shall promulgate a rule binding upon all member states.
   4. The Commission shall not incur obligations of any kind prior to securing the funds adequate to meet the same; nor shall the Commission pledge the credit of any of the member states, except by and with the authority of the member state.
   5. The Commission shall keep accurate accounts of all receipts and disbursements. The receipts and disbursements of the Commission shall be subject to the audit and accounting procedures established under its bylaws. However, all receipts and disbursements of funds handled by the Commission shall be audited yearly by a certified or licensed public accountant, and the report of the audit shall be included in and become part of the annual report of the Commission.

F. Qualified Immunity, Defense, and Indemnification
   1. The members, officers, executive director, employees and representatives of the Commission shall be immune from suit and liability, either personally or in their official capacity, for any claim for damage to or loss of property or personal injury or other civil liability caused by or arising out of any actual or alleged act, error or omission that occurred, or that the person against whom the claim is made had a reasonable basis for believing occurred within the scope of Commission employment, duties or responsibilities; provided that nothing in this paragraph shall be construed to protect any such person from suit and/or liability for any damage, loss, injury, or liability caused by the intentional or willful or wanton misconduct of that person.
   2. The Commission shall defend any member, officer, executive director, employee or representative of the Commission in any civil action seeking to impose liability arising out of any actual or alleged act, error, or omission that occurred within the scope of Commission employment, duties, or responsibilities, or that the person against whom the claim is made had a reasonable basis for believing occurred within the scope of Commission employment, duties, or responsibilities; provided that nothing herein shall be construed to prohibit that person from retaining his or her own counsel; and provided further, that the actual or alleged act, error, or omission did not result from that person's intentional or willful or wanton misconduct.
   3. The Commission shall indemnify and hold harmless any member, officer, executive director, employee, or representative of the Commission for the amount of any settlement or judgment obtained against that person arising out of any actual or alleged act, error or omission that occurred within the scope of Commission employment, duties, or responsibilities, or that such person had a reasonable basis for believing occurred within the scope of Commission employment, duties, or responsibilities, provided that the actual or alleged act, error, or omission did not result from the intentional or willful or wanton misconduct of that person.

SECTION 11. COORDINATED DATABASE

A. The Commission shall provide for the development and maintenance of a coordinated database and reporting system containing licensure, adverse action, and significant investigatory information on all licensed individuals in member states.

B. Notwithstanding any other provision of state law to the contrary, a member state shall submit a uniform data set to the coordinated database on all individuals to whom this compact is applicable as required by the rules of the Commission, including:
   1. Identifying information;
   2. Licensure data;
   3. Significant investigatory information;
   4. Adverse actions against an individual's license;
   5. An indicator that an individual's privilege to practice is restricted, suspended or revoked;
   6. Non-confidential information related to alternative program participation;
   7. Any denial of application for licensure, and the reason(s) for such denial; and
   8. Other information that may facilitate the administration of this Compact, as determined by the rules of the Commission.

C. The coordinated database administrator shall promptly notify all member states of any adverse action taken against, or significant investigative information on, any individual in a member state.

D. Member states contributing information to the coordinated database may designate information that may not be shared with the public without the express permission of the contributing state.

E. Any information submitted to the coordinated database that is subsequently required to be expunged by the laws of the member state contributing the information shall be removed from the coordinated database.

SECTION 12. RULEMAKING

A. The Commission shall exercise its rulemaking powers pursuant to the criteria set forth in this Section and the rules adopted thereunder. Rules and amendments shall become binding as of the date specified in each rule or amendment.

B. If a majority of the legislatures of the member states rejects a rule, by enactment of a statute or resolution in the same manner used to adopt the Compact, then such rule shall have no further force and effect in any member state.

C. Rules or amendments to the rules shall be adopted at a regular or special meeting of the Commission.

D. Prior to promulgation and adoption of a final rule or rules by the Commission, and at least sixty (60) days in advance of the meeting at which the rule will be considered and voted upon, the Commission shall file a Notice of Proposed Rulemaking:
   1. On the website of the Commission; and
   2. On the website of each member state EMS authority or the publication in which each state would otherwise publish proposed rules.

E. The Notice of Proposed Rulemaking shall include:
   1. The proposed time, date, and location of the meeting in which the rule will be considered and voted upon;
   2. The text of the proposed rule or amendment and the reason for the proposed rule;
   3. A request for comments on the proposed rule from any interested person; and
   4. The manner in which interested persons may submit notice to the Commission of their intention to attend the public hearing and any written comments.

F. Prior to adoption of a proposed rule, the Commission shall allow persons to submit written data, facts, opinions, and arguments, which shall be made available to the public.

G. The Commission shall grant an opportunity for a public hearing before it adopts a rule or amendment if a hearing is requested by:
   1. At least twenty-five (25) persons;
   2. A governmental subdivision or agency; or
   3. An association having at least twenty-five (25) members.

H. If a hearing is held on the proposed rule or amendment, the Commission shall publish the place, time, and date of the scheduled public hearing.
    1. All persons wishing to be heard at the hearing shall notify the executive director of the Commission or other designated member in writing of their desire to appear and testify at the hearing not less than five (5) business days before the scheduled date of the hearing.
    2. Hearings shall be conducted in a manner providing each person who wishes to comment a fair and reasonable opportunity to comment orally or in writing.
    3. No transcript of the hearing is required, unless a written request for a transcript is made, in which case the person requesting the transcript shall bear the cost of producing the transcript. A recording may be made in lieu of a transcript under the same terms and conditions as a transcript. This subsection shall not preclude the Commission from making a transcript or recording of the hearing if it so chooses.
    4. Nothing in this section shall be construed as requiring a separate hearing on each rule. Rules may be grouped for the convenience of the Commission at hearings required by this section.

I. Following the scheduled hearing date, or by the close of business on the scheduled hearing date if the hearing was not held, the Commission shall consider all written and oral comments received.

J. The Commission shall, by majority vote of all members, take final action on the proposed rule and shall determine the effective date of the rule, if any, based on the rulemaking record and the full text of the rule.

K. If no written notice of intent to attend the public hearing by interested parties is received, the Commission may proceed with promulgation of the proposed rule without a public hearing.

L. Upon determination that an emergency exists, the Commission may consider and adopt an emergency rule without prior notice, opportunity for comment, or hearing, provided that the usual rulemaking procedures provided in the Compact and in this section shall be retroactively applied to the rule as soon as reasonably possible, in no event later than ninety (90) days after the effective date of the rule. For the purposes of this provision, an emergency rule is one that must be adopted immediately in order to:
    1. Meet an imminent threat to public health, safety, or welfare;
    2. Prevent a loss of Commission or member state funds;
    3. Meet a deadline for the promulgation of an administrative rule that is established by federal law or rule; or
    4. Protect public health and safety.

M. The Commission or an authorized committee of the Commission may direct revisions to a previously adopted rule or amendment for purposes of correcting typographical errors, errors in format, errors in consistency, or grammatical errors. Public notice of any revisions shall be posted on the website of the Commission. The revision shall be subject to challenge by any person for a period of thirty (30) days after posting. The revision may be challenged only on grounds that the revision results in a material change to a rule. A challenge shall be made in writing, and delivered to the chair of the Commission prior to the end of the notice period. If no challenge is made, the revision will take effect without further action. If the revision is challenged, the revision may not take effect without the approval of the Commission.

SECTION 13. OVERSIGHT, DISPUTE RESOLUTION, AND ENFORCEMENT

A. Oversight
    1. The executive, legislative, and judicial branches of state government in each member state shall enforce this compact and take all actions necessary and appropriate to effectuate the compact's purposes and intent. The provisions of this compact and the rules promulgated hereunder shall have standing as statutory law.

2. All courts shall take judicial notice of the compact and the rules in any judicial or administrative proceeding in a member state pertaining to the subject matter of this compact which may affect the powers, responsibilities or actions of the Commission.
3. The Commission shall be entitled to receive service of process in any such proceeding, and shall have standing to intervene in such a proceeding for all purposes. Failure to provide service of process to the Commission shall render a judgment or order void as to the Commission, this Compact, or promulgated rules.

B. Default, Technical Assistance, and Termination
1. If the Commission determines that a member state has defaulted in the performance of its obligations or responsibilities under this compact or the promulgated rules, the Commission shall:
    a. Provide written notice to the defaulting state and other member states of the nature of the default, the proposed means of curing the default and/or any other action to be taken by the Commission; and
    b. Provide remedial training and specific technical assistance regarding the default.
2. If a state in default fails to cure the default, the defaulting state may be terminated from the Compact upon an affirmative vote of a majority of the member states, and all rights, privileges and benefits conferred by this compact may be terminated on the effective date of termination. A cure of the default does not relieve the offending state of obligations or liabilities incurred during the period of default.
3. Termination of membership in the compact shall be imposed only after all other means of securing compliance have been exhausted. Notice of intent to suspend or terminate shall be given by the Commission to the governor, the majority and minority leaders of the defaulting state's legislature, and each of the member states.
4. A state that has been terminated is responsible for all assessments, obligations, and liabilities incurred through the effective date of termination, including obligations that extend beyond the effective date of termination.
5. The Commission shall not bear any costs related to a state that is found to be in default or that has been terminated from the compact, unless agreed upon in writing between the Commission and the defaulting state.
6. The defaulting state may appeal the action of the Commission by petitioning the U.S. District Court for the District of Columbia or the federal district where the Commission has its principal offices. The prevailing member shall be awarded all costs of such litigation, including reasonable attorney's fees.

C. Dispute Resolution
1. Upon request by a member state, the Commission shall attempt to resolve disputes related to the compact that arise among member states and between member and non-member states.
2. The Commission shall promulgate a rule providing for both mediation and binding dispute resolution for disputes as appropriate.

D. Enforcement
1. The Commission, in the reasonable exercise of its discretion, shall enforce the provisions and rules of this compact.
2. By majority vote, the Commission may initiate legal action in the United States District Court for the District of Columbia or the federal district where the Commission has its principal offices against a member state in default to enforce compliance with the provisions of the compact and its promulgated rules and bylaws. The relief sought may include both injunctive relief and damages. In the event judicial enforcement is necessary, the prevailing member shall be awarded all costs of such litigation, including reasonable attorney's fees.

3. The remedies herein shall not be the exclusive remedies of the Commission. The Commission may pursue any other remedies available under federal or state law.

SECTION 14. DATE OF IMPLEMENTATION OF THE INTERSTATE COMMISSION FOR EMS PERSONNEL PRACTICE AND ASSOCIATED RULES, WITHDRAWAL, AND AMENDMENT

A. The compact shall come into effect on the date on which the compact statute is enacted into law in the tenth member state. The provisions, which become effective at that time, shall be limited to the powers granted to the Commission relating to assembly and the promulgation of rules. Thereafter, the Commission shall meet and exercise rulemaking powers necessary to the implementation and administration of the compact.
B. Any state that joins the compact subsequent to the Commission's initial adoption of the rules shall be subject to the rules as they exist on the date on which the compact becomes law in that state. Any rule that has been previously adopted by the Commission shall have the full force and effect of law on the day the compact becomes law in that state.
C. Any member state may withdraw from this compact by enacting a statute repealing the same.
    1. A member state's withdrawal shall not take effect until six (6) months after enactment of the repealing statute.
    2. Withdrawal shall not affect the continuing requirement of the withdrawing state's EMS authority to comply with the investigative and adverse action reporting requirements of this act prior to the effective date of withdrawal.
D. Nothing contained in this compact shall be construed to invalidate or prevent any EMS personnel licensure agreement or other cooperative arrangement between a member state and a non-member state that does not conflict with the provisions of this compact.
E. This Compact may be amended by the member states. No amendment to this Compact shall become effective and binding upon any member state until it is enacted into the laws of all member states.

SECTION 15. CONSTRUCTION AND SEVERABILITY

This Compact shall be liberally construed so as to effectuate the purposes thereof. If this compact shall be held contrary to the constitution of any state member thereto, the compact shall remain in full force and effect as to the remaining member states. Nothing in this compact supersedes state law or rules related to licensure of EMS agencies.

1978 DOT Model EMS Legislation

By 1978, the DOT had over a decade of experience in working towards EMS system development under the Highway Safety Act, however according to the EMS Act, the DHEW was the designated lead federal agency for EMS system development in the United States. Each federal agency had unique EMS system requirements, ultimately contributing to confusion, duplication, and fragmentation of efforts.[160]

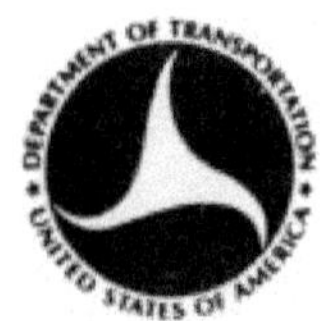

U.S. DEPARTMENT OF TRANSPORTATION
NATIONAL HIGHWAY TRAFFIC SAFETY ADMINISTRATION
WASHINGTON, D.C. 20590

JAN 31 1978 IN REPLY REFER TO:

NTS-13-01

TO: State and Local Officials

This document contains Model State Legislation for a comprehensive Emergency Medical Service (EMS) program. This Model is a revision of EMS Model Legislation developed in 1972 and published as Appendix I of Highway Safety Program Manual #11. This Model contains additional material which has been found to be necessary for a State to have an effective EMS program. As such, it contains reference to both basic and advanced life support procedures along with Federal criteria for uniform care, service identity and system development.

The major purpose of the Model Law is to provide a reference for preparing legislation establishing a statewide EMS program. To accomplish this, the Model provides for a State agency to manage the program and, further, provides this agency with the power to promulate regulations or standards on EMS activities. The agency's management function includes statewide coordination for the planning and implementation of EMS activities at the local/regional levels. The agency's regulatory authority includes EMS personnel training, equipment specifications and placement, necessary communications for rapid response, and standards for the care of injured persons. The agency is provided this regulatory authority to assure that quality life support systems are provided throughout the State.

This model, if adopted and supported by every State, will help continue the advancement toward a nationwide uniform practice of administering EMS activities which would result in bringing uniform emergency medical services to all of the Nation's citizens

Sincerely,

Joan Claybrook
Administrator

Model Legislation for Emergency Medical Services

March 1978

Traffic Safety Programs

Office of Driver and Pedestrian Programs

Enforcement and Emergency Services Division

Preface

The Highway Safety Act of 1966, as amended, requires Governors to be responsible for the administration of their State's highway safety program which includes emergency medical services. Therefore, all pertinent parts of the State government, as well as the citizenry, are responsible for carrying out the program. Also, the actions or inactions of any of the aforementioned parties positively or negatively affect the State's total program efforts. Clearly, Congress did not intend to limit the actions necessary for implementing the program only to those under the Governor's direct control. The legislature, for example, shares responsibility for the program with the Governor. According to the US. Department of Transportation (DOT), the failure of the legislature to enact essential legislation represents a decision on the part of the citizens of the State not to implement the program and to accept unimpeded rates of mortality and morbidity. It is incumbent, then, upon the whole of the State to assume responsibility for an effective and total highway safety program. This includes timely implementation of program elements, such as Standard II, Emergency Medical Services, for developing an effective statewide emergency medical care services (EMS) system.

In view of the widespread national deficiencies in emergency medical services, the States and the citizens cannot afford to abrogate basic provisions of State legislation or other forms of requirement, nor shall they evade enactment of State legislation designed to ensure adequate emergency ambulance service for the sick and injured. The objective of Standard II is to upgrade pre-hospital emergency care throughout the nation by improving training, communications, organization, and equipment in accordance with national uniform standards. For example, DOT views licensing and certification as appropriate tools for a State to use to achieve and maintain a desired level of competence. Rapid transit alone is insufficient support for a seriously ill or injured person whose life might be sustained with proper care; it is important to preclude avoidable death or permanent injury at the scene, in transit, and upon arrival at the hospital.

The States have made commendable progress toward upgrading emergency medical services. It is the intent of this model to help document that progress and to ensure its continuation. It is also a firm hope that it will aid in achieving a nationally uniform high level of care with perpetuity. In this latter regard, it is pertinent to note that exclusions were omitted. The primary reason being that any form of legislation or regulation which is designed to ensure quality emergency medical care can be most ineffective if significant numbers of purveyors are excused. This is both grossly unfair to those who must comply as well as to victims of emergencies who are served by those sub-standard services which result from authorization to evade requirements for providing quality care.

MODEL LEGISLATION

The law is the witness and external deposit of our moral life. It's history is the history of the moral development of the race.

– Oliver Wendell Holmes, Jr.

Section 1–Purpose

This Act establishes a comprehensive emergency medical services (EMS) program in the *(State agency)*. All responsibilities for this program shall be vested in the *(public official)* and such other officers, boards, agencies, organizations, entities, and commissions as shall be specified by law, rules, or regulations adopted pursuant to this Act.

This Act is to encourage and assist in the creation and operation of regional emergency medical services (EMS) entities, and to enable and assist providers of emergency medical services in the delivery of *(adequate) (appropriate) (effective) (quality)* emergency medical services for all the people of *(State)* and the provision of medical care during disaster situations.

Section 2–Definitions

As used in this Act, or in rules and regulations promulgated pursuant to this Act:

"Advanced life support" **shall mean an advanced level of pre-hospital and inter-hospital emergency care that includes basic life support functions (including cardiopulmonary resuscitation (CPR)), plus cardiac monitoring, cardiac defibrillation, telemetered electro-**cardiography, administration of antiarrhythmic agents, intravenous therapy, administration of specific medications, drugs, and solutions, use of adjunctive medical devices, trauma care, and other authorized techniques and procedures;

"Advanced life support personnel" shall mean persons other than physicians engaged in the provision of advanced life support, as defined and regulated by rules and regulations promulgated pursuant to this Act;

"Ambulance" shall mean any publicly or privately owned vehicle that is specifically designed, constructed or modified, and equipped, and is intended to be used for and is maintained or operated for the transportation upon the streets or highways of this State of persons who are sick, injured, wounded, or otherwise incapacitated or helpless.

"Central communications system" shall mean a radio and communications command and control center responsible for accepting calls from the public for emergency medical services, for dispatching emergency medical services personnel and vehicles, for radio coordination of emergency medical services vehicles and personnel, for coordination of medical communications between emergency medical services personnel and public safety agencies, for coordination and management of radio frequencies devoted to biomedical telemetry, and, where applicable, for hospital paging operations;

"Consumer" shall mean a resident of the State who is a recipient or potential recipient of the services provided by an emergency medical services system, who receives no direct or indirect personal, financial, or professional benefit as a result of association with health care or emergency services other than that generally shared by the public at large, and who is not otherwise considered a "provider" within the intent of this Act;

"Disaster situation" shall mean any condition or situation that could be described as "mass casualties," "major emergency," "natural disaster," or "national emergency;"

"Emergency medical services" shall mean the services utilized in responding to the perceived individual needs for immediate medical care in order to prevent loss of life or aggravation of physiological illness or injury;

"Emergency medical technician–ambulance" shall mean persons trained in emergency medical care in accordance with standards prescribed by this Act, or by rules and regulations pursuant to this Act, who provide emergency medical services in accord with their respective levels of training, which may range from basic life support to advanced life support;

"Emergency medical technician–paramedic" shall mean a person trained and authorized to provide advanced life support services;

"Good faith" shall mean *(utilize adjudicated definition issued by highest State court)*;

"Gross negligence" shall mean *(utilize adjudicated definition issued by highest State court)*;

"Local government" shall mean any county, city, *(township, town, village)* in this State;

"Major emergencies" shall mean any emergency events that cannot be resolved through the use of emergency resources that are locally available;

"Mass casualties" shall mean those emergency events that result in ____ or more persons being injured, incapacitated, made ill, or killed;

"Medical community" shall mean the aggregate physician and medical specialist resources located and available within a definable geographic area;

"Medical control" shall mean directions and advice provided from a centrally designated medical facility staffed by appropriate personnel, operating under medical supervision, supplying professional support through radio or telephonic communication for on-site and in-transit basic and advanced life support services given by field and satellite facility personnel;

"Medical emergency" shall mean an unforeseen event affecting an individual in such a manner that a need for immediate medical care (physiological or psychological) is created;

"National emergencies" shall mean any conditions that shall cause the President of the United States to declare a national emergency;

"Natural disaster" shall mean any natural condition or act of God that shall result in disorder, hazard, illness, injury, or death to large numbers of citizens, or that shall present a potential for such disorder, hazard, illness, injury, or death;

"Patient" shall mean an individual who as a result of illness or injury needs immediate medical attention, whose physical or mental condition is such that he/she is in imminent danger of loss of life or significant health impairment, or who may be otherwise incapacitated or helpless as a result or a physical or mental condition;

"Person" shall mean any person, firm, partnership, association, corporation, company, or group of individuals acting together for a common purpose or organization of any kind, including any government agency, other than an agency of the United States government;

"Policy direction" shall mean generalized guidance over goals, objectives, strategies, and financial matters, but shall not extend to routine administration and supervision of personnel;

"Pre-hospital care" shall mean those emergency medical services rendered to emergency patients out of the hospital setting, administered for analytic, stabilizing, or preventive purposes, precedent to and during transportation of such patients to emergency treatment facilities;

"Provider" shall mean a person or the spouse of a person who, as an individual or member of a corporation or organization, whether profit making or nonprofit, on a regular basis gives or offers for sale any supplies, equipment, professional or nonprofessional services, or

is capable of giving or offering for sale supplies, equipment, or services vital or incidental to the functions of an emergency medical services system;

"Public safety personnel" shall mean police officers, firefighters, communications and dispatch specialists, and other public employees charged with maintaining the public safety;

"Region" shall mean, to the greatest extent possible, a geographical area to be of sufficient size, population, and economic diversity so that an efficient and economically feasible emergency medical services system can be established within the boundaries of the said area, taking into consideration existing medical service patterns and health planning areas;

"Regional EMS Advisory Council" shall mean a body or group of individuals, organized and functioning in accordance with Section 5 of this Act, to serve as the policy-making body for its respective regional EMS entity;

"Regional EMS delivery system" shall mean a single entity either private or governmental, either profit making or nonprofit, which possesses the authority and responsibility to organize, direct, administer, provide, and finance all or most of the emergency medical services functions within the entirety of its designated region;

"Regional EMS entity" shall mean a single agency or organization, being a unit of local government, or a public entity administering a compact, a consortium or other regional arrangement, or any other public or nonprofit private entity, which shall be chartered or incorporated by the State, which shall have the capacity and authority to receive and disburse public funds, which shall be organized to accommodate a Regional EMS Advisory Council as its policy-making body, which shall comply with all applicable provisions of this Act, and which shall successfully apply to the *(State official)* for designation as a regional EMS entity;

"State EMS Advisory Council" shall mean the body of individuals appointed by the Governor with the advice and consent of the State Senate, organized and functioning in accordance with Section 4 of this Act, to serve as the advisory body to the *(State agency)* in its administration of the statewide emergency medical services program authorized by this Act;

"Voluntary" shall mean services provided entirely by volunteer personnel;

"Volunteer personnel" shall mean persons who provide services without expectation of remuneration, who do not receive payment for services rendered other than reimbursement for expenses, and who do not depend in any on the provision of such services for their livelihood.

Section 3–Authority of (State agency)

A. The *(State agency)* shall establish and maintain a program for the planning, development, improvement, expansion, and upgrading of emergency medical services throughout the State. The *(State agency)* shall consolidate all State functions relating to emergency medical services, both regulatory and developmental, under the auspices of this program.

B. The *(public official)* shall, after consulting with the State Emergency Medical Services (EMS) Advisory Council, and with such local governments as may be involved, seek the establishment of statewide, regional, and local emergency medical services operations in conformance with the standards established by this Act and by standards, rules, and regulations promulgated pursuant thereto.

C. The *(public official)* shall have full and complete responsibility for supervising and directing the *(State agency)* in its conduct of the program provided for by this Act.

D. Pursuant to the authority of this Act, and of *(other applicable laws)*, the *(State agency)* shall:

(1) Assist in the creation and operation of regional emergency medical services (EMS) entities for the effective and efficient planning, development, coordination, supervision, regulation, monitoring, and/or provision of emergency medical services for all citizens of the States;

(2) In cooperation with State and regional health planning agencies, define the boundaries

of EMS regions and regional EMS delivery systems, to the extent that all areas of the State shall be within defined EMS regions or EMS delivery systems;

(3) In consultation with the State EMS Advisory Council, develop a standardized planning format for regional EMS planning activities;

(4) Review, evaluate, and integrate all regional EMS plans, developed by the regional EMS entities pursuant to this Act, prepare a Statewide EMS Plan, to be completed no later than *(date)*, and publish the said Statewide EMS Plan for distribution to all concerned agencies, entities, and individuals throughout the State. The Statewide EMS Plan, as a minimum, shall contain:

(a) An inventory of emergency medical services resources available within the State for purposes of determining the need for additional services and the effectiveness of existing services;

(b) A statement of goals and specific and measurable objectives for delivery of emergency medical services to all citizens of the State;

(c) Methods to be used in achieving the stated objectives;

(d) A schedule for achievement of the stated objectives;

(e) A method for evaluating the stated objectives; and

(f) Estimated and itemized costs for achieving each of the stated objectives;

(5) Update and republish the Statewide (comprehensive) EMS Plan at least every ____ years;

(6) Develop regional EMS plans for designated EMS regions in the event that no approved regional plan is developed by a regional EMS entity created pursuant to the authority of the Act; provided, that the regional EMS plans thus developed shall conform to the format adopted pursuant to Section 3,D(3) of this Act;

(7) Use all reasonable and lawful means to ensure that all EMS regions and regional EMS delivery systems include an adequate number of health professionals, allied health professionals, and other health personnel, including ambulance personnel, with appropriate training and experience, to provide emergency medical services on a 24-hour basis within the service areas of the regions or systems;

(8) Promulgate and enforce minimum training standards, including certification requirements, for all personnel, whether volunteer or paid, who provide emergency medical services within the State, including public safety personnel; provided, that such training standards shall meet or exceed current standards adopted by the U.S. Department of Transportation and the U.S. Department of Health, Education, and Welfare;

(9) Consistent with Rules of the Federal Communications Commission, design, develop, implement, and coordinate central communications systems to join the personnel, facilities, and equipment of an EMS region or system in a manner that will, as a minimum, provide for medical control of pre-hospital care rendered by ambulance personnel, advanced life support personnel, or other allied health professionals;

(10) Promulgate and enforce standards, rules, and regulations that will ensure all citizens access to emergency medical services through use of either the universal emergency telephone number 911 or a single seven-digit number that is common to an entire region prior to *(date)*;

(11) Use all reasonable and lawful means to ensure that all EMS regions and regional EMS delivery systems include an adequate but appropriate number of necessary ground, air, and water ambulance vehicles and other transportation facilities to meet the individual characteristics of the service areas of the regions or systems;

(12) Promulgate and enforce minimum standards, including inspection, operational, and licensing requirements, for all ambulance vehicles, whether operated by voluntary, commercial, or governmental agencies or organizations; provided, that such standards shall meet or exceed Federal specifications for emergency medical care vehicles (Federal Specification, Ambulance, Emergency Medical Care Vehicle, General Services Administration, KKK-A-1822, January 2, 1974, as amended) and the American College of Surgeons' current recommendations for ambulance equipment (entitled "Essential Equipment for Ambulances").

(13) Promulgate and enforce minimum standards for transportation of both ambulatory and nonambulatory patients who do not need emergency care to appropriate destinations including health care, extended care, and rehabilitation facilities;

(14) Use all reasonable and lawful means to ensure that emergency patients will in all cases be transported from the scene of the medical emergency to the nearest emergency treatment facility that possesses the structural equipment and staff resources to immediately attend to the particular patient's medical needs, with the understanding that in some cases it will be necessary to bypass the closest medical facility;

(15) Use all reasonable and lawful means to ensure that emergency patients, where needed, will have access, including appropriate transportation, to specialized critical medical care units within the service areas of the regions or systems, or, if there are no such units or an inadequate number of them in such service areas, ensure that emergency patients, where needed, will have access to such units in neighboring areas if access is feasible in terms of time and distance;

(16) Use all reasonable and lawful means to ensure that necessary emergency medical services are provided to all patients requiring such services without prior inquiry as to ability to pay;

(17) Design, develop, implement, and coordinate systems that will ensure and provide for transfer of patients to facilities and programs that offer such follow-up care and rehabilitation as are necessary to effect the maximum recovery by the patient; provided, that such systems shall provide a method for ensuring that such transfers are consistent with accepted medical practice to serve the best interests of the patient and are not based on financial considerations alone;

(18) Design, develop, implement, and coordinate a standardized emergency patient data collection system for use throughout the State that records and accumulates all relevant information concerning treatment and care of emergency patients, from initial entry into an EMS system to and including discharge from such system and that utilizes reporting, recording, and informational formats that are consistent with ensuing patient records used in follow-up care and rehabilitation of patients; provided, that all other provisions of applicable law regarding confidentiality shall be respected and preserved in the design, development, implementation, and coordination of the said standardized emergency patient data collection system;

(19) Provide programs of public education and information for informing residents of and visitors to the State of the availability and proper use of emergency medical services, of the value and nature of programs to involve citizens in the administering of prehospital emergency care (including cardiopulmonary resuscitation (CPR)), and of the availability of training programs in emergency care for members of the general public;

(20) Provide for ongoing or periodic comprehensive evaluation of the availability and quality of emergency medical services provided throughout the State, and report annually to the State EMS Advisory Council the content and conclusions of such comprehensive evaluation;

(21) In cooperation with *(State agency with primary responsibility for disaster coordination)*, develop, implement, and coordinate plans to ensure that emergency medical services will be provided at any time mass casualties, major emergencies, natural disasters, or national emergencies occur within the State or affect the people of the State;

(22) In cooperation with appropriate agencies of all adjoining or neighboring States, develop, implement, and coordinate plans and arrangements that will ensure that all necessary emergency medical services, including transfers of patients, are provided without undue concern for State boundaries;

(23) Where specifically authorized by an Act of the *(State Legislature)*, and subject to the provisions of this Act and the Statewide EMS Plan, award grants and contracts to regional EMS entities for purposes of carrying out specific objectives delineated in regional EMS plans;

(24) Within 45 days of their receipt, review and comment on all grant and contract applications for Federal, State, or private funds concerning emergency medical services or related activities, and forward those applications to appropriate agencies, organizations, or funding sources; provided, that an application not acted on by the *(State agency)* within 45 days shall be considered reviewed and favorably commented on.

Section 4–State Emergency Medical Services (EMS) Advisory Council

A. Pursuant to Section 1 of this Act, there shall be a comprehensive emergency medical services (EMS) program. In the (*State agency*), all responsibility for this program shall be vested in the (*public official*) and such other officers, boards, agencies, organizations, entities, and commissions as shall be specified by law, rules, or regulations adopted pursuant to this Act.

B. There shall be established with the *(State agency)* a State Emergency Medical Services (EMS) Advisory Council, composed of ____ members.

C. Membership on the State EMS Advisory Council shall be by appointment of the Governor with the advice and consent of the State Senate.

D. The State EMS Advisory Council shall include three (3) licensed practicing physicians with regular and frequent involvement in the provision of emergency care, and one representative from each of the following groups: (a) fire protection organizations; (b) law enforcement agencies; (c) hospitals; (d) ambulance service organization; (e) emergency care nurses; and (f) emergency medical technicians. There shall also be _____ members who are consumers, with at least one of said consumers to be appointed from Regional Emergency Medical Services (EMS) Councils established pursuant to Section 6 of this Act.

E. State agencies and private, nonprofit service agencies may participate as non-voting exofficio members of the State EMS Advisory Council, subject to the discretion of the Chairperson of the said Council.

F. At least one provider member of the State EMS Advisory Council shall be appointed from each Regional EMS Council. Provider members of the State EMS Advisory Council may be recommended to the Governor by their respective Regional EMS Councils, by provider groups, or both.

G. Of the members first appointed to the State EMS Advisory Council by the Governor, ____ members shall be appointed for a term of two years, and ____ members for a term of three years. An equal number of consumer and provider members shall be selected for the first two year term. Subsequent appointees shall serve three year terms.

H. Per diem allotments to members of the State EMS Advisory Council, and schedules for reimbursement of members' expenses, shall be established by the *(State legislature)*.

I. ____ members shall constitute a quorum for the transaction of business by the State EMS

Advisory Council, more than half of whom shall be consumers. The Chairperson shall be a consumer elected annually from the membership of the Council. The Council shall meet at least four times annually at the call of the Chairperson or the *(public official)*.

J. All meetings of the State EMS Advisory Council shall be conducted in open, public sessions, at such hours and in such locations, and subject to methods of notification, which will encourage and facilitate attendance by interested persons.

K. The State EMS Advisory Council shall:

(1) Approve or disapprove a proposed Statewide EMS Plan, as prepared by the *(State agency)*, pursuant to Section 3,D(4) of this Act; provided, that if any such proposed Statewide EMS Plan is not disapproved by the State EMS Advisory Council within 45 days of its submission to the Council in open meeting, it shall be considered approved;

(2) Approve or disapprove any proposed revisions to the Statewide EMS Plan, as prepared by the *(State agency)*, pursuant to Section 3,D(5) of this Act; provided, that if any such proposed revision to the Statewide EMS Plan is not disapproved by the State EMS Advisory Council within 45 days of its submission to the Council in open meeting, it shall be considered approved;

(3) Advise the *(State agency)* on all aspects of its responsibilities pursuant to Section 3 of this Act, including the format and content of any standards, rules, or regulations promulgated by the *(State agency)*;

(4) Serve as the Statewide focal point for discussion, inquiry, and investigation of any and all complaints and/or grievances concerning emergency medical services, or any aspect thereof, which are brought to the Council's attention from any source;

(5) Oversee the *(State agency)* in the conduct of its enforcement of this Act, or any standards, rules, and regulations promulgated pursuant thereto;

(6) Review and comment on all proposals to apply and/or applications for Federal, State, local, and private funds (under either grants or contracts) which may be prepared, developed, and submitted to funding sources or agencies by regional EMS entities within the State.

Section 5–Regional Emergency Medical Services (EMS) Advisory Councils

A. Pursuant to Section 3,B of this Act, the *(public official)* shall, after consulting with the State Emergency Medical Services (EMS) Advisory Council, and with such local governments as may be involved, seek the establishment of Statewide, regional, and local emergency medical services operations in conformance with the standards established by this Act and by standards, rules, and regulations promulgated pursuant thereto.

B. Pursuant to Section 3,D(1) of this Act, the *(State agency)* shall assist in the creation and operation of regional emergency medical services (EMS) entities for the effective and efficient planning, development, coordination, supervision, regulation, monitoring, and/or provision of emergency medical services for all citizens of the State.

C. Regional entities are defined in Section 2 of this Act.

D. Each regional EMS entity officially designated by the *(State official)* shall function under the policy direction of a Regional EMS Advisory Council

E. Each Regional EMS Advisory Council shall:

(1) Be formally and officially established as the policy making body for its respective regional EMS entity;

(2) Be acknowledged by resolution of the elected representatives of at least two-thirds of the county and municipal governments located within the designated service area of its respective regional EMS entity;

(3) Provide the opportunity for council membership to representatives of the following organizations, groups, professions, occupations, services, and/or disciplines, as well as consumers: (a) local governments; (b) fire protection organizations; (c) law enforcement agencies; (d) licensed practicing physicians with regular and frequent involvement in the provision of emergency care; (e) emergency care nurses; (f) mental health professionals; (g) emergency medical technicians and other allied health practitioners; (h) providers of ambulance services, including both paid and volunteer services; (i) hospitals; provided, that consumers shall comprise at least ____ percent of the total number of Council members.

(4) Meet with adequate frequency to provide policy direction to the respective regional EMS entity, and to ensure that adequate information is transmitted from the regional EMS entity and the Regional EMS Advisory Council to the organizations, groups, professions, occupations, services, and/or disciplines, and consumers represented by the respective Council members;

(5) Conduct all council meetings in open, public sessions, at such hours and in such locations, and subject to methods of notification, that will encourage and facilitate attendance by interested persons;

(6) Cooperate with the respective regional EMS entity in the development of a regional EMS plan, and provide for public hearings on such a regional plan, with ample opportunity for public and professional response and contribution to the plan;

(7) Formally adopt a regional EMS plan within one year of official designation of the respective regional EMS entity;

(8) Cooperate with the regional EMS entity as it assists the *(State agency)* in the design, development, implementation, and coordination of the State's standardized emergency patient data collection system, and utilize information accumulated and reported through the said system for development and updating of the respective regional EMS plan, as well as maintenance or improvement of EMS services within the respective region;

(9) Serve as the regional focal point for discussion, inquiry, and investigation of any and all complaints and/or grievances concerning emergency medical services, or any aspect thereof, within the respective region or service area;

(10) Upon determination that corrective or punitive action is necessary or appropriate with regard to any matter related to emergency medical services within the respective region, direct a formal notice to the *(State agency)*, stating the nature of the problem, a description of the inquiry undertaken by the Regional EMS Advisory Council, a summary of conclusions, and recommended corrective or punitive measures to be taken or initiated by the *(State agency)*;

(11) Review and approve all applications for Federal, State, local, and private funds (under either grants or contracts) which may be prepared, developed, and submitted to funding sources or agencies by the respective regional EMS entity.

Section 6—Regional Emergency Medical Services (EMS) Entities

A. Pursuant to Section 3,B of this Act, the *(public official)* shall, after consulting with the State Emergency Medical Services (EMS) Advisory Council, and with such local governments as may be involved, seek the establishment of statewide, regional, and local emergency medical services operations in conformance with the standards established by this Act and by standards, rules, and regulations promulgated pursuant thereto.

B. Pursuant to Section 3,D(1) of this Act, the *(State agency)* shall assist in the creation and operation of regional emergency medical services (EMS) entities for the effective and efficient planning, development, coordination, supervision, regulation, monitoring, and/or provision of emergency medical services for all citizens of the State.

C. Regional EMS entities are defined in Section 2 of this Act.

D. Eligible regional EMS entities may apply to the *(State agency)* for official designation on forms or in a format approved by that *(agency)*. The intent of such application is to determine the fitness and ability of the applicant entities to serve in accord with the definition in Section 2 of this Act.

E. Official designation of regional EMS entities, or denial of any application for designation, shall be made by the *(public official)* and shall be communicated in writing to applicants within ninety (90) days of application.

F. Official designation of regional EMS entities shall be made by *(public official)* after appropriate evaluation and investigation of applicants, including an evaluation of staff and organizational resources and competencies, a determination of the applicant's ability to function appropriately within the entire area previously defined as an EMS region or regional EMS delivery system service area, and after consultation with the State EMS Advisory Council and with such local governments as may be involved.

G. Pursuant to the authority of this Act, and of *(other applicable laws)*, regional EMS entities shall:

(1) Seek and obtain official designation as a regional EMS entity;

(2) Function under the policy direction of a Regional EMS Advisory Council, as authorized by Section 4 of this Act;

(3) Within one year of official designation, develop a regional EMS plan that addresses, as a minimum, all EMS system components enumerated in Federal Emergency Medical Services Systems published criteria, and that contains, as a minimum: (a) an inventory of emergency medical services resources available within the EMS region or regional EMS delivery system service area for purposes of determining the need for additional services and the effectiveness of existing services; (b) a statement of goals and specific and measurable objectives for delivery of emergency medical services to all citizens of the EMS region or regional EMS delivery system services area; (c) methods to be used in achieving the stated objectives; (d) a schedule for achievement of the stated objectives; (e) a method for evaluating the stated objectives; and (f) estimated and itemized costs for achieving each of the stated objectives;

(4) Apply for and receive Federal, State, local, and private funds (under either grants or contracts) for planning, development, coordination, supervision, monitoring, improvement, and/or provision of emergency medical services within the designated area of the respective regional EMS entity;

(5) Assist the *(State agency)* in the design, development, implementation, and coordination of the State's standardized emergency patient data collection system, including the distribution of report forms, supervision of data collection, accumulation and auditing of reported information, cooperation with the *(State agency)* in statewide assimilation of reported information, distribution of periodic reports developed by the *(State agency)*, and use of the reported information for development and updating of the regional EMS plan, as well as maintenance or improvement of emergency medical services;

(6) Cooperate with the *(State agency)* in its efforts to carry out the authority and responsibility defined and enumerated in Section 3,D of this Act;

(7) Provide necessary and reasonable staff services for the respective Regional EMS Advisory Council;

(8) Provide an authorized delegate to all meetings of the State EMS Advisory Council;

(9) Provide convenient and appropriate office facilities that can serve as a regional focal point for EMS planning, development, and coordination functions.

H. Where deemed appropriate, the *(State agency)*, after consultation with the respective Regional EMS Advisory Council, may assign one or more employees of the *(State agency)* to serve as staff to the regional EMS entity for purposes of carrying out the intent and provisions of this Act.

I. Where deemed appropriate, competitive applications for designation as a regional EMS entity may be solicited by the *(public official)*.

J. Where deemed appropriate, the *(public official)*, after consultation with the State EMS Advisory Council, and subject to conditions and provisions of grants and contracts, may discontinue the official designation of a regional EMS entity where the best interests of emergency medical services in the respective region or regional EMS delivery system service area would be served by such action.

Section 7–Advanced Life Support Services

In authorizing the promulgation and enforcement of rules and regulations pursuant to this Section, it is the intent of this Act to respond to a critical shortage of professionally trained medical and nursing personnel for the delivery of fast and efficient life support skills to the ill and injured at the scene of medical emergencies, and during transport to a health care facility. Improved emergency medical services are required to reduce mortality during the first critical minutes immediately following an accident or the onset of a serious medical condition, and to reduce morbidity among survivors of medical emergencies. Within the goals of this Act, in authorizing the *(State agency) (Board) (Commission) (Medical authority) (etc.)* to promulgate and enforce rules and regulations, is the provision of the best and most effective emergency medical care, and compliance with national standards for advanced life support.

A. Notwithstanding any other provision of law, advanced life support personnel may be authorized to provide advanced life support services as defined by rules and regulations promulgated by the *(State agency) (Board) (Commission) (Medical authority) (etc.)*. Rules and regulations promulgated pursuant to this authority shall, as a minimum:

(1) Provide descriptive titles and define minimum prerequisites for advanced life support personnel;

(2) Define and authorize training programs for advanced life support personnel; provided, that all such training programs shall meet or exceed the performance requirements of the Training Program for the Emergency Medical Technician Paramedic, developed for the U.S. Department of Transportation under Contract No. DOT-HS-5-01207 (April 1976);

(3) Define and authorize appropriate advanced life support functions to be performed by advanced life support trainees and personnel;

(4) Specify minimum operational requirements that will ensure medical control over all advanced life support services;

(5) Specify minimum testing and certification requirements and provide for certification of all advanced life support personnel;

(6) Specify continuing education and periodic recertification requirements for all advanced life support personnel;

(7) Provide for the decertification of advanced life support personnel under specified circumstances and where it is determined that the best interests of the public would be served by such action;

(8) Require cooperation and compliance with regional and statewide standardized emergency patient data collection systems.

B. Advanced life support personnel, trained, certified, and functioning pursuant to the rules and regulations authorized by this Section, and agencies, organizations, institutions, corporations, or entities of State or local government, sponsoring, authorizing, supporting, financing, or supervising the functions of advanced life support personnel, shall be subject to all other provisions of this Act, and all other rules and regulations promulgated pursuant to the authority of this Act.

Section 8–Immunity from Liability

A. No person, certified and authorized pursuant to this Act or rules and regulations promulgated pursuant to this Act, shall be liable for any civil damages for any act or omission in connection with their training or in connection with services rendered outside a hospital where the life of a patient(s) is in immediate danger, unless the act or omission is inconsistent with the said person's training, and unless the act or omission was the result of gross negligence or willful misconduct.

B. No agency, organization, institution, corporation, or entity of State or local government that sponsors, authorizes, supports, finances, or supervises the functions of emergency medical services personnel certified and authorized pursuant to this Act, including advanced life support personnel, shall be liable for any civil damages for any act or omission in connection with sponsorship, authorization, support, finance, or supervision of such emergency medical services personnel, where the act or omission occurs in connection with their training or with services rendered outside a hospital and where the life of a patient(s) is in immediate danger, unless the act or omission is inconsistent with the training of the said emergency medical services personnel, and unless the act or omission was the result of gross negligence or willful misconduct.

C. No principal, agent, contractor, employee, or representative of an agency, organization, institution, corporation, or entity of State or local government that sponsors, authorizes, supports, finances, or supervises any functions of emergency medical services personnel certified and authorized pursuant to this Act, or rules and regulations promulgated pursuant to this Act, including advanced life support personnel shall be liable for any civil damages for any act or omission in connection with such sponsorship, authorization, support, finance, or supervision of such emergency medical services personnel, where the act or omission occurs in connection with their training, or occurs outside a hospital where the life of a patient(s) is in immediate danger, unless the act or omission is inconsistent with the training of the said emergency medical services personnel, and unless the act or omission was the result of gross negligence or willful misconduct.

D. No physician who in good faith arranges for, requests, recommends, or initiates the transfer of a patient from a hospital to a critical medical care facility in another hospital, shall be liable for any civil damages as a result of such transfer where sound medical judgment indicates that the patient's medical condition is beyond the care capability of the transferring hospital, or the medical community in which that hospital is located, and where the physician has confirmed that the transferee facility possesses a more appropriate level of capability for treating the patient's medical needs, and where the physician has secured a prior agreement from the transferee facility to accept and render necessary treatment to the patient.

Section 9–General Provisions

A. All standards, rules, and regulations promulgated pursuant to this Act shall be promulgated (and enforced) in compliance with *(any applicable statutory or Constitutional provision concerning promulgation (and enforcement) of standards, rules, and regulations).*

B. A local government may contract to obtain ambulance services for the use and benefit of its residents and may pay for the entire cost or any part thereof from funds that may be available. A local government that is a party to its share of the cost by special *(taxes) (assessments)* created, levied, collected, and annually determined in accord with procedures set forth in *(applicable State laws)*.

C. Authority for patient management in a medical emergency shall be vested in that licensed or certified person at the scene of the emergency who has the highest degree of training and/or certification specific to the provision of emergency medical care. If a licensed or certified person is not available at the scene of the emergency, the authority shall be vested in the most appropriately trained representative of other public safety agencies at the scene, and shall be effective until relieved by a person with a higher and more appropriate degree of training and certification specific to the provision of emergency medical care.

D. Authority for the management of the scene of a medical emergency shall be vested in appropriate public safety agencies. The scene of a medical emergency shall be managed in a manner designed to minimize the risk of death or health impairment to the patient and to other persons who may be exposed to the risks as a result of the emergency condition, and priority shall be placed upon the interests of those persons exposed to the more serious risks to life and health. Public safety personnel shall ordinarily consult emergency medical services personnel or other authoritative medical professionals at the scene in the determination of relevant risks.

E. Neither this Act nor rules and regulations promulgated pursuant to this Act shall apply to emergency medical services vehicles or personnel from another State or nation that render requested assistance in this State in a disaster situation, or that operate from a location outside this State and occasionally transport patients into this State for needed medical care. No emergency medical services vehicles nor personnel from another State or nation may be utilized to pick up and transport patients within this State without first complying with this Act and all standards, rules, and regulations promulgated pursuant to this Act.

F. The driver of an emergency medical services vehicle, when operating such vehicle under emergency conditions or a reasonable belief that an emergency condition does in fact exist, may exercise the privileges and be subject to the constraints prescribed by *(applicable State law)*.

G. The *(State agency)* may revoke any license, certificate, or other authorization provided for by this Act, or by rules and regulations promulgated pursuant to this Act, for failure to comply with, or for violation of, any of the provisions of this Act, or rules and regulations promulgated thereunder, but only after appropriate warning has occurred and reasonable time has been allowed for compliance in accord with procedural standards to be established by the *(State agency)*. Any person who wishes to appeal such a revocation must appeal to the *(State agency)* within ____ days of the revocation. Hearing shall thereafter be held in accord with *(applicable State law, or procedural standards to be established by the State agency)*. Within ____ days after conclusion of the hearing, the *(State agency)* shall issue a written decision that shall include a statement of findings as to the revocation. The written decision shall be promptly transmitted to the appellant by the *(State agency)*.

H. Upon revocation of any license, certificate, or other authorization provided for by this Act, or by rules and regulations promulgated pursuant to this Act, the person whose license, certificate, or other authorization has been revoked shall immediately cease to engage in the activity for which the license, certificate, or other authorization was issued.

I. No employer shall employ nor permit any employee to perform any services for which a license, certificate or other authorization is required by this Act, or by rules and regulations promulgated pursuant to this Act, unless and until the person so employed possesses all licenses, certificates, or authorizations that are so required.

J. Standards, rules, regulations, or requirements promulgated by the *(State agency)* pursuant to Section 3,D of this Act shall, as a minimum:

(1) Provide a fee structure for application and/or licenses, permits, certificates, or authorizations that may be required; provided, that agencies of State or local governments shall be exempt from paying fees;

(2) Require provider of emergency medical services to obtain and maintain policies of insurance, or acceptable means of self-insurance, in amounts and types of coverage as shall be deemed necessary by the *(State agency)*;

(3) Provide for all licenses, permits, certificates, or authorizations to be renewed and reissued annually, except that certification of *(specified classes of emergency medical services personnel)* shall be subject to renewal every ____ years;

(4) Provide that all licenses, permits, certificates, or authorizations issued by the *(State agency)* shall not be transferable;

(5) Provide for semiannual inspections of all emergency medical services vehicles and ambulance service facilities where said vehicles and/or facilities are subject to regulations by the *(State agency)*;

(6) Provide minimum equipment, maintenance, and operational standards for vehicles routinely used, or designated as available for use in providing pre-hospital emergency care and life support, but that are not designed for, nor capable of, transporting emergency patients;

(7) Provide for minimum staffing requirements for all emergency care vehicles, including the requirement that no ambulance vehicle shall be allowed to operate while transporting a patient or patients unless at least one certified emergency medical technician is attending to the patient(s);

K. Pursuant to the authority of Section 3,D(12) of this Act, the *(State agency)* may set standards for regulate the use of descriptive words, phrases, symbols, and/or emblems that represent or denote that a service is available or may be provided. The authority of the *(State agency)* to regulate the use of such descriptive devices shall specifically extend but not be limited to their use of the purpose of advertising, promoting, or selling the services rendered by an emergency services operation or emergency medical services personnel, including advanced life support personnel.

L. No person shall furnish, operate, conduct, maintain, advertise, or otherwise be engaged in or profess to be engaged in the provision of any form of emergency medical services which is regulated by this Act, or by rules and regulations promulgated pursuant to this Act, until and unless the said person is fully licensed, permitted, certified, and/or authorized by the *(State agency)* to engage in the provision of emergency medical services for which a valid and current license, permit, certificate, and/or authorization is issued.

M. No person or agency, public or private, shall advertise or disseminate information leading the public to believe that the person or agency provides emergency medical services, including advanced life support services, unless that person or agency does in fact provide such services in compliance with the provisions of this Act, or rules and regulations promulgated pursuant to this Act, and unless such services are provided on a continual basis of 24 hours per day, 7 days per week.

N. Any vehicle subject to licensing, permit, certificate, or authorization pursuant to this Act, or by rules and regulations promulgated pursuant to this Act, may be impounded where it is determined that the said vehicle is being used without the required license, permit, certificate, or authorization. Authority for impoundment and release of any vehicle so impounded shall be vested in the *(State agency)*. At the request of the *(State agency)*, the *(police agencies)* shall assist in impounding any vehicle which shall be deemed subject to this

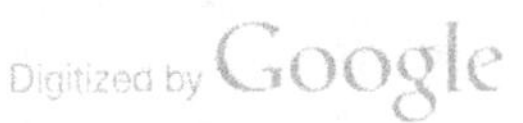

provision. The registered owner(s) of any vehicle so impounded shall be liable for any fees and charges accrued as a result of the impoundment of said vehicle.

O. Any vehicle that is licensed, permitted, certified or authorized pursuant to this Act, or by rules and regulations promulgated pursuant to this Act, shall not be required to meet subsequently modified vehicle design standards or specifications as long as the said vehicle is continuously used in accordance with the said license, permit, certificate, or authorization, or until the said vehicle's title of ownership shall be transferred.

P. Nothing in this Act, nor in rules and regulations promulgated pursuant to this Act, shall be construed to authorize any medical treatment or transportation of a person who objects thereto on religious grounds.

Q. Any person who shall violate this Act, or rules and regulations promulgated pursuant to this Act, shall be guilty of a misdemeanor.

R. If any provision of this Act, or rules and regulations promulgated pursuant to this Act, or the application of any such provision to any person or circumstance, shall be held invalid for any reason, the remainder of this Act, or of the said rules and regulations, shall not be affected thereby.

S. This Act shall become effective *(______________)*.

☆U.S. GOVERNMENT PRINTING OFFICE: 1978-261-238/37

CONGRESSIONAL INQUIRY SUMMARY (1977)[a]

Due to the long-term impacts on the development of the EMS system, the summary from the Committee on Appropriations inquiry[161] is printed here.

A REPORT TO

THE COMMITTEE ON APPROPRIATIONS

U.S. HOUSE OF REPRESENTATIVES

on

EMERGENCY MEDICAL SERVICES SYSTEMS

in the

UNITED STATES

Surveys and Investigations Staff

February 1978

[a] Inquiry initiated in 1977, written in 1978, and part of 1979 congressional record.

220

SUMMARY AND RECOMMENDATIONS

A. Summary

The Investigative Staff has reviewed the Emergency Medical Services (EMS) Systems programs of both the Department of Health, Education, and Welfare (HEW) and the Department of Transportation (DOT) and evaluated the relationship of these agencies with respect to EMS systems development in the United States. The EMS program was also reviewed at the State level, particularly with regard to the roles of the State EMS coordinator and the Governor's Representative.

The investment by HEW and DOT in the Federal program to develop 300 EMS regions in the United States by 1985 could exceed \$800 million. HEW's emergency medical services system development program has received nationwide support from State, local, and private organizations. It has resulted in improved emergency medical care in many sections of the country. Despite these successes, there are problems with the EMS systems development as there is a need for improved control over and evaluation of this program by HEW, and better coordination and cooperation at both the Federal and State levels.

The Division of Emergency Medical Services (DEMS), within the Health Services Administration (HSA), was created to administer the EMS systems development program of HEW.

1. Long-Range Plans Call for Full Development of the 300 EMS Regional Systems at a Total HEW Grant Cost of \$475 Million

As envisioned by DEMS officials, the program for full development of the 300 EMS regional systems (HEW grant cost of about \$475 million) will require another 3-year extension of the EMS Systems Act with Section 1203 and 1204 funding provided through FY 1985. To date the HEW EMS systems program has not been evaluated and the Investigative Staff believes that there are questions which need to be studied before the program is extended. Some areas which require study include:

- -- The nationwide effect on systems development that an anticipated reduction in DOT Section 402 funding will have.
- -- Whether EMS regional systems capable of providing advanced life support can be developed wall-to-wall throughout the United States. Evidence indicates that many regions will be unable to develop or support such a system.

221

-- Whether the EMS systems which have already received the maximum 5 years of HEW systems grants will continue to operate as systems. If the regions reviewed by the Investigative Staff are typical, many will not.

2. Administrative Problems Impair Effectiveness of HEW's EMS Program

DEMS administers the EMS systems development program of HEW.

a. Inadequate Guidance Provided for Systems Development

HEW lacks a formal structured system (current written procedures and instructions, manuals, etc.) for providing program guidelines to States, regions, and local bodies. In the absence of a formal HEW system, the development of an EMS systems program has, to a large extent relied on the Director of DEMS to personally provide information on program direction at all levels. Typically, because of noted internal shortcomings and limited staffing, planning is on a short-term ad hoc basis (less than 6 months), not in writing, and usually not coordinated with the central office staff and HEW regional personnel. The Director of DEMS is also called on to provide technical assistance, conduct national symposia, regional workshops, and travel extensively to personally provide information on EMS priorities and program changes.

State EMS officials do not always have ready access to the Director of DEMS. Much of the program information is received thirdhand via the grapevine--by word of mouth from other participants in the programs. Complaints were made that the HEW regional offices were often not aware of program changes made by the Director of DEMS, and so the regional offices were unable to provide proper and timely guidance to program participants. In particular, the officials criticized HEW's failure to publish revised regulations and guidelines reflecting the changes made by amendments to the EMS Systems Act in 1976.

As a result of these deficiencies, there has been a fragmented, uncoordinated departmental approach to implementing a viable, standardized EMS program. A further fallout of the department's informal approach to the program has been the creation of dissatisfaction and confusion among the program participants at the operational levels.

b. DEMS Central Office Was Not Provided Sufficient Staffing to Properly Administer the EMS Program

If the EMS grant program is to continue beyond FY 1979, there is a need for a permanent and adequately staffed

DEMS central office. Although DEMS was delegated responsibility for administering the EMS program for HEW, no permanent positions have been budgeted for this purpose. Since FY 1975, requests for permanent staffing and additional personnel have been rejected by either the Secretary of HEW or OMB. Legislative changes in 1976 provided additional administrative central office responsibilities with no increase in personnel. This shortage of personnel has impaired the management of the EMS program. As previously mentioned, the Director of DEMS traveled a total of 106 days during FY 1977 providing onsite technical assistance. His extended absence from the central office, together with the personnel shortage, added to the backlog of unfinished business. Thus, the central office was operating shorthanded with an increased workload, and mounting unfinished administrative responsibilities. The following areas suffered from lack of attention:

-- Reports required by Congress were not prepared, or were submitted late.

-- A suitable data bank for purposes of making evaluations of EMS was never started.

-- Support of the Interagency Committee on Emergency Medical Services was inadequate.

-- The EMS program monitoring effort was limited primarily to review of written quarterly and annual reports.

-- The clearinghouse functions were reduced to an information response activity.

3. <u>HEW Research Unresponsive to Needs of Developing Systems</u>

The National Center for Health Service Research (NCHSR), Health Resources Administration (HRA), is responsible for developing and administering EMS research projects under Section 1205 of the EMS Systems Act of 1973.

a. Most EMS research projects awarded were long-term, multiyear studies, the results of which are not timely in meeting the current needs of the developing systems. Timeliness of information is critical because the capital investment for EMS systems development is being made now. NCHSR officials have exhibited the "purest" point of view and have not generally funded short-term projects addressing immediate high priority problems because technically they consider these projects to be analyses as opposed to research.

b. NCHSR has denied grant proposals because of design weaknesses without considering the merit of the research proposed for study or the possibility of offering design assistance. As a result, proposals submitted by persons involved with EMS systems development are denied and grants are awarded to academically oriented medical centers, which write well-designed research proposals concerned with problems peripheral to those of the developing systems.

c. The Interagency Committee on EMS was not monitoring the Federal EMS research effort nor making suggestions to HEW concerning the type of EMS research that was needed.

4. <u>HEW Training Programs Have Created Confusion</u>

Within HEW, both DEMS and HRA conduct programs which provide funds for training emergency medical technicians (EMT's). These programs were not well coordinated and have created confusion and dissatisfaction at the State and local levels. State EMS officials criticized the HRA program for not complementing EMS systems development, for its lack of coordination with State EMS personnel, and for the manner in which the program was administered. The Investigative Staff believes that both DEMS and the State EMS coordinators should have more control over short-term EMT training programs.

5. <u>DOT Reluctant to Accept HEW Leadership Role in EMS</u>

DOT and HEW conduct EMS programs under separate laws, DOT under the Highway Safety Act of 1966, and HEW under the Emergency Medical Services Systems Act of 1973, as amended.

The DOT program emphasizes the <u>prehospital</u> functions of EMS, particularly as they relate to highway accident victims. The HEW program includes the prehospital EMS functions and focuses on the development of comprehensive regional systems capable of providing the wide range of emergency medical care. The two programs have overlapping features and there is a need for better coordination.

Since 1974, HEW and DOT have been trying to develop a Memorandum of Understanding clarifying their respective roles in EMS development. HEW, as the lead agency for EMS, wants DOT's programs to be coordinated with and approved by HEW. DOT is reluctant to relinquish the leadership role derived from its earlier association with emergency medical care, established in the late 1960's and early 1970's, and actively resents having to coordinate any of its programs with HEW. Constant bickering between the two agencies has had an adverse affect on the national EMS program.

6. DOT Has Little Control Over State's Use of DOT Highway Safety Funds

The Highway Safety Act provided, under Section 402, Federal formula grants to help States develop and operate a highway safety program. DOT established 18 uniform highway safety standard programs around which State highway safety programs were to be developed. Standard 11, titled "Emergency Medical Services," outlines DOT requirements for a State EMS program.

The decision on how Section 402 funds should be allocated and spent within the 18 uniform standard program areas is left to the State. Neither the DOT central office nor DOT regional offices have much influence over the State's decision. For this reason, there is little if any coordination between HEW and DOT concerning Section 402 funding.

7. State EMS Officials Oppose the Proposed Deletion of EMS as a Required Part of the Highway Safety Program

In July 1977, the Secretary of Transportation issued a report to Congress entitled "An Evaluation of the Highway Safety Program." The report recommended that the present 18 uniform highway safety standard programs be replaced with a reduced number of uniform requirements. Standard 11, Emergency Medical Services, along with 11 other standards would no longer be a mandatory requirement of a State's highway safety program. State EMS officials were adamant in their opposition to this change. They believed, as did many DOT officials, that it would result in a significant decrease in Section 402 funds allocated for EMS. Section 402 funding for EMS in 1977 totaled approximately $17 million, as compared to HEW EMS systems grants which totaled about $33 million. Section 402 funding plays an important role in many State's EMS programs.

8. The Department of Labor (DOL) Failed to Coordinate its EMS Training Activities

DOL, at the time of this report, could provide only fragmented and inconclusive information concerning the extent of its support for EMS training. DOL support is provided primarily under the Comprehensive Employment and Training Act (CETA). Preliminary responses from only four regional offices showed that over $10 million was spent on this program during the period FY 1974 through FY 1977. The overall magnitude of this program appears substantial. Our review of one DOL program, the EMT apprenticeship program, disclosed that it had not been properly coordinated with other Federal and State EMS programs. The need for a DOL EMT apprenticeship program was questioned by State EMS officials who believed that it duplicated existing State and Federal programs. It is possible that other DOL training programs suffer from the same deficiencies.

9. Interagency Committee on Emergency Medical Services (IAC-EMS) Failed to Coordinate Federal EMS Programs

The IAC-EMS was established under Section 1209 of the EMS Systems Act. Its purpose is to coordinate and provide for communications and exchange of information among all Federal programs and activities relating to EMS. This Committee has not been effective in coordinating the Federal EMS program in a number of areas:

a. The IAC-EMS has not satisfied Congressional reporting requirements. These include an evaluation and report on adequacy, technical soundness, and redundancy of all Federal programs and activities relating to EMS; development of a comprehensive Federal EMS funding and resource-sharing plan; and a report describing the sources of Federal support available for the purchase of vehicles and communication support equipment.

b. State EMS coordinators criticized the IAC-EMS for not addressing or seeking answers to critical problems faced by EMS providers at the State level. The officials said there is a need for State representation on the IAC-EMS.

c. The IAC-EMS review of Federal EMS activities has, at best, been superficial. There is a reluctance on the part of Federal agencies to coordinate their EMS programs with the IAC-EMS. Agencies (especially DOT and HEW) jealously guard what they consider to be their own "turf."

d. The IAC-EMS has operated without adequate staffing and, therefore, meetings have not been properly planned and coordinated. Although required to meet four times a year, the IAC-EMS met only twice during CY 1977.

10. EMS is a State and Local Responsibility

The success of the Federal EMS program is dependent upon how well the programs are executed at the State and local levels. DOT and HEW programs were not always well managed or coordinated at this level and Federal program requirements were not always met.

a. Continuation of Regional EMS Systems is Dependent Upon State Support

Should Federal funding end, State support will be necessary to keep EMS systems intact. EMS regions are not political entities with direct taxing authority and must rely on the local governments participating in the system for financial and other support.

The degree of support that the EMS regions might receive is unknown. In view of the competing demands for limited tax dollars, it appears doubtful, however, that adequate financial help will be forthcoming in many areas. As a consequence, the future of many in-place EMS systems will be in jeopardy, unless the States decide to actively support the program.

b. State Health Department is the Lead Agency for EMS

Within the State health department, the State EMS coordinator is responsible for developing a statewide EMS program. The State EMS coordinator assesses EMS needs statewide; works extensively with regions developing EMS systems; and, in most States, determines how DOT funds made available for EMS by the Governor's Representative will be spent.

c. Governor's Representative Controls the Use of DOT Highway Safety Funds

The day-to-day operation of the highway safety program in each State is handled by a Governor's Representative. He determines how funds provided by DOT under Section 402 of the Highway Safety Act of 1966 will be spent. Standard 11, Emergency Medical Services is just one of 18 uniform highway safety standards competing for his attention.

d. Uncoordinated EMS Programs Exist in Some States

In 9 of the 28 States in which EMS programs were reviewed by the Investigative Staff, two separate EMS programs were run at the State level, both funded through Federal grant programs. In these States, the Governor's Representative does not rely on the State EMS coordinator's assessment of EMS needs but instead makes an independent evaluation. This allows local governments which do not wish to be part of the regional EMS system to circumvent State and HEW program requirements and still obtain Federal funding. In addition, the independent assessment of EMS needs is duplicative and creates confusion at the State level.

e. Requirement for State EMS Plans by DOT and HEW Cause Confusion

Both DOT and HEW require a State EMS plan. The DOT plan is primarily an inventory of prehospital resources. The HEW plan details the establishment, operation, and expansion of regional EMS systems. DOT and HEW officials have not enforced or clarified their requirements for a State EMS plan. Development of a State plan requires extensive coordination and a considerable resource commitment. For these reasons, most State plans were

227

either not completed or are outdated. Many States consider their current DEMS grant application to be the updated State EMS plan, satisfying both DOT and HEW requirements.

f. Complexity of HEW Systems Grants Limits Use in Some Regions--DOT Funding More Flexible

Rural and "have not" regions are at a distinct disadvantage when applying for funding under Sections 1202, 1203, and 1204 of the EMS Systems Act of 1973. These regions lack the necessary resources to develop an EMS grant application, and the hospitals, facilities, and medical personnel required for systems development. In addition, they lack a sufficient financial base to guarantee continuance of the program when Federal funding ends. As an alternative, DOT Section 402 funds have been used to purchase ambulances and EMS equipment in these regions. Section 402 funding requires only identification of the problem and the Governor's Representative's approval.

g. Standard Recordkeeping Requirements Not Supported by State and Local EMS Officials

DEMS grant guidelines required that EMS systems establish standardized medical recordkeeping systems which cover patient treatment from initial entry into the system through discharge. Standard recordkeeping is necessary to provide data for program evaluation and management purposes. However, there is considerable resistance at the local level to standardized recordkeeping. Hospital administrators are reluctant to handle the extra paperwork or to provide information because of patient confidentiality and the possiblity of malpractice suits. In addition, the costs of gathering and compiling information are considered prohibitively high by State and local officials. As a result, adequate data bases do not exist for evaluation purposes.

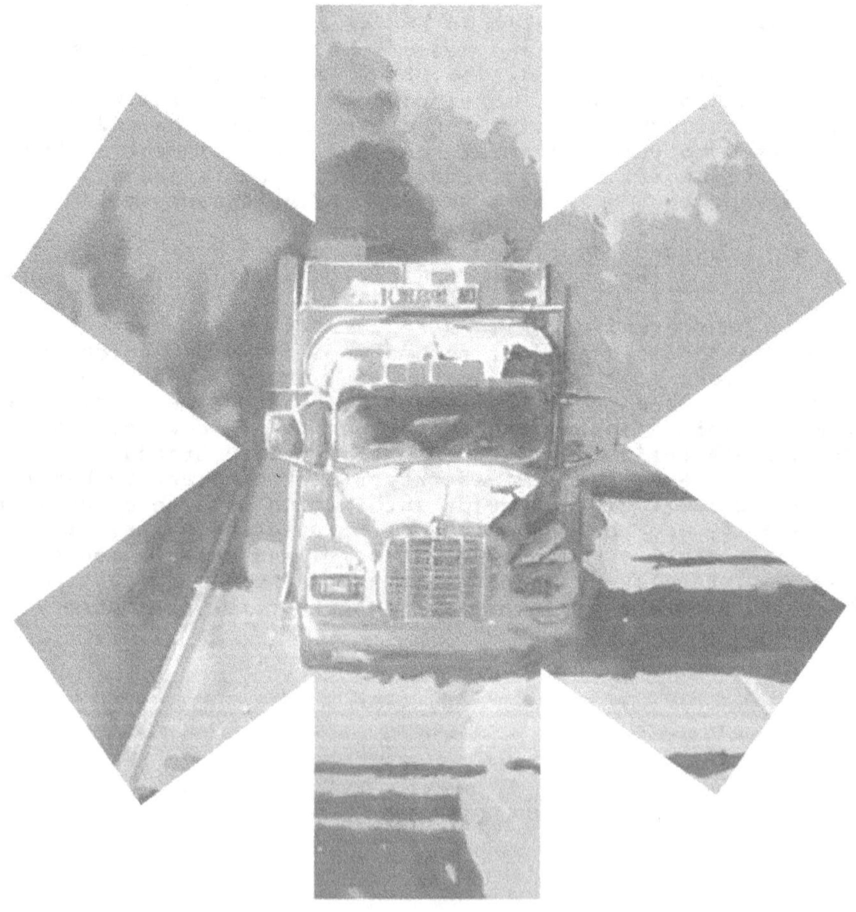

INDEX

GLOSSARY

AAA: American Ambulance Association

AAMS: Association of Air Medical Services

AAOS: American Academy of Orthopedic Surgeons

ACEP: American College of Emergency Physicians

ACLS: Advanced Cardiac Life Support

ACPE: American College of Paramedic Executives

ACS: American College of Surgeons

AHA: American Heart Association

ALS: Advanced Life Support

AMA: American Medical Association

AMRF: African Medical & Research Foundation

ARC: American Red Cross

ATS: American Trauma Society

BCCTPC: Board for Critical Care Transport Paramedic Certification

BLM: Bureau of Land Management

CAAHEP: Commission on Accreditation of Allied Health Education Programs

CAT: Computer Adaptive Testing

CCP: Critical Care Paramedic

CDPHE: Colorado Department of Public Health & Environment

CoAEMSP: Committee on Accreditation of Emergency Medical Services Professions

CQI: Continuous Quality Improvement

CSG: Council of State Governments

DARPA: Defense Advanced Research Projects Agency

DHEW: Department of Health, Education & Welfare

DHHS: Department of Health & Human Services (Also, HHS)

DHS: Department of Homeland Security

DLC: Driver License Compact

DOT: Department of Transportation

EDI: Equity, Diversity & Inclusion

EMAC: Emergency Management Assistance Compact

EMS: Emergency Medical Services

EMSC: Emergency Medical Services for Children

EMT: Emergency Medical Technician

EMTALA: Emergency Medical Treatment and Labor Act

ENA: Emergency Nurses Association

FBI: Federal Bureau of Investigation

FEMA: Federal Emergency Management Agency

FICEMS: Federal Interagency Committee on EMS

FSMB: Federation of State Medical Boards

FTO: Field Training Officer

HIPAA: Health Insurance Portability & Accountability Act

HRSA: Health Resources & Services Administration

IACP: International Association of Chiefs of Police

IAED: International Academies of Emergency Dispatch

IAEMSC: International Association of EMS Chiefs

IAFC: International Association of Fire Chiefs

IAFF: International Association of Fire Fighters

IBSC: International Board of Specialty Certifications

ICEMSPP: Interstate Commission for EMS Personnel Practice

IMLC: Interstate Medical Licensure Compact

JEMS: Journal of Emergency Medical Services

JRCEP: Joint Review Committee on Education Programs

LEIE: List of Excluded Individuals, Entities

MASH: Mobile Army Surgical Hospital

NAEMSE: National Association of EMS Educators

NAEMSP: National Association of EMS Physicians

NAEMT: National Association of EMTs

NAS: National Academy of Sciences

NASA: National Aeronautics and Space Administration

NASEMSD: National Association of State EMS Directors

NASEMSO: National Association of State EMS Officials

NCIC: National Center for Interstate Compacts

NCLEX: National Council Licensure Examination

NCSBN: National Council of State Boards of Nursing

NEMSCD: National EMS Coordinated Database

NEMSID: National EMS Identification Number

NEMSIS: National EMS Information System

NEMSMA: National EMS Management Association

NFIRS: National Fire Incident Reporting System

NFPA: National Fire Protection Association

NFS: National Forest Service

NHTSA: National Highway Traffic Safety Administration

NLC: Nurse Licensure Compact

NPDB: National Practitioner Data Bank

NRC: National Research Council

NREMT: National Registry of EMTs

NSC: National Standard Curriculum

PANCE: Physician Assistant National Certifying Examination

PHTLS: Pre-Hospital Trauma Life Support

PTSD: Post-Traumatic Stress Disorder

REPLICA: Recognition of EMS Personnel Licensure Interstate Compact

TCCC: Tactical Combat Casualty Care

UASI: Urban Areas Security Initiative

UMIS: Universal Medical Identification Symbol

USFA: United States Fire Administration

COMPANION WEBSITE

www.ems-history.com

Readers are warmly invited to delve further into the rich array of resources available on this book's companion website, found at **www.ems-history.com.** This platform not only provides direct access to most documents referenced within this book but also serves as an expansive resource hub for EMS Managers, Leaders, and State EMS Officials. It hosts an impressive collection of insightful videos, offers direct connections to national EMS organizations, presents accessible congressional records, and much more. To enrich their understanding and extend their knowledge, readers are encouraged to visit this comprehensive companion website.

About the Author

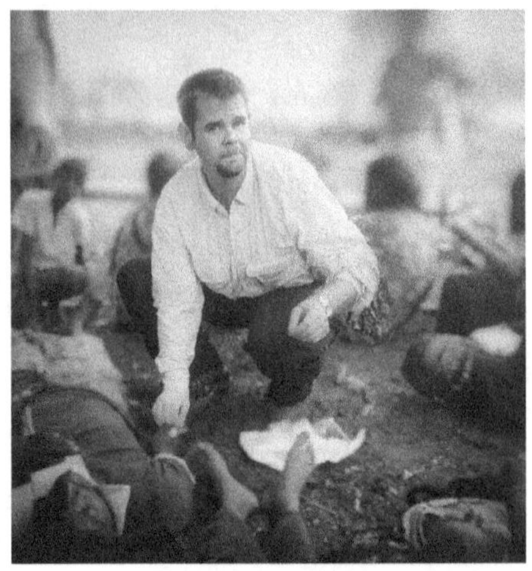

Donnie Woodyard Jr., MAML, NRP, has an extensive three-decade-long career in the field of Emergency Medical Services. His journey started in high school when he volunteered as an EMT in Pearisburg, Virginia. This initial experience sparked his interest in EMS, leading him to become a Paramedic at the age of 19 upon graduating from Sinclair Community College in Dayton, Ohio. Pursuing higher education, Donnie acquired another undergraduate degree from Indiana University and a Master's Degree in Management and Leadership from Liberty University. He is currently working on his Doctorate degree in Public Administration.

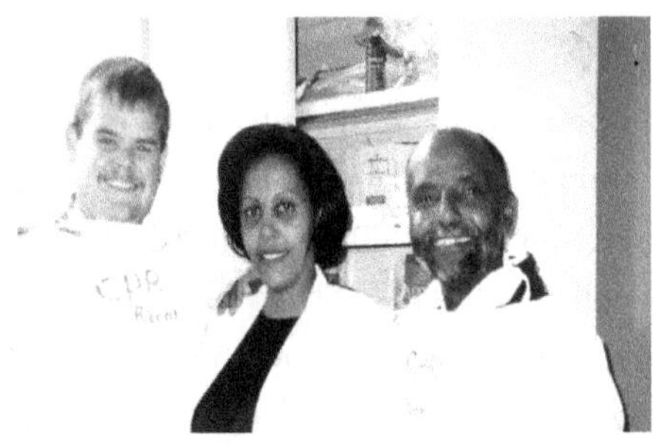

In 1999, Donnie achieved certification as a Critical Care Paramedic through a combined program by the University of Maryland Baltimore County and Loyola University. This achievement was attained during his pre-med studies at Cedarville University. He also holds an IBSC Board Certification as a Wilderness Paramedic. Over his lengthy career, Donnie has taken on multiple EMS leadership roles, serving as an EMS Chief in volunteer and salaried positions, an EMS instructor, and the Paramedic Program Director for a Community College and a hospital-based Paramedic program.

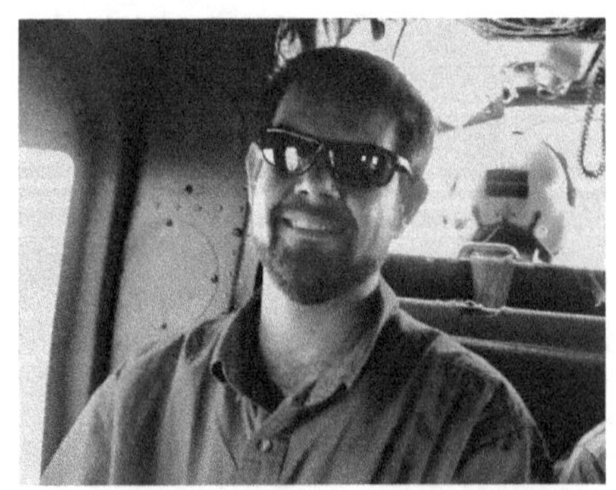

Previously, Donnie served on the Board of Directors for the National Association of State EMS Officials and was an ex-officio member of the Colorado Emergency Medical Practice Advisory Council. He also served in critical state leadership roles, including the State EMS Director for Louisiana and Chief of the Emergency Medical & Trauma Services Branch for the State of Colorado. As the Chief Operating Officer for the National Registry of EMTs, Donnie initiated several technological advancements including the National EMS ID Number, the NREMT mobile app, and the National EMS Coordinated Database.

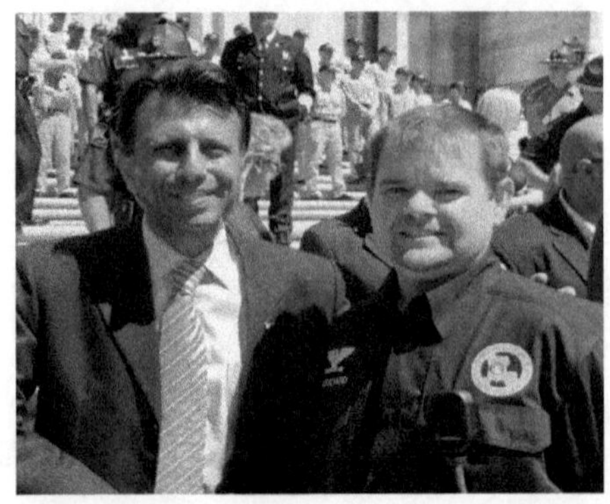

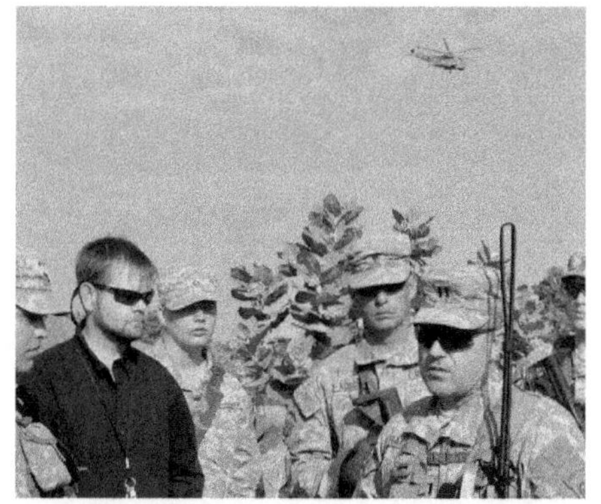

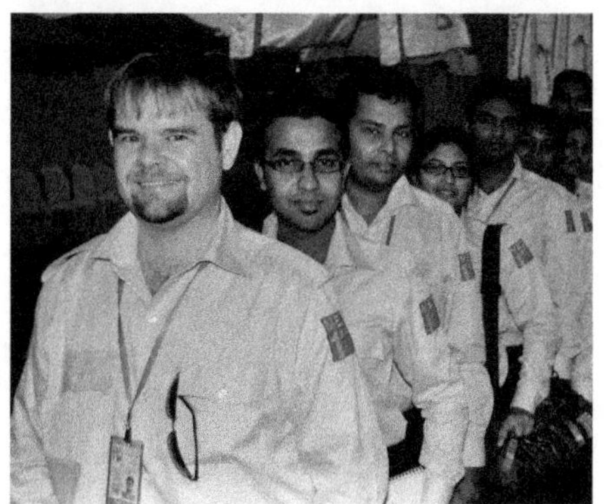

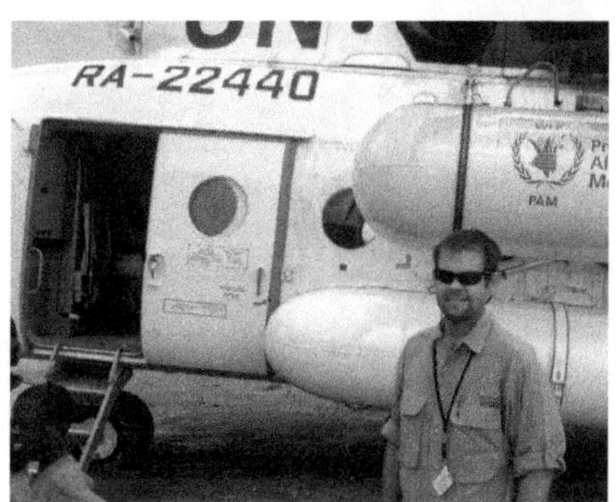

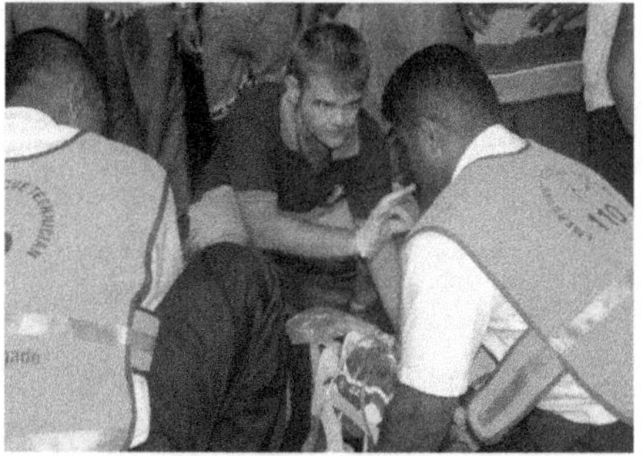

Donnie's contributions have been integral to implementing the EMS Compact as Colorado's Commissioner. He was elected to serve as the Chair of the Executive Committee for the Interstate Commission for EMS Personnel Practice after serving as Vice Chair. In 2023, he was appointed as the full-time Executive Director for the EMS Compact.

Donnie's influence extends beyond national boundaries. He is recognized for establishing the modern EMS System in Sri Lanka and advising on EMS and trauma system designs in several South Asian countries. He has authored, edited, or consulted on EMS textbooks published in Sinhala, Tamil, Khmer, and Bengali languages.

Beyond his work in EMS, Donnie is a skilled Scuba Dive Master, with over 800 dives to his credit. He is also an airplane pilot and currently serves as a Squadron Commander with the United States Air Force Auxiliary – Civil Air Patrol. His commitment to public service is further exemplified by his humanitarian work, having participated in disaster, war, and medical response aid missions in many countries including Haiti, Sri Lanka, Ethiopia, and Bangladesh.

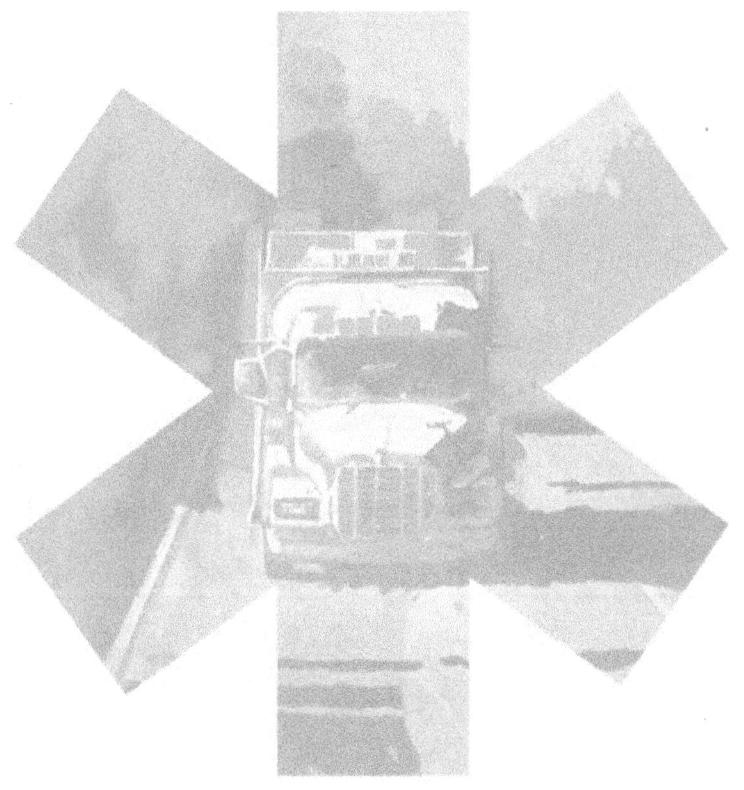

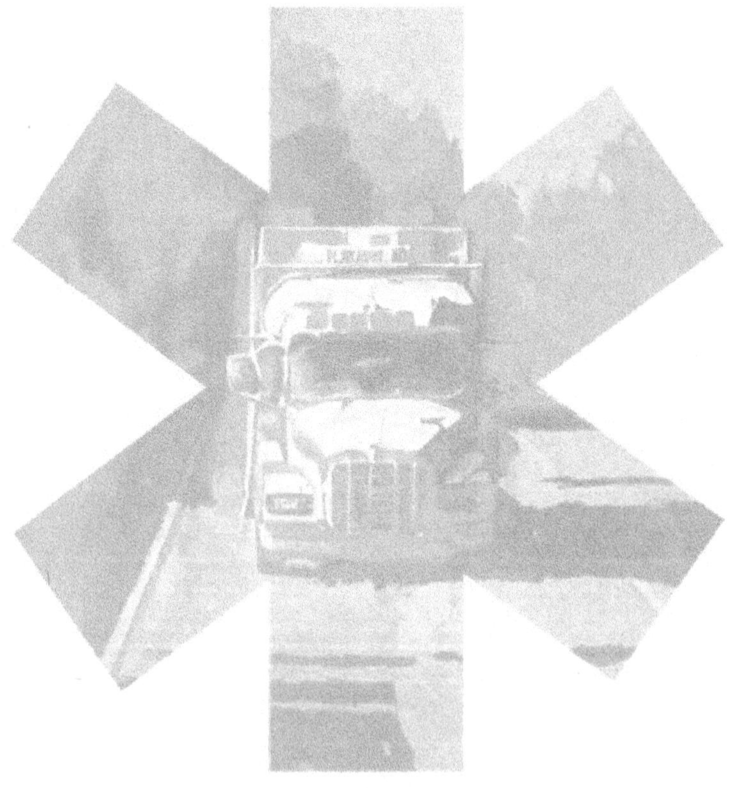

ENDNOTES: REFERENCES & CITATIONS

[1] Baron Larrey, D. J. (1814). Memoirs of Military Surgery, and Campaigns of the French Armies, on the Rhine, in Corsica, Catalonia, Egypt, and Syria; at Boulogne, Ulm, and Austerlitz; in Saxony, Prussia, Poland, Spain, and Austria.
[2] Barkley, K. T. (1978). The Ambulance: The Story of Emergency Transportation of Sick and Wounded Through the Centuries. Hicksville, NY: Exposition Press.
[3] National Library of Medicine, Image: A023560
[4] General Photograph Collection. (n.d.). Curtiss JN-4D 'Jenny' air ambulance [Photograph]. Fort Sam Houston, San Antonio, Texas. Office of Information, Aerospace Medical Division, Air Force Systems Command, Brooks AFB, Texas. Identifier: 075-0912.
[5] Johnson Publishing Company. (1960, January 28). Jet Magazine, 17(14), 64 pages. ISSN 0021-5996.
[6] Bledsoe, B. E., & Wesley, A. K. (2007). History of aeromedical transport. In K. Curtis & C. Ramsden (Eds.), Emergency and Trauma Care for Nurses and Paramedics (2nd ed., pp. 589-598). Pearson Education.
[7] President's Committee for Traffic Safety. (1966). Highway Safety Action Program. U.S. Government Printing Office.
[8] National Academy of Sciences (NAS) and National Research Council (NRC). (1966). Accidental death and disability: The neglected disease of modern society. National Academies Press.
[9] National Traffic and Motor Vehicle Safety Act, Pub. L. No. 89-563, 80 Stat. 718 (1966).
[10] Highway Safety Act of 1966, Pub. L. No. 89-564, 80 Stat. 731 (1966).
[11] President Johnson. (1966, September 9). Remarks at the Signing of the National Traffic and Motor Vehicle Safety Act and the Highway Safety Act.
[12] Farrington, J. D. (1967). Death in a ditch. Bulletin of the American College of Surgeons, 52(3), 121-130.
[13] Highway Safety Act of 1966 (PL 89–564). *Legislative History*. Washington DC: U.S. Government Printing Office; 1967:2741–2765. (pg. 2755)
[14] National EMS Information System (NEMSIS), (2022) NHTSA Office of EMS, Department of Transportation, 2020 Data Report.
[15] Roles and Resources of Federal Agencies in Support of Comprehensive Emergency Medical Services. (1972). United States: U.S. Health Services and Mental Health Administration, Special Projects Office, Emergency Medical Services.
[16] Simpson, A. T. (2013). Transporting Lazarus: Physicians, the State, and the Creation of the Modern Paramedic and Ambulance, 1955–73. *Journal of the History of Medicine and Allied Sciences, 68*(2), 163–197. http://www.jstor.org/stable/24672078
[17] University of Pittsburgh School of Medicine Magazine. (2004, February). Vol. 6, Issue 1.
[18] Photograph album (dismantled), 1905-1983. Papers of Nancy L. Caroline, 1905-2007, MC 531; Vt-139; DVD-2, PD.1-PD.5., Box: | PHOTOGRAPHS, Box 161. Schlesinger Library, Radcliffe Institute.
[19] Andrews, R. B. (1975). Methodologies for the Evaluation and Improvement of Emergency Medical Services Systems: Final Report. United States: U.S. Department of Transportation, National Highway Traffic Safety Administration.

[20] Wedworth-Townsend Paramedic Act, Cal. Health & Safety Code §§ 1480-1481 (1970).
[21] Compendium of State Statutes on the Regulation of Ambulance Services: Operation of Emergency Vehicles, and Good Samaritan Laws. (1969). United States: U.S. Government Printing Office.
[22] State Statutes on Emergency Medical Services. (1972). United States: U.S. Division of Emergency Health Services.
[23] Emergency Medical Services Systems Act of 1973, Pub. L. No. 93-154, 87 Stat. 594 (1973).
[24] Boyd, D.R., Cowley, R.A. Comprehensive regional trauma/Emergency Medical Services (EMS) delivery systems: The United States experience. *World J. Surg.* **7**, 149–157 (1983).
[25] Emergency Medical Services Amendments, 1976: Hearing Before the Subcommittee on Health of the Committee on Labor and Public Welfare, United States Senate, Ninety-fourth Congress, Second Session, on S. 2548 ... January 23, 1976. (1976). United States: U.S. Government Printing Office.
[26] Hull, J. A. (1979). Emergency Medical Services Communications System Technical Planning Guide. United States: Department of Commerce, National Telecommunications and Information Administration.
[27] Highway/transit Proposals: Hearings Before the Subcommittee on Surface Transportation of the Committee on Public Works and Transportation, House of Representatives, Ninety-fifth Congress, First [-second] Session. (1977). United States: U.S. Government Printing Office.
[28] Kohler, S. (2007). The Emergency Medical Services Program of the Robert Wood Johnson Foundation (Case 42). In Casebook for The Foundation: A Great American Secret. New York: PublicAffairs.
[29] The Effect of Emergency Medical Systems on Prehospital Cardiovascular Care: An Evaluation of Studies and an Inventory of Data Bases. (1981). United States: National Highway Traffic Safety Administration.
[30] Omnibus Budget Reconciliation Act of 1981, Pub. L. No. 97-35, 95 Stat. 357 (1981).
[31] Effective Oct 1, 1981. Title 42, The public health and welfare. (1982). United States: U.S. Government Printing Office.
[32] U.S. Congress. (1990). Trauma Care Systems Planning and Development Act of 1990 (Public Law 101-590). U.S. Government Printing Office.
[33] U.S. Government Printing Office. (1969). Basic Training Program for Emergency Medical Technician-Ambulance: Concepts and Recommendations. Washington, D.C.
[34] American Medical Association. (1959). Summary report on national emergency medical care. Chicago.
[35] American Medical Association. (1963). Universal Medical Identification Symbol. Journal of the American Medical Association, 186(1), 56.
[36] National Traffic and Motor Vehicle Safety Act, Pub. L. No. 89-563, 80 Stat. 718 (1966).
[37] Highway Safety Act of 1966, Pub. L. No. 89-564, 80 Stat. 731 (1966).
[38] Savas E. Simulation and cost-effectiveness analysis of New York's emergency ambulance service. *Management science.* 1969; 15(12):B-608-B-627.
[39] Becker, L. R. (1991). An EMS history primer: A synopsis of ambulance and rescue service history in the United States. St. Louis, MO: Mosby Lifeline.
[40] Boyd, David R. (September 2015). "A trauma surgeon's journey". Journal of Trauma and Acute Care Surgery. 79 (3): 497–514.
[41] Departments of Labor, and Health, Education, and Welfare Appropriations for 1969: Hearings, Ninetieth Congress, Second Session. (1968). United States: U.S. Government Printing Office. (343)

[42] National Traffic and Motor Vehicle Safety Act, Pub. L. No. 89-563, 80 Stat. 718 (1966).
[43] Highway Safety Act of 1966, Pub. L. No. 89-564, 80 Stat. 731 (1966).
[44] Emergency Medical Services Systems Authorization: Hearing Before the Subcommittee on Health and the Environment of the Committee on Interstate and Foreign Commerce, House of Representatives, Ninety-sixth Congress, First Session, on H.R. 3039 ... H.R. 3124 ... H.R. 2212 ... March 21, 1979. (1979). United States: U.S. Government Printing Office.
[45] U.S. Government Printing Office. (1969). Basic Training Program for Emergency Medical Technician-Ambulance: Concepts and Recommendations. Washington, D.C.
[46] Farrington JD. The seven years' war. Bull Amer Coll Surg 1973; 58:15–22. 59th Annual Clinical Congress of the American College of Surgeons.
[47] Institute of Medicine. (2007). Emergency Medical Services: At the Crossroads. Washington, DC: The National Academies Press.
[48] Emergency Medical Services: Recommendations for an Approach to an Urgent National Problem: Proceedings of the Airlie Conference on Emergency Medical Services, Airlie House, Warrenton, Virginia, May 5-6, 1969
[49] Weekly Compilation of Presidential Documents. (1974). United States: Office of the Federal Register, National Archives and Records Service, General Services Administration.
[50] Medical Requirements for Ambulance Design and Equipment. (1970). United States: U.S. Government Printing Office.
[51] Safar, P. (2000). From Pittsburgh to Vienna: An Autobiographical Memoir (Careers in Anesthesiology, Vol. V). Park Ridge, Illinois: Wood Library-Museum of Anesthesiology. ISBN 1-889595-06-1.
[52] Safar, P., Esposito, G., & Benson, D.M. (1971). Ambulance Design and Equipment for Mobile Intensive Care. *Archives of Surgery*, 102.
[53] American Medical Association. (1963). Universal Medical Identification Symbol. Journal of the American Medical Association, 186(1), 56.
[54] Universal Medical Identification Symbol. *Am J Dis Child.* 1964;107(5):439. doi:10.1001/archpedi.1964.02080060441001
[55] FBI Law Enforcement Bulletin. (1966). United States: Federal Bureau of Investigation, U.S. Department of Justice.
[56] Wiegenstein, J. G. (1972). AMA star of life needs to be recognized. Journal of the American College of Emergency Physicians, 1(3), 15-17.
[57] Becker, L. R. (1991). An EMS history primer: A synopsis of ambulance and rescue service history in the United States. St. Louis, MO: Mosby Lifeline.
[58] United States Patent and Trademark Office, serial number 72454410 and registration number 1020230.
[59] United States Department of Transportation. (1974). Highway Safety Program Manual, Volume 11: Emergency Medical Services (p. IV-61).
[60] Emergency Medical Services. (1974). United States: The Administration.
[61] Public Health Reports. (1974). United States: U.S. Department of Health, Education, and Welfare, Public Health Service, Health Resources Administration.
[62] Emergency Medical Services Systems Act of 1973, Pub. L. No. 93-154, 87 Stat. 594 (1973).
[63] Departments of Labor and Health, Education, and Welfare Appropriations for 1979: Hearings Before a Subcommittee of the Committee on Appropriations, House of Representatives, Ninety-fifth Congress, Second Session, Subcommittee on the Departments of Labor and Health, Education, and Welfare. (1978). United States: U.S. Government Printing Office. (255-)

---

64 Progress, But Problems in Developing Emergency Medical Services Systems: Health Services Administration, Department of Health, Education, and Welfare: Report to the Congress. (1976). United States: U.S. General Accounting Office.
65 American Economic Policy in the 1980s. (2007). United States: University of Chicago Press.
66 Departments of Labor, Health, Education, and Welfare, and related agencies appropriations for 1981: hearings before a subcommittee of the Committee on Appropriations, House of Representatives, Ninety-sixth Congress, second session. (1980). (n.p.): U.S. Government Printing Office.
67 Omnibus Budget Reconciliation Act of 1981, Pub. L. No. 97-35, 95 Stat. 357 (1981).
68 Departments of Labor, Health and Human Services, Education, and related agencies appropriations for fiscal year 1986: hearings before a subcommittee of the Committee on Appropriations, United States Senate, Ninety-ninth Congress, first session, on H.R. 3424 (1985). United States: U.S. Government Printing Office.
69 Departments of Labor and Health, Education, and Welfare Appropriations for 1979: Hearings Before a Subcommittee of the Committee on Appropriations, House of Representatives, Ninety-fifth Congress, Second Session, Subcommittee on the Departments of Labor and Health, Education, and Welfare. (1978). United States: U.S. Government Printing Office.
70 Institute of Medicine. (2007). Emergency Medical Services: At the Crossroads. Washington, DC: The National Academies Press.
71 National Highway Traffic Safety Administration. (1996). EMS Agenda for the Future. (34)
72 Andrews, R. B. (1975). Methodologies for the Evaluation and Improvement of Emergency Medical Services Systems: Final Report. United States: U.S. Department of Transportation, National Highway Traffic Safety Administration.
73 National Emergency Medical Services Advisory Council. (2009, April 16). Committee: Education/Workforce. Report Number: 001-EDW-05-FINAL. Title: Standardized Certification, Licensure, and Credentialing.
74 Department of Transportation and Related Agencies Appropriations for Fiscal Year 1985: Architectural and Transportation Barriers Compliance Board. (1984). United States: U.S. Government Printing Office.
75 Institute of Medicine. 2007. Emergency Medical Services: At the Crossroads. Washington, DC: The National Academies Press. https://doi.org/10.17226/11629.
76 National Highway Traffic Safety Administration. (1996). EMS Agenda for the Future: A Systems Approach. Retrieved from https://www.ems.gov/pdf/education/EMSAgendaWeb.pdf.
77 EMS Education Agenda for the Future: A Systems Approach. (2000). Prehospital emergency care, 4(4), 365–366.
78 Dawson, D. E. (2006). National Emergency Medical Services Information System (NEMSIS). Prehospital Emergency Care, 10(3), 314-316. https://doi.org/10.1080/10903120600724200
79 Emergency Medical Services: Recommendations for an Approach to an Urgent National Problem: Proceedings of the Airlie Conference on Emergency Medical Services, Airlie House, Warrenton, Virginia, May 5-6, 1969
80 SAFETEA-LU, Pub. L. No. 109-59, § 10202, 119 Stat. 1144 (2005), codified at 42 U.S.C. § 300d-4.
81 Federal Interagency Committee on Emergency Medical Services, 42 U.S.C. § 300d-4.
82 Omnibus Budget Reconciliation Act of 1981, Pub. L. No. 97-35, 95 Stat. 357 (1981).

---

[83] U.S. Congress. (1990). Trauma Care Systems Planning and Development Act of 1990 (Public Law 101-590). U.S. Government Printing Office.
[84] Moving Ahead for Progress in the 21st Century Act (MAP-21), Pub. L. No. 112-141, § 31108, 126 Stat. 405 (2012), codified at 42 U.S.C. § 300d-4.
[85] Pub. L. No. 89–563, 80 Stat. 718 (1966).
[86] National Highway Traffic Safety Administration. (2007). National EMS Scope of Practice Model.
[87] National Highway Traffic Safety Administration. (2009). National EMS Education Standards.
[88] America Burning: The Report. (1973). United States: U.S. Government Printing Office.
[89] Proclamation 4332—Emergency Medical Services Week, 1974 (November 5, 1974).
[90] Jesse C. Baumgartner, Sara R. Collins, and David C. Radley, *Racial and Ethnic Inequities in Health Care Coverage and Access, 2013–2019* (Commonwealth Fund, June 2021). https://doi.org/10.26099/spz0-mk34
[91] Lewis, J. F., Zeger, S. L., Li, X., Mann, N. C., Newgard, C. D., Haynes, S., Wood, S. F., Dai, M., Simon, A. E., & McCarthy, M. L. (2019). Gender Differences in the Quality of EMS Care Nationwide for Chest Pain and Out-of-Hospital Cardiac Arrest. *Women's health issues: official publication of the Jacobs Institute of Women's Health*, *29*(2), 116–124.
Andra M. Farcas, Anjni P. Joiner, Jordan S. Rudman, Karthik Ramesh, Gilberto Torres, Remle P. Crowe, Travis Curtis, Rickquel Tripp, Karen Bowers, Megan von Isenburg, Robert Logan, Lauren Coaxum, Gilberto Salazar, Michael Lozano Jr., David Page & Ameera Haamid (2022) Disparities in Emergency Medical Services Care Delivery in the United States: A Scoping Review, Prehospital Emergency Care
[92] Young MF, Hern HG, Alter HJ, Barger J, Vahidnia F. Racial differences in receiving morphine among prehospital patients with blunt trauma. J Emerg Med. 2013;45(1):46-52. doi:10.1016/j.jemermed.2012.07.088.
[93] Crowe RP, Krebs W, Cash RE, Rivard MK, Lincoln EW, Panchal AR. Females and Minority Racial/Ethnic Groups Remain Underrepresented in Emergency Medical Services: A Ten-Year Assessment, 2008-2017. Prehosp Emerg Care. 2020 Mar-Apr;24(2):180-187. doi: 10.1080/10903127.2019.1634167. Epub 2019 Jul 24. PMID: 31225772.
[94] Mitchell H. W. (1965). Ambulances and emergency medical care. *American journal of public health and the nation's health*, *55*(11), 1717–1724. https://doi.org/10.2105/ajph.55.11.1717
[95] Doeksen, G. A., Frye, J., & Green, B. (1975). Economics of rural ambulance service in the Great Plains. Economic Development Division, Economic Research Service, U.S. Department of Agriculture. AER No. 308.
[96] Progress, But Problems in Developing Emergency Medical Services Systems: Health Services Administration, Department of Health, Education, and Welfare: Report to the Congress. (1976). United States: U.S. General Accounting Office.
[97] Data Presentation. Colorado Department of Public Health & Environment (2023). Presented to the EMS Sustainability Task Force on April 13, 2023.
[98] Blue Ribbon Commission to Study Emergency Medical Services in the State, State of Maine. (2023). 130th Legislature Second Regular Session, Hillary Risler, Legislative Analyst Daniel Tartakoff, Principal Analyst Office of Policy & Legal Analysis.
[99] National EMS Advisory Council. (2016). Committee Report and Advisory Final as of December 2, 2016. Finance Committee. *EMS Funding and Reimbursement.* U.S. Department of Transportation.

---

[100] Mitchell H. W. (1965). Ambulances and emergency medical care. American journal of public health and the nation's health, 55(11), 1717–1724. https://doi.org/10.2105/ajph.55.11.1717

[101] Doeksen, G. A., Frye, J., & Green, B. (1975). Economics of rural ambulance service in the Great Plains. Economic Development Division, Economic Research Service, U.S. Department of Agriculture. AER No. 308.

[102] American Ambulance Association, "EMS Structured for Quality: Best Practices in Designing, Managing and Contracting for Emergency Ambulance Service," McLean, VA, American Ambulance Association, 2008.

[103] American Ambulance Association, "EMS Structured for Quality: Best Practices in Designing, Managing and Contracting for Emergency Ambulance Service," McLean, VA, American Ambulance Association, 2008.

[104] U.S. Government Accountability Office (GAO), "Ambulance Providers: Costs and Expected Medicare Margins Vary Greatly," Report to Congressional Committees, GAO-07-383, May 2007.

[105] Public Law No: 116-260, 116th Cong., 2d sess. (2020).

[106] Blue Ribbon Commission to Study Emergency Medical Services in the State, State of Maine. (2023). 130th Legislature Second Regular Session, Hillary Risler, Legislative Analyst Daniel Tartakoff, Principal Analyst Office of Policy & Legal Analysis.

[107] U.S. Congress. (2021). American Rescue Plan Act of 2021, Pub. L. No. 117-2.

[108] Rockwood, C. A., Mann, C. M., Farrington, J. D., Hampton, O. P., & Motley, R. E. (1976). History of emergency medical services in the United States. The Journal of Trauma, 16(4), 299-308

[109] Departments of Labor, and Health, Education, and Welfare Appropriations for 1969: Hearings, Ninetieth Congress, Second Session. (1968). United States: U.S. Government Printing Office. (343)

[110] National Association of State EMS Officials. National EMS Scope of Practice Model 2019 (Report No. DOT HS 812-666). Washington, DC: National Highway Traffic Safety Administration.

[111] National EMS Scope of Practice, pg. 11

[112] (2017) Clinical Credentialing of EMS practitioners, Prehospital Emergency Care, 21:3, 397-398, DOI: 10.1080/10903127.2017.1282565

[113] Department of Transportation and Related Agencies Appropriations for Fiscal Year 1985: Architectural and Transportation Barriers Compliance Board. (1984). United States: U.S. Government Printing Office.

[114] Emergency Medical Services: Recommendations for an Approach to an Urgent National Problem: Proceedings of the Airlie Conference on Emergency Medical Services, Airlie House, Warrenton, Virginia, May 5-6, 1969

[115] Training of Ambulance Personnel: And Others Responsible for Emergency Care of the Sick and Injured at the Scene and During Transport; Guidelines and Recommendations. (1968). United States: U.S. Government Printing Office.

[116] "Committee on Emergency Medical Services, Division of Medical Sciences, National Academy of Sciences, National Research Council. (1968). Training of Ambulance Personnel and Others Responsible for Emergency Care of the Sick and Injured at the Scene and During Transport: Guidelines and Recommendations. Washington, D.C.

[117] Emergency Medical Services: Recommendations for an Approach to an Urgent National Problem: Proceedings of the Airlie Conference on Emergency Medical Services, Airlie House, Warrenton, Virginia, May 5-6, 1969

118 Page 17, Proceedings of the Airlie Conference on Emergency Medical Services, Airlie House, Warrenton, Virginia, May 5-6, 1969
119 Health Resources Statistics. (1976). United States: U.S. Department of Health, Education, and Welfare, Public Health Service, Office of Health Research, Statistics, and Technology, National Center for Health Statistics. (Page 312)
120 Rocco V Morando's personal account recorded in 2005.
121 Rockwood, C. A., Mann, C. M., Farrington, J. D., Hampton, O. P., & Motley, R. E. (1976). History of emergency medical services in the United States. The Journal of Trauma, 16(4), 299-308
122 American Educational Research Association, American Psychological Association, & National Council on Measurement in Education. (2014). Standards for Educational and Psychological Testing. Washington, DC: American Educational Research Association.
123 Ashish R. Panchal, Madison K. Rivard, Rebecca E. Cash, John P. Corley Jr., Marjorie Jean-Baptiste, Kirsten Chrzan & Mihaiela R. Gugiu (2022) Methods and Implementation of the 2019 EMS Practice Analysis, Prehospital Emergency Care, 26:2, 212-222, DOI: 10.1080/10903127.2020.1856985
124 Seo DG. Overview and current management of computerized adaptive testing in licensing/certification examinations. J Educ Eval Health Prof. 2017 Jul 26;14:17. doi: 10.3352/jeehp.2017.14.17. PMID: 28811394; PMCID: PMC5676016.
125 Rockwood, C. A., Mann, C. M., Farrington, J. D., Hampton, O. P., & Motley, R. E. (1976). History of emergency medical services in the United States. The Journal of Trauma, 16(4), 299-308.
126 National Highway Traffic Safety Administration, Office of EMS. (2009, January). National Emergency Medical Services Education Standards (Report No. DOT HS 811 077A).
127 McSwain, Norman. (May 2014). Personal interview. McSwain, Norman. (2023). Norman McSwain Full CV. Retrieved from https://mcswaintraumaeducation.com/wp-content/uploads/2022/04/McSwain-full-CV-Revised-8-2015-v1-PDF.pdf
128 Joint Review Committee on Educational Programs for the EMT-Paramedic. (1978). Essentials for EMT-Paramedic Program Accreditation. Adopted by the American Medical Association Council on Medical Education.
129 Caroline, N. L. (1985). Emergency medical technician-paramedic: National standard curriculum. Washington, DC: U.S. Department of Transportation, National Highway Traffic Safety Administration.
130 Higher Education Amendments of 1992, Pub. L. No. 102-325, 106 Stat. 448 (1992).
131 Nationally Recognized Accrediting Agencies and Associations: Criteria and Procedures for Listing by the U.S. Commissioner of Education and Current List. (1978). United States: Department of Health, Education, and Welfare, Office of Education, Bureau of Higher and Continuing Education, Division of Eligibility and Agency Evaluation.
132 Health Resources Statistics. (1976). United States: U.S. Department of Health, Education, and Welfare, Public Health Service, Office of Health Research, Statistics, and Technology, National Center for Health Statistics.
133 Nurse Training Act of 1964, Pub. L. No. 88-581, 78 Stat. 908 (1964).
134 National Highway Traffic Safety Administration. (2000, June). The EMS Education Agenda for the Future (DOT HS 809042).
135 U.S. Census Bureau. (2019). American Community Survey: 2019.
136 U.S. Census Bureau. (2022). Urban and Rural Classification.
137 AAA/Avesta 2019 Ambulance Industry Employee Turnover Study
138 Articles of Confederation. (1777). Article VI.

---

[139] Michael L. Buenger & Richard L. Masters, The Interstate Compact on Adult Offender Supervision: Using Old Tools to Solve New Problems, 9 Roger Williams University Law Review 1 (2003)
[140] Virginia v. Tennessee, 148 U.S. 503 (1893).
[141] Buenger, M. L., Litwak, J. B., McCabe, M. H., & Masters, R. L. (2016). The evolving law and use of interstate compacts (2nd ed., pp. 42–48). ABA Publishing.
[142] Emergency Management Assistance Compact. (1996). Pub. L. No. 104-321.
[143] Donaho BA. The Pew Commission Report: nursing's challenge to address it. ANNA J. 1997 Oct;24(5):507-12. PMID: 9392732.
[144] Reforming Health Care Workforce Regulation: Policy Considerations for the 21st Century : Report of the Taskforce on Health Care Workforce Regulation. (1995). United States: Pew Health Professions Commission.
[145] Virginia v. Tennessee, 148 U.S. 503 (1893).
[146] Colorado House Bill 15-1015. (2015). Recognition of EMS Personnel Licensure Interstate Compact.
[147] Health Insurance Portability and Accountability Act of 1996, Pub. L. No. 104-191, 110 Stat. 1936 (1996).
[148] Emergency Medical Treatment and Labor Act, 42 U.S.C. § 1395dd (1986).
[149] United States Reports. (1889). Dent v. West Virginia, 129 U.S. 114. Library of Congress.
[150] Hawker v. New York, 170 U.S. 189 (1898).
[151] National Association of EMS Officials. (2010). State Emergency Medical Services System Models Project: Model State EMS System Lead Agency. Falls Church, VA.
[152] MN Stat § 169.686 (2016)
[153] 75 PA Cons Stat § 3121 (2022)
[154] Health Care Quality Improvement Act of 1986, Pub. L. No. 99-660, 100 Stat. 3743 (1986).
[155] Hawker v. New York, 170 U.S. 189 (1898).
[156] EMS Agenda 2050: A People-centered Vision for the Future of Emergency Medical Services. (2019). United States: National Highway Traffic Safety Administration.
[157] Graphic as originally printed in the EMS Agenda 2050: A People-centered Vision for the Future of Emergency Medical Services. (2019). United States: National Highway Traffic Safety Administration.
[158] Srikameswaran, A. (2002, March 31). Dr. Peter Safar: A life devoted to cheating death. Post-Gazette. Retrieved from https://old.post-gazette.com/lifestyle/20020331safar0331fnp2.asp
[159] Selected Bibliography of Scientific Publications and Programmatic Reports for the U.S.A. Bicentennial Emergency Medical Services and Traumatology Conference, May 10-12, 1976, Baltimore, Md. (1976). United States: U.S. Department of Health, Education, and Welfare, Public Health Services Administration, Bureau of Medical Services, Division of Emergency Medical Services.
[160] Model Legislation for Emergency Medical Services. (1978). United States: (n.p.).
[161] Departments of Labor and Health, Education, and Welfare and Related Agencies Appropriations for Fiscal Year 1979: Hearings Before a Subcommittee of the Committee on Appropriations, United States Senate, Ninety-fifth Congress, Second Session. (1978). United States: U.S. Government Printing Office.

www.ingramcontent.com/pod-product-compliance
Lightning Source LLC
LaVergne TN
LVHW081321110826
845149LV00007B/1564
9798988525400